ALCOHOL AND MORAL REGULATION

Public attitudes, spirited measures
and Victorian hangovers

Henry Yeomans

First published in Great Britain in 2014 by

Policy Press
University of Bristol
6th Floor
Howard House
Queen's Avenue
Clifton
Bristol BS8 1SD
UK
Tel +44 (0)117 331 5020
Fax +44 (0)117 331 5367
e-mail pp-info@bristol.ac.uk
www.policypress.co.uk

North American office:
Policy Press
c/o The University of Chicago Press
1427 East 60th Street
Chicago, IL 60637, USA
t: +1 773 702 7700
f: +1 773-702-9756
e:sales@press.uchicago.edu
www.press.uchicago.edu

British Library Cataloguing in Publication Data
A catalogue record for this book is available from the British Library

Library of Congress Cataloging-in-Publication Data
A catalog record for this book has been requested

ISBN 978 1 44730 993 2 hardcover

Cover design by Policy Press
Cover image: taken from: http://www.demondrink.co.uk/
Image supplied by: Livesey Collection, University of Central
Lancashire.
Printed and bound in Great Britain by CPI Group (UK) Ltd,
Croydon, CR0 4YY
The Policy Press uses environmentally responsible print partners

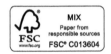

Contents

List of figures   v

List of abbreviations   vi

Acknowledgements   vii

one   **Thinking about drinking**   1

Introduction   1

The 'rational' explanation   3

The 'ebb and flow' of the drink problem   6

Moral regulation   12

Morality, regulation and moral regulation   17

Methods   21

two   **Temperance and teetotalism**   **35**

Introduction   35

The 'second necessity of life'   36

Classical virtues and Georgian excesses   36

The 'temperance reformation'   42

The Beer Act 1830   55

Reflections   58

three   **Balancing acts or spirited measures?**   **65**

Introduction   65

'A new moralising subtext'   66

The split personality of Victorian temperance   66

Legal impacts of the temperance movement   72

Attitudinal or heuristic impacts of the temperance movement   81

The legacy of the temperance movement   88

four   **The apogee of the temperance movement**   **97**

Introduction   97

Drink as a national problem   98

Responses to war   100

Post-war: what now?   112

The apogee of the temperance movement   121

five	**An age of permissiveness?**	**129**
	Introduction	129
	New frontiers, 1921–45	130
	The growth of targeted regulation	145
	Conclusion	158
six	**Alcohol, crime and disorder**	**167**
	Introduction	167
	The narrative of deregulation	167
	Acceptable in the 1980s?	171
	The 'new culture of intoxication'	176
	The attitudinal heritage of Victorian temperance	183
	Conclusion	192
seven	**Health, harm and risk**	**203**
	Introduction	203
	Drink, health and moral health until the 1960s	204
	Debates about alcohol and health, 2003–10	218
	Good health!	231
eight	**Conclusion: spirited measures and Victorian hangovers**	**243**
	Conspectus	243
	Public attitudes and alcohol regulation	243
	Alcohol and moral regulation	248
	Moral inheritance	251
	Bibliography	255
	Index	269

List of figures

2.1   'The Village Holiday' by David Wilkie, 1809–11   45
3.1   Envelope issued by The Temperance Society, 1851   68
3.2   F. Allen & Sons' Cocoa Chocolate and Confectionery   86
       Works London, circa 1880

List of abbreviations

AA   Alcoholics Anonymous
AHA   Alcohol Health Alliance
BAPT   British Association for the Promotion of Temperance
BL   British Library
CCB   Central Control Board
COETS   Church of England Temperance Society
DORA   Defence of the Realm Act
DPPO   Designated Public Place Order
FASD   foetal alcohol spectrum disorder
IAS   Institute of Alcohol Studies
MP   Member of Parliament
MUP   minimum unit pricing
NCA   National Council on Alcoholism
SOB   Strength of Britain Movement
TCT   total consumption theory
US   United States
VD   venereal disease

Acknowledgements

Much of this book is based on my doctoral thesis so thanks, first and foremost, to Kim Stevenson and Adrian Barton for their expert supervision. Thanks also to Judith Rowbotham and Jason Lowther for their extensive constructive input as examiners. Many others deserve thanks for providing help, advice or guidance at various points in the process of producing this book. They include, but are not limited to: Chas Critcher, Annemarie McAllister, Helen Cooper, Paul Jennings, Zoe James, Nigel Firth, Rachel MacLean, Peter Ramsey, Iain Channing and Jen Hendry. It must also be acknowledged that my doctoral research was funded by the Economic and Social Research Council.

Some of the findings of this broad research project have already been published in the journals *Sociological Research Online*, *Sociology and Law, Crime and History*, and the edited collection *Moral Panics in the Contemporary World*. Chapter endnotes are used throughout the book to highlight where content touches on or overlaps with my other publications.

I would also like to thanks my partner, Maria, and my family for continual support and inspiration. Cheers!

Finally, I would like to dedicate this book to peace, love and Plymouth Argyle.

ONE

Thinking about drinking

Introduction

In April 2011, French riot police threatened to go on strike in response to government plans to ban officers from consuming alcoholic drinks while on duty. The riot control force – Compagnies Républicaines de Sécurité – were accustomed to consuming wine, beer, cider or perry with their lunch and unions reacted furiously to attempts to alter this hitherto acceptable practice.[1] In July of the same year, the Russian government passed legislation that vastly increased restrictions on the sale of beer. Previously, most types of beer were classified as foodstuffs rather than alcohol and subject to little legal regulation. The British press covered this event in a bemused fashion; the *Daily Telegraph* reported that Russian President Dmitry Medvedev had 'signed a bill that confirms what the rest of the world has known for centuries: that beer is in fact alcoholic'.[2] Similarly, the threatened strike by the French riot police was depicted in a humorous manner, which reproduced the popular stereotype of the French as a people whose love of wine is matched only by their passion for industrial action. But once the amusement subsides, some intriguing questions remain. Must all alcoholic drinks be legally regulated? Is drinking necessarily antonymical to proper public conduct and the maintenance of good social order? And more generally, how do we understand alcohol and how do these understandings shape its regulation?

While the raising of quizzical eyebrows in the direction of our European neighbours makes for entertaining news stories, the clear waters of the English Channel can also be used to reflect on British attitudes towards alcohol. Part of the value of these stories, particularly in the French case, comes from the strangely permissive relationship with alcohol that some other countries appear to possess. This situation starkly contrasts the British context in which alcohol is a consistent and prolific source of public anxiety. In 2005, the relaxation of statutory controls on opening times for licensed premises provoked widespread alarm about national drinking alleged to be already 'out of control'.[3] More recently, health professionals have waged a high-profile campaign against the 'collateral damage' of 'passive drinking', which includes violence, vandalism, accidents and ill-health.[4] It has been claimed that 'drink companies spread liver disease as surely as mosquitoes do malaria'[5] and journalists have asserted that 'this is now a matter of life and, increasingly, death'.[6] It is routine to hear that Britain is in the grip of a 'crisis',[7] a 'plague'[8] or 'an epidemic, bringing death, violence and shame in its wake'.[9] Consistent with this shrill discursive tone, laws surrounding drinking are relatively strict in England and Wales. In 1944, George Orwell attacked restrictive drink laws and, inspired by the existence of more relaxed regulations in France and other countries, demanded more liberty for the 'downtrodden' British.[10] A very similar situation, however, exists today. Who can sell alcohol and who can buy it (in terms of age) are strictly controlled by licensing legislation, and when this transaction can take place is decided by local authorities. The price of drink is shaped by excise duties and the conduct of people after drinking is subject to a myriad of regulations concerning public behaviour, driving and other activities. Attitudinally and legally, alcohol is taken very seriously in Britain.

Alarmed public attitudes and strict laws are indicative of a widespread perception that alcohol and drinking are grave threats. This is connected to a strong public belief that current behavioural problems are the advent of recent history. The supposition that drinking used to be restrained or controlled is inferred by the assertion that it is *now* 'out of control' and a tantamount belief in worsening social conditions is inherent within the idea of a drinking 'epidemic'. Former Prime Minister Tony Blair clearly distinguished current problems from any historical antecedents by describing heavy drinking as a 'new British disease'.[11] This sense of 'presentism'[12] is reinforced by specific, pervasive concerns about binge drinking, a consumptive practice ubiquitously associated with the under-25s.[13] This generational profiling again implies that the 'crisis' is new and separate from the actions of older generations, either now or when they were young. Problematic drinking is cast as an emergent behavioural form and, given its association with various types of serious 'collateral damage', it is positioned within a bigger narrative of national decline or social disintegration. A variety of further legal restrictions, such as a ban on new licensed premises in so-called 'binge towns',[14] a higher legal purchase age of 21[15] or a minimum unit price for all alcoholic drinks,[16] are then demanded in an effort to halt or mitigate the perceived deterioration. This conception of a downward social trajectory situates drinking in chronological perspective by advancing the conception that we are living in uniquely troublesome times.

Current problems with drink are seen to be unmatched in history in terms of both their form and seriousness. But even a brief glance at history reveals the erroneous nature of this idea. Past examples of heavy consumption include the port-drinking excesses of aristocratic Georgian dinner parties or the 19th-century practice of 'Saint Monday', which entailed workers elongating their weekends largely for the purposes of drinking. Notably, average consumption in the early 21st century is lower than at other points in modern history, such as the late 19th century.[17] British history further abounds with instances of public disquiet about alcohol use. The Georgian 'gin panics' and the Victorian temperance movement were vivid historical manifestations of mass anxiety about alcohol consumption. The idea that either heavy drinking or concerns about heavy drinking are recent occurrences is, therefore, a fallacy. So, rather than asking why the French and Russians have for so long tolerated certain drinking practices, it might be useful to consider how public discourse on alcohol in Britain has come to be characterised by a contrasting sentiment of acute public unease.

This book investigates how the way in which we currently think about and try to regulate drinking has developed historically in England and Wales. Public discourse is a publicly aired series of communications and, following a dictionary definition, an attitude is a 'settled way of thinking or feeling about something'.[18] 'Public attitudes' are thus defined here as ways of thinking or feeling that are expressed in public. The term 'public anxiety' is also used fairly frequently in the coming pages to denote the specific type of public attitude to alcohol, characterised by fear, alarm or trepidation, which has already been outlined. So, taking contemporary anxious public attitudes to alcohol as its object of enquiry, this book explains how we got to where we are now. It examines publicly expressed attitudes and attempts to regulate drinking through time in order to produce a historically grounded account of the 'drink problem' in England and Wales.[19]

The 'rational' explanation

The Russian, French and historical examples cited allude to significant historic and cross-national variation in how alcohol is understood and regulated. Of course, the public unease that typifies the British relationship with alcohol could have arisen because social problems resulting from drinking in this country are indeed especially bad. This was certainly the implication when Chief Medical Officer for England, Sir Liam Donaldson, diagnosed in 2009 that 'England has an alcohol problem'.[20] Similarly, when health professionals Moriarty and Gilmore wrote of a contemporary 'epidemic of binge drinking',[21] they effectively distanced current drinking habits from past practices. Such statements provide 'expert' confirmation for wider populist alarm about drinking. Public anxieties are thus rationalised and calls for new remedial regulation are legitimated. This position has been labelled variably an 'objectivist',[22] pragmatic[23] or 'rational' model for understanding how social problems are governed.[24] All monikers refer to a standpoint that posits the existence of an objective, real and unambiguous connection between the level of alcohol consumption or alcohol-related harm and the social reaction to these phenomena, as manifested in either public attitudes or legal regulation. Inflamed public concerns about alcohol and comparatively rather strict drink laws are thus explained as the straightforward result of a particularly acute and/or worsening national drink problem.

Plant and Plant utilise the rational model although, recognising that Britain has a long history of anxieties about drinking, they do not conform to its cruder 'presentist' versions. Drawing on Greenfield and Giesbrecht, they use this historical perspective to describe a chronological pattern of alcohol problems that can be summarised thus: the problem behaviour increases, the government intervenes with restrictive measures, the problem behaviour lessens, restrictions are relaxed as problems are forgotten, and then the problem rises again.[25] Understandings of alcohol are thus said to result from a straightforward comprehension of the objective level at which drinking and drink-related harm have been occurring and regulation derives simply and unequivocally from these rational, impartial assessments of consumption and harm. Sheron et al adopt a similar position in asserting that 'UK history demonstrates that it is relatively straightforward for governments to either encourage or control alcohol consumption at a population level'.[26] They attribute historical peaks and troughs in consumption exclusively to fluctuations in the extent and form of legal regulation and cite two examples as evidence of this mono-causal relationship. It is claimed, first, that the 'gin epidemic' of the 18th century was brought to an end by new restrictions contained within the Gin Act 1751 and, second, that the 19th-century increase in consumption, cirrhosis and alcoholism was 'eventually curtailed by the Defence of the Realm Act (DORA) at the outbreak of World War One'.[27] Behaviour, in this case consumption and harm, is thus explained as an effect of legal regulation just as attitudes and regulation are, in turn, determined by behaviour.

The rational model thus reduces ontological connections between behaviour, attitudes and regulation to simple, deterministic relationships. But the historical examples cited by Sheron et al do not withstand scrutiny. Warner et al's research found that the Gin Act 1751 and other pieces of Georgian legislation had only a very limited impact on levels of spirits consumption.[28] It is well established that average drinking began to decline in the late 1890s, well before DORA,[29] and Jennings' research suggests that drunkenness was also declining around the turn of the 20th century.[30] These difficulties are magnified if the contemporary context is considered. Evidence on consumption and harm in the present day fails to provide strong grounds for the claim that an 'epidemic' or 'crisis' is ongoing. There are substantial data showing that alcohol consumption rose for most of the second half of the 20th century[31] and that liver disease mortality is on an upward trajectory.[32] But, in 2004, the World Health Organization ranked average British alcohol consumption as below the average for the European Union.[33] Moreover, surveys on consumption and data on alcohol sales have actually recorded a sustained reduction in average drinking since the early 2000s.[34] Research does suggest that heavy sessional consumption (or binge drinking) among young people is more common in Britain than most European countries,[35] but there is evidence that this habit is also declining.[36] Rates of liver cirrhosis and alcohol-related cancer are also much higher in France, Germany and Italy than in Britain.[37] Furthermore, while it is very difficult to measure alcohol-related crime specifically, the best data on overall national crime suggest that it has been falling since the mid-1990s.[38] Current anxieties about alcohol do not appear, therefore, to be based on any simple, rational comprehension of levels of alcohol consumption or alcohol-related harm.

The ontological relationship between actual behavioural trends and the formulation of specific types of regulation is also distant. Across history, different countries have employed a variety of legal means to address drink problems. Prohibition, free trade, state monopolies on the alcohol trade, rationing, anti-spirits legislation and harm reduction are among the many strategies that have been employed to address perceived problems with excessive consumption in different national and chronological settings.[39] Crucially, the selection of a particular regulatory strategy is driven by more than an unmediated comprehension of the objective nature of the problem faced. Schrad examined how, in the 1910s, Russia, Sweden and the United States (US) sought to manage drinking using divergent means of prohibition and state monopoly, ultimately highlighting the importance of political and cultural factors in producing differing national policies.[40] So, the proposition that relationships between attitudes, regulation and behaviour are straightforward and rational thus runs contrary to a wealth of historical and contemporary evidence. Drink habits are not produced exclusively by legal frameworks just as attitudes and regulation surrounding alcohol do not result from levels of consumption or harm in any direct, mechanistic way. There is clearly some distance between objective behavioural trends and subjective understandings of these trends. The question remaining is if public alarm and action against drink do not stem directly from a worsening or particularly British problem with alcohol, where do they come from? Why is Britain such a fertile breeding ground for public anxiety about alcohol?

The 'ebb and flow' of the drink problem

While not necessarily employing it, a fair amount of social science research on drinking refrains from confronting the rational model directly. Criminologists tend to investigate the connection of drinking to violence and disorder in the context of recent social changes such as the increasing marketisation of drinking and drunkenness, the rise of late-modern forms of consumption or the state's apparent retreat from the task of providing security in the night-time economy.[41] It could be inferred from these analyses that public drunkenness and related crime and disorder are indeed new issues or, at least, new variants of older problems. A number of scholars pursuing explanations of drinking and other social problems have, however, deviated markedly from the rational model. American sociologist Joseph Gusfield states that social problems are 'historical occurrences which emerge or disappear without any necessary relationship to the conditions of their existence'.[42] Reinforcing this perspective, Hunt notes that the 'gin panics' of the 18th century occurred at a time when arrests for drunkenness were declining[43] and Reinarman documents how US attitudes to drink-driving became increasingly disapproving at a time when instances of the offence appeared relatively scarce.[44] This section explores how factors other than consumption and harm have impacted on conceptions of a 'drink problem' in England and Wales over time.

Alcoholic drinks have played a central role in British society for hundreds of years. They were available in pre-Roman times and, after the Roman conquest, taverns were established to provide wine on trade routes across Britain. The English began using hops to brew beer in the 15th century and, by the 18th century, drink could be purchased in taverns, inns and alehouses.[45] The Assize of Bread and Ale 1267 ranked beer as the 'second necessity of life' and created a system of pricing that, by tying the price of beer to the price of grain, sought to ensure that the nation's favourite drink was always available at affordable prices.[46] Furthermore, the True Making of Malt Act 1548 sought to promote the proper manufacturing of beer by condemning swift brewing, poor barrels and other hindrances to overall quality.[47] Beer continued to be a socially ubiquitous substance for many centuries. Burnett reports that Queen Elizabeth I drank beer at breakfast, an average of three pints per day was given to children at Christ's Hospital and St Bartholomew's Hospital in the 17th century, and many workers were paid purely in beer, even after this practice was outlawed in 1887.[48] In 1660, diarist Samuel Pepys described his first encounter at breakfast time with that modern emblem of Britishness, the cup of tea, being much more accustomed to drinking wine or ale at that time of day.[49] Alcohol was once regarded as a normal part of life and beer was widely consumed on an everyday basis, during work and other activities.

Concerns about excessive drinking certainly existed during medieval and early modern periods. Legislation – such as the Alehouse Act 1552, which required drink-sellers to obtain a licence from a magistrate, and The Act to Repress the Odious and Loathsome Sin of Drunkenness 1606 – demonstrates the existence of perceived alcohol problems and attempts to deal with them through regulation. But many scholars believe that drinking was not the focus of mass, sustained public alarm until the reaction of social elites to spirit-drinking in Georgian London instigated social unease and a number of Gin Acts. Warner has described these events as an early version of the modern 'drug scare'[50] and Borsay suggests that they were 'perhaps the first drink-related "moral panic"'.[51] Drawing on Warner, Nicholls and others, Critcher relates the 'gin panics' to concerns about maintaining public order and disciplining lower social classes, as well as counteracting the opportunities for excessive consumption afforded by an efficient, industrial means of production (of, in this case, spirits).[52] While coloured by such dilemmas, which soon became typical of modern societies, the 'gin panics' remained geographically concentrated in London and tailed off markedly in the 1750s. The emergence of the temperance movement from the late 1820s onwards coincided with a period during which drinking emerged as a major national issue. By the second half of the 19th century, alcohol was the subject of extensive public discussion and a significant amount of legislative activity. From the near-hysteria about drink during the First World War to the Mass Observations[53] in the inter-war years, drinking habits continued to attract significant public and political attention into the 20th century. In the post-war years, issues of youth violence, antisocial behaviour, ill-health, addiction and driving have become focal points for disquiet about drinking. Alcohol consumption is now a consistent, high-profile concern within public discourse and political action.

This rough sketch suggests that the 18th century and particularly the 19th century are crucial periods for understanding the advent of the 'drink problem' in England and Wales. So why might drinking have changed from being an occasional source of anxiety to the object of a borderline social neurosis around this time? While industrialisation and urbanisation initiated deep and pervasive social change, how people understood and sought to regulate the social world around them also shifted. Research by Malcolmson, Roberts and others has explored how popular leisure and other aspects of social life were affected by moral reform campaigns during the 18th and 19th centuries.[54] Some of these campaigns might relate to the civilizing process, identified by Elias, which was well established by this point. Unlike in the medieval period, eating from communal dishes, bodily functions and nudity had become evidence of coarseness or sources of shame, which helped to erect an 'invisible wall' of personal manners between one human body and another.[55] The promotion of these codes of etiquette created a 'social constraint towards self-constraint'.[56] Foucault also describes how, in the 19th century, new surveillance-based technologies were increasingly used to inculcate certain forms of discipline within individual subjects, thus contributing to the regulation of behaviour.[57] The disciplinary mechanisms, for Foucault, were part of a wider 'bio-politics', which subjects individual bodies to forms of state or political power.[58] The rise of urban, industrial, capitalist modernity saw the development and maturation of social processes, which engendered the tighter regulation of individual behaviour.

While Elias and Foucault do not relate their analyses to drinking in England and Wales, some historical studies have tackled these issues more directly. Greenaway examines political developments pertaining to drinking from 1830 until the turn of the 21st century. The Beer Act 1830, which removed the need for beer-sellers to be licensed by a magistrate, was examined in reference to government attempts, in the absence of strong opposition, to free up the market in beer, reduce spirits consumption and resuscitate cereal prices.[59] The beliefs and actions of key political personalities, such as William Gladstone, are also examined.[60] Greenaway's focus on the 'high politics' of drink usefully maps the parliamentary and partisan contours of debates about alcohol since 1830.[61] Baggott's and Thom's respective books provide some complement to Greenaway's work by highlighting a range of other significant actors in the policy-making process from the post-war period onwards. These include the civil service, industry lobby groups, charities, professional medical bodies, temperance groups and public opinion.[62] Both authors are concerned with the interaction of different stakeholders in the formulation and implementation of alcohol policies. They also recognise how the ideas, beliefs and values articulated by various agents are entwined with their actions. Baggott, for example, argues that the principle of liberty, as something counterposed to state action, held sway over political decision making in the 1960s, 1970s and 1980s and thus acted as an obstacle for the advancement of serious alcohol control policies.[63] Thom examines the decline of the 'moral model' for treating alcoholism, which was bound up with religious and temperance ideas, and its replacement, in the 20th century, with the 'medical model'.[64]

Nicholls' *The Politics of Alcohol* is broader and examines political debates about alcohol from the early modern period onwards. Nicholls asserts that public debates about alcohol 'have always been about other cultural issues'.[65] The temperance movement, for Nicholls, was related partly to changing forms and amounts of alcohol consumption, but also to contention over the legitimate limits of state action and the proper ambit of personal liberty in Victorian society.[66] Nicholls also follows Warner in depicting the Georgian 'gin panics' as less about spirits drinking and more about the maintenance of social order in the face of an expanding, unruly metropolitan populace.[67] Drink as a social problem, therefore, is either affected by ulterior ideas and beliefs or, using Nicholls' argument that 'explicit social anxieties reveal implicit ones',[68] is a surrogate for the discussion of deeper political questions. Consumption and harm are not, therefore, the only significant factors. Historians and social scientists have identified a range of historical factors, from various policy stakeholders to the dilemmas of government, which have influenced how alcohol and drinking are understood and regulated.

With regards to the 19th century specifically, another potentially important factor can be identified. Harrison and Shiman both examine the rise of the temperance movement from the late 1820s, its subsequent division into prohibitionist and moral suasionist strands, and its demise at the end of the 19th century following the Liberal defeat in the 1895 General Election.[69] Both authors explore how, despite middle-class beginnings and bourgeois ethics,[70] the temperance movement became popular with the working class. Shiman goes on to argue that this class profile indicated that the movement was not a simple bourgeois effort to impose sober discipline on workers, but also offered the sort of fraternity and social opportunities that newly urbanised areas were lacking.[71] Such was the popularity and influence of this social movement that Harrison argues it 'forced society to recognize drunkenness as a serious evil'.[72] Shiman equally emphasises how, in the Victorian period, drunkenness came to be consistently recognised as a serious social problem and no longer 'treated with the good-hearted tolerance of former times'.[73]

These historians thus add credence to the idea that anxieties about alcohol have become more frequent and severe since the 19th century. Interestingly, they also suggest that the British temperance movement may have been a crucial agency in altering public perceptions of the 'drink problem'.

This point is strengthened by the apparent hardening of attitudes to alcohol in other countries where temperance movements were potent. Levine identifies nine 'temperance cultures' in which large-scale, abstinence-based social movements occurred.[74] These are Australia, Britain, Canada, Finland, Iceland, New Zealand, Norway, Sweden and the USA. Interestingly, while non-temperance France remains more permissive towards drinking,[75] these temperance countries are now usually regarded as 'ambivalent cultures' characterised by conflict between drinkers and those who wish to regulate their drinking.[76] This conflict is likely connected to the comparatively restrictive alcohol laws that these 'temperance cultures' have implemented in recent history. Although varying somewhat between areas, Australia and New Zealand generally required licensed premises to cease serving drinks at 6pm between the First World War and the 1960s. Sweden, which pioneered state management of the drinks trade, still retains a state monopoly over off-sales of alcohol. Finland and Norway have similar state monopolies, as do most provinces of Canada. Although varying between different drinks, the United Kingdom and the Nordic countries also impose comparatively very high levels of excise duties on the sale of alcohol.[77] While the US's famous experiment with prohibition ended in 1933, it still retains a number of 'dry counties' and one of the world's highest legal purchase ages for alcohol of 21.[78] Comparatively speaking, it seems that countries that were home to abstinence-based temperance movements have also played host to a variety of restrictive alcohol laws in recent history.

So, there are certainly discernible fluctuations within the 'drink problem' in England and Wales that are not bound up simply with levels of consumption and harm. Various scholars have identified the importance of 'high politics', the wider policy-making process, deeper political principles and dilemmas as well as a number of agents, including the civil service, popular campaigns and drinks industry lobby groups. As mentioned earlier, Reinarman dismissed the idea that any measurable change in behaviour was responsible for increasing concerns about drink-driving in the US in the late 20th century. Instead, he attributed the inflated salience of the issue to the 'moral entrepreneurship' of the Mothers Against Drunk Drivers campaign group.[79] Reinarman subsequently echoes Gusfield in asserting that social problems have careers that 'ebb and flow' in a manner that is not dictated by the 'objective' manifestation of the behaviours thought to constitute them.[80] From this constructionist perspective, it is imperative to examine how certain behaviours come to be understood and described as social problems. In addition to policy and political issues examined in existing literature, this section has identified the British temperance movement as a potentially noteworthy phenomenon in relation to explaining the 'ebb and flow' of the 'drink problem' in England and Wales. The chronological and international coincidence of temperance movements with heightened public anxieties about drink and the existence of rigorous legal restrictions certainly warrants further investigation.

Several authors have already taken views on alcohol as a social problem that are informed by social constructionism and sociological approaches more broadly. The work of Gusfield, Valverde and Sulkunen is particularly noteworthy: Gusfield has made extensive study of temperance and the 'drink problem' in the US; Valverde has examined expert discourse around alcohol in North America and Europe; and Sulkunen has focused on how the social conditions of late modernity have precluded the possibility of serious alcohol control policies being enacted in Britain and the Nordic countries.[81] The work of all three authors has some relevance to public attitudes to alcohol (which will be discussed further in coming chapters), although none focuses intensively on England and Wales. Despite the evident changeability of the 'drink problem' over time, its non-reducibility to consumption and harm, and its connection to various political, cultural and economic factors (as highlighted by a number of academics), no dedicated formative investigation has previously been attempted of public attitudes and the regulation of alcohol in England and Wales.

This section has underlined the need to concentrate empirical attention on how the manner in which alcohol is currently understood and regulated has developed through time. A specific objective concerning the influence of the temperance movement over relevant historical developments has also been added. The key questions this book addresses can now be identified as:

- How have current public attitudes to alcohol been formed through time?
- How has the current system of alcohol regulation developed through time?

- What role, if any, has the temperance movement had in shaping public attitudes to the regulation of alcohol?

The book is historically oriented yet it is also informed by the questions, concepts and theories of social science, such as social constructionism. It constitutes something of a genealogical 'history of the present'. The next section will explore the conceptual tools utilised in more depth.

Moral regulation

The configuration of drinking behaviour, public attitudes and the regulation of alcohol warrant further empirical attention. The construction of attitudes and regulation is seriously neglected by proponents of the rational model and, despite the existence of good research on transnational drink issues and the political and policy dimensions of alcohol in Britain, the ideas, beliefs and values that underpin anxieties about alcohol are not currently well understood. With regards to England and Wales, this project aims to develop a comprehension of the 'drink problem' that does not merely conflate attitudes with behaviour, reaction with action or subjective with objective. Moreover, it explores the relation of this heuristic dimension to regulatory responses to drink. This book uses the concept of 'moral regulation' to explore this subject area further.

The concept of 'moral regulation' originates with Durkheim, to whom it constituted a set of shared values, social roles and moral boundaries that provide social cohesion, thus protecting against the normlessness of anomie.[82] In the 1980s, Corrigan and Sayer borrowed Durkheim's concept but put it to work in a distinctly Marxist arena by emphasising that shared values in capitalist society inevitably embody bourgeois beliefs and interests. They defined moral regulation as 'a project of normalizing, rendering natural, taken for granted, in a word "obvious", what are in fact ontological and epistemological premises of a particular and historical form of social order'.[83] Moral regulation was therefore transformed from a means to enhance social integration into a tool for consolidating or reproducing the status quo. Corrigan and Sayer examined the development of the British state, which, it was proposed, resulted from a bourgeois cultural revolution over several centuries. Summarising their theory, Ruonavaara postulated that for different forms of the state to exist, they must be animated and legitimised by a particular moral ethos.[84] Moral regulation thus creates a social environment amenable to the development of certain societal orders by justifying particular legal regulations and legitimising forms of political, economic and social domination. For Corrigan and Sayer, attitudes can be connected to a longer-term project of generating or reproducing certain forms of social order.

Various theorists have expanded on Corrigan and Sayer. Ruonavaara has argued that moral regulation is also carried out by non-state actors, such as religion and the media, who do not necessarily act in the state's interest.[85] Hunt's definition of moral regulation projects as a 'form of politics in which some people act to problematise the conduct, values or culture of others and seek to impose regulation upon them' supports this wider view of agency.[86] Hunt focuses on the moral discourse of campaigning social movements and also employed a more Foucauldian concentration on the construction of knowledge and the ethical subjectivity of individuals.[87] Self-government, how people see themselves and what, if anything, they decide to do about it, becomes pertinent. As well as providing legitimation for aspects of social order, moral regulation also encompasses efforts to alter people's perceptions in order to engender self-reformation of behaviour. 'Moral regulation' is thus a diffuse and varied concept; it embodies a plethora of social actors, including social movements, as well as a concern for self-formation. Large swathes of social action relating to ongoing efforts to compel people to behave differently are encapsulated by moral regulation. Moral regulation, in this analysis, refers to the process through which social actors both decide and attempt to alter the behaviour of other people. It is best described as a social relation as it is less about how and why individuals alter their own behaviour and, as Ruonavaara describes, more about how individuals and groups seek to alter each other's conduct.[88]

Hunt notes that employing the concept of moral regulation thus pitches empirical enquiries somewhere on the interface between what Foucault calls the 'government of the self' and the 'government of others'.[89] In this respect, moral regulation projects occupy a similar conceptual area to the notion of a 'moral panic'. A moral panic has been defined as an exaggerated or disproportionate reaction to a social phenomenon that is seen to be, in some fashion, threatening.[90] Following Cohen, anxiety about structural social change is directed towards and becomes fixed on a certain type of behaviour and the people who engage in it. These people become 'folk devils' and social notables leap on the 'moral barricades' in order to issue condemnations.[91] Social anxiety and moral panic have been used to explain some historical instances of alarm about drinking. In the early 1960s, Gusfield highlighted the causal importance of status anxiety within the emerging middle class in producing the US temperance movement.[92] More recently, Borsay's discussion of the Georgian 'gin panics' cited contextual factors, such as rapid urbanisation, increasing working-class affluence and concerns about the breakdown of the family, as factors instrumental in producing the social unease that came to be directed at the consumption of spirituous liquor.[93] The concept of a 'moral panic' can be connected to how attempts to govern the drinking of others arise.

But the utility of the 'moral panic' concept is limited by its reliance on social anxiety as an explanation for outbursts of alarm about certain groups or types of behaviour. In his study of the Black Act 1723, Thompson criticises the idea that this repressive law, which condemned many people to death for relatively minor criminal offences, could be explained simply by the wave of public concern unleashed by social unrest. A widespread perception of crisis may have led to a consensus that something needed to be done, but '[i]f we agree that "something" needed to be done this does not entail the conclusion that *anything* might be done'.[94] Hunt explains how the notion of anxiety is limited in its capacity to explain the nuances of certain public reactions. Why, to use Cohen's example, did social anxieties in the 1960s become fixed on youth culture? Or, to return to Thompson's example, why were poaching and the felling of trees seen as potent threats to the dominant social order in the 18th century? An empirical focus on problematisation helps to remedy this explanatory problem. For Hunt, empirical enquiry should focus on the discursive formations through which a social problem is identified, agitators are recruited and support is mobilised. His research on sexual purity movements of the 18th and 19th centuries highlights this process of problematisation by examining the target, discourse, agency and tactics of these social movements in addition to their political context.[95] The concept of 'moral regulation', partly constituted by the discursive process of problematisation, thus offers a more promising explanatory matrix than moral panic approaches.

The work of Hunt and other moral regulation scholars typically examines problematisation and attempts at behavioural regulation over the course of centuries, rather than years or decades. This conception of moralisation as a long-term process again means that moral regulation conflicts with moral panic approaches, which are classically episodic. In Cohen's words, moral panics rise up 'every now and then'[96] before submerging again as some form of social equilibrium is reached or restored. Each panic, therefore, appears as an exceptional, temporary state. This depiction has been disputed by, among others, Rowbotham and Stevenson who have argued that moral panics are not episodic but a regular, if not routine, feature of social life.[97] The idea that outbursts of public alarm are exceptional events also contradicts the historical consistence and pervasiveness of anxiety about alcohol already described. While the contours of the debate have shifted, drinking has hardly ceased to be a public issue for any serious amount of time since the 19th century. It seems unlikely that these recurrent or endemic concerns about drinking are merely a succession of independent, unrelated moral panics. By contrast, taking a long-term view of how target groups or behaviours are identified, how these targets are discursively constructed, how agitators are recruited and how public support is mobilised may shed light on why alcohol has become such a persistent source of public anxieties in England and Wales. Concentration on singular episodes of moral panic is less useful than moral regulation's discursive orientation towards the construction of social problems over long periods of time.

However, although anxieties about alcohol have a long history that could be studied developmentally, there were and are high points of concern within these extended processes. It has already been noted that drinking was the object of borderline hysteria during the First World War and, indeed, Greenaway calls this episode a 'moral panic'.[98] Some of the restrictions on sales of alcohol introduced by the government to tackle the threat of drink to the war effort were made permanent by the Licensing Act 1921 and retained until as late as the early 21st century.[99] As well as representing a peak in public alarm about alcohol, this short period of time was also crucially formative with regard to the legal rules governing the trade in alcohol. Recognising historical fluctuations within discourse and regulation, some social scientists have tried to reformulate moral regulation. Hier has referred to 'the volatility of moralization'[100] and has used volatility as a substitute for moral panics, a way to denote 'sensational, inflammatory, and spectacular discourses that articulate moral transgressions on the part of diverse individuals and/or social groups'.[101] Critcher, meanwhile, has retained the 'moral panic' concept, arguing that such events are significant and require their own conceptual identity. He does, however, argue that moral panics are an extreme and temporary form of moral regulation, high points within an established current of moral concern. Moral panics are thus a constituent part of longer-term processes of moral regulation.[102] The 'ebb and flow' of the drink problem over time, as well as the existence of important formative moments, means that Critcher's synthesis of episodes and processes is appropriate for studying this topic.

There is a problem lurking within Critcher's conceptual synthesis. Moral panic studies commonly rest on a comparison of the perceived to the actual; a disproportionate reaction being irrational and hence indicative of panic. This neat separation of the imagined and the real might jar epistemologically with more relativist-influenced researchers. But much social science research is oriented towards the development of accurate, valid knowledge about social reality and the elimination of misrepresentations. Notably, the influential 'realist' approach holds that there is a social reality independent of human perception and research must seek to understand or uncover it.[103] Hunt does not reject the possibility of separating the perceived and the actual, but he does shun the concept of 'moral panics' for implying a 'negative normative judgment' about responses to some social problems.[104] Worried about prejudicing empirical enquiries from the outset and keen to distance his work from conspiracy theory, Hunt warns against the automatic 'ascription of irrationality to projects of moral regulation'.[105] Critcher adopts an alternative position and claims that social science must have a political purpose. If research and learning is not to be used to discern reality from representation, he argues, then what exactly is the point?[106] While Hunt is right to stress that research should not begin on the grounds that its object is essentially irrational, it does not seem unreasonable to suppose that the term 'moral panic' might be used if research findings do suggest a specific social reaction to have been disproportionate or exaggerated. The term 'moral panic', denoting an extreme episode within longer-term processes of moral regulation, is therefore used sparingly in this book and always supported with reference to analysis of available evidence.

Within this conceptual synthesis, it is worth clarifying matters with regard to the persistent issue of social structure and human agency within historical social science. Succinctly, this tension revolves around whether individuals are masters of their own social destiny or products of deterministic social forces. Cohen's version of the moral panic emphasises personal agency through its focus on the people who ensure that the '"moral barricades" are manned'.[107] Foucault, by contrast, draws on the structuralist tradition in his view that human beings have no direct authorship over their own actions, as knowledge is socially constructed and individuals are socially constituted.[108] While attributing much importance to extra-individual social forces, the simultaneous recognition of the role of agency in projects of moral regulation is apparent in, for example, Hunt's concentration on the beliefs and actions of social movements and Corrigan and Sayer's assertion that the consciousness of the subordinated must be taken seriously.[109] It is suggested here that the consideration of human agency and social structure are not mutually exclusive and that the tension between them is a false dichotomy. Elias explains that:

> plans and actions, the emotional and rational impulses of individual people, constantly interweave in a friendly and hostile way. This basic tissue resulting from many single plans and actions of men can give rise to changes and patterns that no individual person has planned or created. From this interdependence of people arises a social order sui generis, an order more compelling and stronger than the will and reason of the individual people composing it.[110]

Elias thus rejects a concentration on either the atomised, free-thinking individual or monolithic, faceless social structures, alternatively promoting the non-dichotomous study of social relations. Society is composed of individuals but is simultaneously something more than just the sum of individuals who constitute it. Elias' figurational approach promotes the study of social relations, how people interact and interdepend, as a solution to the problem of agency and structure.

It is helpful, therefore, to understand moral regulation as a social relation. It refers to how individuals and groups see the world and seek to change it; how they problematise specific groups or certain behaviours and attempt regulation as a solution. Moral regulation incorporates individual and group agency as well as more impersonal political, cultural and economic frameworks within its conceptual purview. To summarise its other uses, moral regulation's connection to discursive formations, such as problematisation, suggests that it can go beyond explanations of the 'ebb and flow' of the 'drink problem' that rely on the vague notion of social anxiety. Its processual, long-term focus, albeit punctuated with shorter-term episodes of interest, also offers an appropriate rubric with which to challenge presentist representations of the 'drink problem' in England and Wales. Drawing particularly on the innovations of Hunt, Critcher and Ruonavaara, the concept of 'moral regulation' provides a suitable means with which to further the study of understandings and regulation of alcohol.[111]

Morality, regulation and moral regulation

So, moral regulation, as a conceptual lens, zeroes attention in on the discursive process of problematisation, the salience of agency and the significance of long-term developments. Thus far, however, limited exploration of *how* individuals and social groups may seek to alter the behaviour of others has been made. When translated into social action, what does the impulse to reform other people's conduct look like?

Most obviously, moral regulation may involve legal regulation. A government may, for example, pass legislation that criminalises morally undesirable behaviour and thus makes it possible for its perpetrators to be prosecuted and punished. That government might be acting in order to maintain and legitimise the existing social order or, perhaps, is acting on the instigation of a social movement. But various scholars have emphasised that regulation is far broader than law alone and refers to a whole gamut of mechanisms through which people's behaviour may be influenced. In the early 1990s, Ayres and Braithwaite depicted forms of regulation as a pyramid, with criminal justice, the most serious and least commonly used sanction, positioned above various 'softer' mechanisms for control, including persuasion and forms of self-regulation.[112] Rose and Miller made a parallel argument insisting that political power extends beyond the overt activities of the state and is apparent throughout economic activity, social life and individual conduct. Personal autonomy, they proposed, is not the antithesis of political power but has become a component in its operation as 'education, persuasion, inducement, management, incitement, motivation and encouragement' may shape individual actions into a more socially desirable form.[113] The identification of agency as diffuse and often non-state shows that much moral regulation literature embodies the idea of regulation as varied and sometimes 'soft'. This is reinforced by Ruonavaara's emphasis on efforts to persuade people to voluntarily adopt approved behavioural codes and thus reform their own behaviour.[114] Moral regulation, therefore, involves coercive legal regulation as well as extra-legal efforts to govern individual behaviour, which may be persuasive or softer.

The supposition that morality may affect the law is a little controversial. For some, the prospect is welcome. In the mid-20th century, Lord Devlin argued against the decriminalisation of gay sex by insisting that the existence of society is predicated by certain moral commonalities and so it is legitimate for the law to uphold these.[115] A century earlier, J.S. Mill took an opposing view and rallied against 'the spirit of puritanism',[116] which he saw as encouraging the legal imposition of religious and moral principles on individuals who do not share these principles. Specifically citing the temperance movement as imbued with exactly this spirit, Mill argued that 'the only purpose for which power can be rightfully exercised over any member of a civilized community, against his will, is to prevent harm to others'.[117] Mill's harm principle was invoked by H.L.A. Hart in response to Devlin.

In some ways, Hart sought to extricate morality from the ambit of law by positioning moral issues, such as sex, outside the boundaries of legitimate state action.[118] Legal positivists, such as Hart, also insist that the law grants and imposes *legal* rights and duties rather than necessarily *moral* ones.[119] However, legal positivists do generally accept that the creation of statutory law may entail the moral values of the legislature becoming law[120] and Hart also recognised that there was a 'penumbra of uncertainty'[121] surrounding much legislation, which means, in certain legal cases, that judges are required to make moral judgments about the principle or spirit of the law.[122] The law does not, therefore, exist in a social vacuum and is shaped by the attitudes of the people who devise and enforce it. While some liberals see it as unwelcome, it is difficult to reject the premise that the formulation and interpretation of law can have some connection to morality.

Of course, this assertion must be founded upon a definition of morality. Dictionaries tend to define morality in reference to the distinction between right and wrong.[123] Durkheim elaborated by describing morality as comprised of norms, rules, values, beliefs and ideals, which society either obliges or desires people to act in concert with. In terms of content, Durkheim located morality within actions that are altruistic, oriented at goals beyond individual egoism and motivated by concern for the social or common good.[124] More contentiously, Durkheim and some other social scientists believe that morality is something that is consensual or common to most members of a given society,[125] or something that brings solidarity by strengthening social bonds.[126] Without going into exhaustive depth here, it is enough to note that the author has reservations about this definition. To return to the example of homosexual relations, it is apparent that this was a divisive issue in the 1950s and 1960s, when it was debated by Devlin and Hart, and recent political controversy around gay marriage shows that, to some extent, it remains so today. Similarly, abortion, often constructed as a moral issue in reference to either women's rights or the sanctity of life, has become a crucial battleground within the US 'culture wars'.[127] This is not to refute the suggestion that moral debates may forge solidarity; instead, it is to assert that, as moral issues can also engender conflict, consensus or solidarity are not *always* components of morality. Hunt offers a preferable position by describing how any division of behaviour into acceptable and unacceptable necessarily has a moralising effect. Morality simply entails a normative judgment that a certain action is not consistent with how people *should* behave.[128] This academic definition leaves aside the troubling issue of consensus and defines morality in a manner closer to the dictionary definitions.

Wiener, drawing on Humphries, relates this point to the law. He states that 'law is not simply a corpus of practical rules, but a part of the ongoing "discourse about good and bad states of society"'.[129] The law directly concerns the designation of acceptable and unacceptable forms of conduct and, following Hunt, this overriding normative composition means that the law is inherently moral. This does not mean that legal regulation and moral regulation are coterminous; indeed, the promotion of self-reform or self-regulation has already been highlighted as a crucial form of non-legal moral regulation. Additionally, while the state possesses a monopoly on the legitimate use of coercion, it is usual (in liberal democracies at least) for it to refrain from the enforcement of morals on people. Emsley argues that the police, at least, prefer to 'act by consent' rather than by coercion.[130] To elaborate, the police are tasked, among others things, with enforcing laws on drink-driving by detecting offences and sending offenders to the courts for punishment. The state, however, does not rely on detection and punishment of infraction, or the deterrent function that publicising detection and punishment may exercise, as sufficient guarantors of lawfulness. Rather, regular government-sponsored anti-drink-driving campaigns aim to further promote compliance with the law by persuading people that drink-driving is dangerous and unacceptable. Corrigan and Sayer cite Samuel Taylor Coleridge emphasising the importance of governmental legitimacy: 'Hobbes has said that laws without the sword are but bits of parchment … but without the laws the sword is but a piece of iron.'[131] As described earlier, Corrigan and Sayer specify that moral regulation performs the function of 'rendering natural' or legitimate particular interventions in people's lives and thus producing consent to particular forms of governance. Moral regulation ensures that drink-driving restrictions and other legal regulations are widely accepted and so, as is generally the case in modern Western countries, the Hobbesian sword of governmental coercion can remain largely sheathed.

Morality, therefore, consists of a normative designation of behaviour as either right or wrong and regulation constitutes a swathe of legal and non-legal attempts to shape people's behaviour. Moral regulation, then, is the coincidence of these two phenomena; an attempt, through variable means, to alter other people's behaviour on the basis that their existing conduct is believed to be, in some sense, wrong. The concept incorporates recognition of the strong moral components of legal regulation while simultaneously enabling a broader discursive focus on extra-legal forms of regulation. It is, therefore, a useful tool with which to further knowledge of how alcohol is understood and regulated. It must be noted that the continued occurrence of both drinking and drunkenness places some limit on the extent to which any effort to morally regulate drinking could be said to be successful. The focus of this book is not, however, on drinking behaviour itself but on how that behaviour is understood and how efforts to regulate it are made. As Rose and Miller stress, 'Whilst we inhabit a world of programmes, that world is not itself programmed. We do not live in a governed world so much as a world traversed by the "will to govern".'[132] The issue at stake here is the will to govern drinking rather than its impact on behaviour. How have moral impulses to regulate drinking developed historically and how do they relate to the governance of drinking?

Methods

The need for a historical discourse analysis of the development of both public attitudes and alcohol regulation in England and Wales has been identified. The concept of 'moral regulation' has also been acknowledged as a useful tool for advancing knowledge of this area, albeit tempered with a valuation of short-term historical episodes and human agency, which is partly borrowed from moral panic theory. Methodologically, this book is constituted primarily by an analysis of law and public discourse that covers the 18th century onwards. Although simple content analysis is occasionally employed, the research is principally qualitative in nature.

A variety of sources are used to investigate public discourse relating to alcohol. Most extensively, press sources are utilised. Partly this is because recent advances in digitisation have meant that vast newspaper archives are now available online. These valuable resources have not yet been fully explored for their content pertaining to drinking. Hence, systematic searches of the British Library's (BL's) *Catalogue of Nineteenth Century Newspapers*, consisting of 49 local and national newspapers,[133] and its *Burney Collection* of 18th-century sources have been conducted. The archives of *The Times*, *The Guardian/Observer* and *UK Press Online* (which includes the *Daily Express*, *Sunday Express*, *Daily Mirror*, *Sunday Mirror* and other newspapers) have also been systematically examined, as has *Lexis Nexis*' collection of the main national newspapers from 1985 onwards. Using these digital resources allowed for thousands of news sources to be incorporated into this research. As well as availability, the press was also studied as it forms a significant part of public discourse. First, the press depicts historical events. Rowbotham and Stevenson have shown that Victorian newspapers were a generally reliable source of reportage on legal developments[134] but, even in the absence of reliability, press reports are still likely to provide useful evidence on how certain events were contemporaneously depicted.[135] Second, the press functions as a forum for the expression of opinion. These opinions may belong to journalists, editors or the owners of the newspaper, but the views of prominent public figures are often discussed and, particularly through letters sections, the views of some members of the public are also evidenced. Third, it is clear that certain publications can take a particular stance and campaign on certain issues. Newspapers or television channels can be discursive agents themselves, as well as sources of information and forums for debate. It must be acknowledged that the press is one aspect of public discourse and attempts are not made to look at, for example, novels or television shows. This is due to the focus here on efforts to regulate alcohol, rather than wider representations of drinking, to which press coverage of contemporaneous phenomena will be pertinent.

The press is thus a convenient and crucial source of information on public attitudes to alcohol. It is also a problematic source of data as reportage might be either inaccurate or unreliable. It is essential to follow the prescriptions in methodological literature to scrutinise each source according to its origins and purpose, the accuracy of its content, whether its meaning is clear and whether it is typical of its kind.[136] It is also important to clarify that, while analysed with reference to public attitudes, press sources are not relied on in this study as a proxy for public opinion. It cannot be presumed that the press either represents or determines public opinion in any straightforward way. The press is studied for its function in helping to construct an arena in which certain social issues are communicated to an audience; for what Bingham argues is its importance in creating the 'public sphere'.[137] Rather than analysing certain historical newspapers in order to retrospectively poll the opinions of its readership, this book aims to understand how alcohol was represented and debated in public forums through time. It is about attitudes expressed in public conversation, not public opinion. This public focus means that analysis may well be skewed towards dominant interests who, at any point in time, held a privileged position within public discourse.[138] It is further apparent that this book addresses mainly male drinking. This was unintended and results from a historical situation where public discourse on drinking is usually oriented towards more traditionally male issues such as violence, disorder, industrial productivity and military efficiency. Female drinking has been a public concern at some points in history but, at many other points, has been confined more to familial, medical or psychiatric domains, which are not always amenable to public scrutiny or intervention.[139]

This desire to account for *public* attitudes is also the reason why political or personal sources are not heavily used. Diaries or memoirs might reveal interesting attitudes towards alcohol but they do not form part of public conversation unless they were expressed publicly. Similarly, parliamentary debates are not studied through their minutes (available through *Hansard*) but, largely, through how they were reported in the press at the time. Public discourse is distinct from parliamentary discourse as well as public opinion. Some non-press sources are used to help gauge the character of publicly expressed attitudes to alcohol. These sources relate primarily to the public actions of certain campaign or pressure groups, such as Victorian temperance societies or contemporary public health groups. An exhaustive analysis of the actions of such groups is not attempted but they are investigated when, as active discursive agents, their efforts to morally regulate the use of alcohol gain some significance (as evidenced in wider public discourse). Hence, some sources are taken from BL's Evanion Catalogue of Victorian Printed Ephemera, the Royal Mail Archive and the publications of the Royal College of Physicians. Some visual sources, such as advertisements and artworks, are further included. Visual resources were not, however, systematically researched and have been identified indirectly by primary or secondary sources used. Hence, they are used to illustrate wider points that have been evidenced through a range of other sources.

Data on public discourse will provide evidence pertaining to public attitudes to alcohol and, potentially, 'softer' forms of regulation also, given that persuasion can be used to promote self-reform of behaviour. The principal remaining source of evidence for this enquiry is law – the 'hard' regulation. Hence, considerable use of legislation relating to the sale and consumption of alcohol is analysed. Legislation is analysed in reference to the forms of regulation it established (or attempted to establish) in addition to being assessed for its qualitative symmetry to public attitudes. This latter task allows for the normative judgments that underpin legal regulation to be interrogated and for the moral ethos that animated forms of legal regulation, as in Corrigan and Sayer's work, to be considered. The enforcement of law, by courts, police or other agencies, is not directly analysed here and is studied only in so far as it featured in public discourse at any point in time. Partly this is due to time constraints but also due to the concentration here on, to return to Rose and Miller's term, the 'will to govern' drinking. The performative aspects of those attempts at governance relate more closely to the behavioural aspects of the 'drink problem', which are not the priorities of this study.[140]

The breadth of source material poses a problem in terms of how much can feasibly be examined. This problem is exacerbated by the timeframe of this study. The developmental focus of moral regulation, as well as the desire to understand whether the 19th century was indeed the turning point it initially appears, means that concentrating on the 18th century onwards is necessary. It is simply not viable to produce a comprehensive study of press, legal and other sources that spans three hundred years. The paucity of available press sources from the 18th century means a long-term focus on that period is possible (and is conducted in Chapter Two), but the same cannot be said for subsequent centuries. Research has generally been conducted, therefore, in a longitudinal manner with detailed analysis of public discourse and relevant law conducted at certain points throughout history. These points have been selected to embody either heightened public debates about alcohol and/or significant regulatory moments, such as the passage of an important legislation through Parliament. While intervening periods are not studied intensively, a certain amount of primary source material from them is studied and secondary literature is also used to ensure that important events and processes are not overlooked. As well as being practical, this episodic approach to the study of historical development corresponds to the conceptual underpinnings of this study. If, following Critcher and Hier, there are short-term high points within the long-term processes of moralisation, then it seems logical that they should be studied. This is particularly pertinent given the socio-legal focus of this book as said high points of concern also tend to coincide with significant legal reforms.

Chapter Two spans from 1700 to 1840. As noted, this timeframe is enabled by the shortage of 18th-century sources. Sources for the 19th century are more plentiful and so data collection was concentrated around the period from 1828 to 1840. The emergence of the British temperance movement, its distinctiveness from earlier efforts to morally regulate drinking and its relationship to the liberalising Beer Act 1830 are addressed. The next two chapters form something of an impact assessment as they examine the relationship of the temperance movement, at different points in its lifespan, to changing legal regulations. Chapter Three focuses on the new forms of drink regulation established between 1864 and 1872, with a particular concern for the Licensing Act 1872 – the basis of much current alcohol regulation. Chapter Four examines the fascinating period from 1914 to 1918, during which time a host of new restrictions on drinks sales were pioneered and various authorities urged citizens, for the good of the nation, to abstain from alcohol for the duration of the war. It further investigates the post-war alcohol settlement, which made the wartime closure of licensed premises in the morning and afternoon permanent. In both chapters, the temperance movement's crucial formative impact on public attitudes to alcohol and attempts to regulate drinking will be highlighted. Across Chapters Two, Three and Four the concept of 'moral regulation' is further elucidated and explicitly related to historical developments.

The subsequent chapters embody a slight change of tack. This is partly related to their concentration on the inter-war years onwards, during which time the temperance movement was in terminal decline in Britain. But it will also become apparent that they concern the advent of discursive and regulatory frameworks more indicative of the contemporary 'drink problem'. Chapter Five examines the emergence of youth, drink-driving and female drinking as major public concerns in the inter-war and post-war years. It includes intensive studies of 1923 and 1961–65, as these periods coincide with significant legal reforms, as well as the Second World War, a period in which surprisingly little regulatory change occurred. Chapters Six and Seven are thematically arranged. Chapter Six examines the burgeoning association of alcohol with crime and disorder throughout the late 20th and early 21st centuries. Detailed studies, which correspond chronologically to legal changes, are made of 1985, 1988 and 2003. Chapter Seven concentrates on issues of health, harm and risk and, after some focus on the 1960s and 1980s, focuses on public attitudes to alcohol and campaigns for regulatory change from around 2007 onwards. Both chapters examine the various regulatory mechanisms, both legal and extra-legal, which constitute current attempts to morally regulate the use of alcohol. In both chapters, the qualitative affinity between recent moral regulation projects and their Victorian antecedents is also stressed.

It must be emphasised that this book is not a comprehensive history of alcohol laws or attitudes to alcohol. Nor is it an entirely comprehensive exploration of the nuances of temperance through time. It does, however, aim to identify and explain the key formative moments in the construction of the contemporary 'drink problem' in England and Wales. Its unique focus on public attitudes and regulation, as well as extensive use of press sources over such a long timeframe, mean that new light is shed on some hitherto shady areas of history. This book, for instance, includes the first systematic analysis of the 'pledge' campaign mounted during the First World War as well as significant analysis of the 'drink problem' in the often overlooked period 1939–45. Additionally, the concept of 'moral regulation' gives the book a critical edge, which helps enable some of the sacred cows that are revered in other studies of this subject area to be slaughtered. For example, the idea that the British temperance movement achieved very little is disputed in Chapter Three, the notion that the 1950s and 1960s ushered in a 'normatively neutral' age of permissiveness is challenged in Chapter Five, contemporary attempts to separate moral and medical conceptions of drinking are confronted in Chapter Seven and the emphasis placed on de-regulation by many scholars of current alcohol governance is attacked in Chapter Six. Ultimately, a fuller comprehension of how the way in which we understand and seek to regulate alcohol in England and Wales has developed through history will be fostered. The sort of cross-national differences noted at the beginning of this chapter may continue to be amusing but, by the end of the book, they will hopefully be less puzzling.

Notes

[1] 'France Riot Police Face Beer and Wine Meal Ban', *BBC News*, 22 April 2011.

[2] 'Russia Finally Accepts that Beer is Alcoholic', *Daily Telegraph*, 21 July 2011.

[3] Kelly, Lorraine 'Booze Britain: It's a Plague', *The Sun*, 2008, 29 February.

[4] Donaldson, Sir Liam, *Annual Report of the Chief Medical Officer 2008: On the State of Public Health*, London: Department of Health, 2009, p 5.

[5] Gilmore, Anna, and Colin, Jeff, 'Drink Companies Spread Liver Disease as Surely Mosquitoes do Malaria', *The Guardian*, 21 February 2011.

[6] Linklater, Magnus (2009) 'The Terrible Cost of Not Raising Drink Prices', *The Times*, 17 March.

[7] 'Alcohol Pricing: Government Accused of Weak Leadership', *BBC News*, 13 March 2013.

[8] Kelly, 'Booze Britain'.

[9] Ibid.

[10] Orwell, George, 'As I Please', *Tribune*, 18 August 1944.

[11] 'Alcohol the "New British Disease"', *BBC News*, 20 May 2004.

[12] Hunt, Alan, *Governing Morals: A Social History of Moral Regulation*, Cambridge: Cambridge University Press, 1999, p 196.

[13] See: UK Government, *Safe. Sensible. Social.*, London: Department of Health, 2007.

[14] Johnston, Lucy, 'Ban Alcohol in Binge Towns', *Sunday Express*, 22 March 2009.

[15] 'Profile: Chief Constable Peter Fahy', *BBC News*, 18 August 2007.

[16] See: Donaldson, *Annual Report*.

[17] Harrison, Brian, *Drink and the Victorians*, London: Faber and Faber, 1971, pp 66-72; Plant, Martin, and Plant, Moira, *Binge Britain*, Oxford: Oxford University

Press, 2006, p 29; Wilson, George B., *Alcohol and the State*, London: Nicholson and Watson, 1940, pp 331–335.

[18] 'Attitude', *Oxford Dictionaries*, http://oxforddictionaries.com/definition/english/attitude?q=attitudes

[19] While I sometimes refer to Britain or the British in this book, the focus here is on the legal jurisdiction of England and Wales. The book will likely hold some relevance for those interested in the 'drink problem' in other parts of the British Isles, but no specific attempts are made to investigate drinking in other areas. Those interested in attitudes and the regulation of alcohol in Scotland are directed towards: McLaughlin, Patrick M., 'Responding to Drunkenness in Scottish Society: A Socio-Historical Study of Responses to Alcohol Problems', unpublished PhD thesis, University of Stirling, 1989.

[20] Donaldson, *Annual Report*, p 22.

[21] Moriarty, Kieran, and Gilmore, Ian T., 'Licensing Britain's Alcohol Epidemic', *Journal of Epidemiology and Community Health*, 2006, vol 60, p 94.

[22] Goode, Erich, and Ben-Yehuda, Nachmann, 'Grounding and Defending the Sociology of Moral Panic', in Hier, Sean (ed) *Moral Panic and the Politics of Anxiety*, Abingdon: Routledge, 2011, pp 29–36.

[23] Wiener, Martin, *Reconstructing the Criminal*, Cambridge: Cambridge University Press, 1990.

[24] Thom, Betsy, *Dealing with Drink: Alcohol and Social Policy from Treatment to Prevention*, London: Free Association Books, 1999, p 11.

[25] Plant and Plant, *Binge Britain*. See also: Greenfield, T.K., and Giesbrecht, N.A., 'Views of Alcohol Control Policies in the 2000 National Alcohol Survey: What News for Alcohol Policy Development in the US and its States?', *Journal of Substance Use*, 2007, vol 12 (6), pp 429–445.

[26] Sheron, Nick, Hawkey, Chris, and Gilmore, Ian, 'Projections of Alcohol Deaths – a Wake Up Call', *The Lancet*, 2011, vol 377 (9774), pp 1297–1299.

[27] Ibid, p 1298.

[28] Warner, Jessica, Her, Minghao, Gmel, Gerhard, and Rehm, Jurgen, 'Can Legislation Prevent Debauchery? Mother Gin and Public Health in 18th Century England', *American Journal of Public Health*, 2001, vol 91 (3), pp 375–384.

[29] Plant and Plant, *Binge Britain*, p 29; Wilson, *Alcohol and the State*, pp 331–335.

[30] Jennings, Paul, 'Policing Drunkenness in England and Wales from the Late Eighteenth Century to the First World War', *The Social History of Alcohol and Drugs*, 2012, vol 26 (1), pp 69–92.

[31] Plant and Plant, *Binge Britain*, p 29.

[32] Sheron et al, 'Projections of Alcohol Deaths'.

[33] WHO (World Health Organization), *Global Status Report on Alcohol*, Geneva: WHO, 2004, www.who.int/substance_abuse/publications/global_status_report_2004_overview.pdf, pp 11–12.

34 Office for National Statistics, *General Lifestyle Survey*, Newport: Office for National Statistics, 2013; Whalley, Rachel, 'Drinking Alcohol', in Fuller, Elizabeth (ed) *Smoking, Drinking and Drug Use among Young People in England 2011*, London: NatCen Social Research, 2012, pp 121-152; 'Alcohol Consumption "Continues to Fall"', *BBC News*, 3 September 2010.

35 Hibell, Bjorn, Guttormsson, Ulf, Ahlström, Salme, Balakireva, Olga, Bjarnason, Thoroddur, Kokkevi, Anna, and Kraus, Ludwig, *The 2007 ESPAD Report*, Stockholm: European School Survey Project on Alcohol and Other Drugs, 2007.

36 Measham, Fiona, and Ostergaard, Jeanette, 'The Public Face of Binge Drinking: British and Danish Young Women, Recent Trends in Alcohol Consumption and the European Binge Drinking Debate', *Probation Journal*, 2009, vol 56, pp 415-434.

37 WHO, *Global Status Report on Alcohol*, p 57.

38 Office for National Statistics, 'Crime in England and Wales: Year Ending December 2012', 2013, www.ons.gov.uk/ons/dcp171778_307458.pdf

39 Room, Robin, 'Addiction and Personal Responsibility as Solutions to the Contradictions of Neoliberal Consumerism', in Bell, Kirsten, McNaughton, Darlene, and Salmon, Amy (eds) *Alcohol, Tobacco and Obesity*, Abingdon: Routledge, 2011, pp 47-58.

40 Schrad, Mark Lawrence, *The Political Power of Bad Ideas*, Oxford: Oxford University Press, 2010.

41 Hadfield, Phil, *Bar Wars: Contesting the Night in Contemporary British Cities*, Oxford: Oxford University Press, 2006; Hayward, Keith, and Hobbs, Dick, 'Beyond the Binge in Booze Britain: Market-led Liminalisation and the Spectacle of Binge Drinking', *British Journal of Sociology*, 2007, vol 58 (3), pp 437-456; Winlow, Simon, and Hall, Steve, *Violent Night*, Oxford: Berg, 2006.

42 Gusfield, Joseph, *Contested Meanings: The Construction of Alcohol Problems*, Wisconsin, WI: University of Wisconsin Press, 1996, p 12.

43 Hunt, *Governing Morals*, p 38.

44 Reinarman, Craig, 'The Social Construction of an Alcohol Problem: The Case of Mothers Against Drunk Drivers and Social Control in the 1980s', *Theory and Society*, 1988, vol 17 (1), pp 91-120.

45 Barr, Andrew, *Drink: A Social History*, London: Pimlico, 1988; Brown, Pete, *Man Walks into Pub*, London: Pan Macmillan, 2004; Burnett, John, *Liquid Pleasures*, London: Routledge, 1999; Hames, Gina, *Alcohol in World History*, Abingdon: Routledge, 2012, pp 33-45; Jennings, Paul, *The Local: A History of the English Pub*, Stroud: History Press, 2007.

46 Burnett, *Liquid Pleasures*, p 111.

47 Wilson, *Alcohol and the Nation*, p 94.

48 Burnett, *Liquid Pleasures*, pp 112-124.

49 Ibid, p 1.

50 Warner, Jessica, *Craze: Gin and Debauchery in an Age of Reason*, London: Profile, 2004, p 7.

51 Borsay, Peter, 'Binge Drinking and Moral Panics: Historic Parallels?', (2007) *History and Policy*, www.historyandpolicy.org/papers/policy-paper-62.html (accessed 11 June 2011).

52 Critcher, Chas, 'Drunken Antics: The Gin Craze, Binge Drinking and the Political Economy of Moral Regulation', in Hier, Sean (ed) *Moral Panics and Politics of Anxiety*, London: Routledge, 2011, pp 171-189. See also: Nicholls, James, *The Politics of Alcohol*, Manchester: Manchester University Press, 2009; Warner, *Craze*.

53 The Mass Observation was a social research project, begun in the 1930s, which examined everyday life. It included a number of observations of pubs and drinking behaviour.

54 Malcolmson, Robert W., *Popular Recreations in English Society 1700–1850*, Cambridge: Cambridge University Press, 1979; Roberts, M.J.D., *Making English Morals*, Cambridge: Cambridge University Press, 2004.

55 Elias, Norbert, *The Civilizing Process*, Oxford: Blackwell, 1994, p 56.

56 Ibid, p 443.

57 Foucault, Michel, *Discipline and Punish*, London: Penguin, 1991.

58 Foucault, Michel, *Security, Territory, Population: Lectures at the College de France 1977–78*, Palgrave: Basingstoke, 2007, p 120.

59 Greenaway, John, *Drink and British Politics*, Basingstoke: Palgrave, 2003, p 21.

60 Ibid, pp 29-34.

61 Ibid, pp 1-2.

62 Baggott, Rob, *Alcohol, Politics and Social Policy*, Aldershot: Gower, 1990; Thom, *Dealing with Drink*.

63 Baggott, *Alcohol, Politics and Social Policy*, pp 157-158.

64 Thom, *Dealing with Drink*.

65 Nicholls, *Politics of Alcohol*, p 260.

66 Ibid, pp 96-108.

67 Ibid, pp 34-50. See also: Warner, *Craze*.

68 Ibid, p 255.

69 Harrison, *Drink and the Victorians*; Shiman, Lilian Lewis, *Crusade Against Drink*, Basingstoke: Macmillan, 1988. Although Harrison's timeframe extends only until 1872, his final chapter 'The End' comments on the drink problem after that date and into the early years of the 20th century.

70 Shiman, *Crusade Against Drink*, p 4; Harrison, *Drink and the Victorians*, pp 393-396.

71 Shiman, *Crusade Against Drink*, pp 1-5 and pp 244-248. In this respect, Shiman's analysis of the social function of organised temperance for the working class parallels E.P. Thompson's examination of Methodism in the same period. Dorn, by contrast, tied the temperance movement to state concerns for social control over the working class. See: Thompson, E.P., *The Making of the English Working Class*, Middlesex: Penguin, 1980; Dorn, Nicholas, *Alcohol, Youth and*

the State: Drinking Practices, Controls and Health Education, Beckenham, Kent: Croon Helm, 1983.

72 Harrison, *Drink and the Victorians*, p 28.

73 Shiman, *Crusade Against Drink*, p 244.

74 Levine, Harry, 'Temperance Cultures: Concern about Alcohol in Nordic and English-Speaking Countries', in Lader, Malcolm, Edwards, Griffith, and Drummon, D. Colin (eds) *The Nature of Alcohol and Drug-Related Problems*, Oxford: Oxford University Press, 1993, pp 16-36.

75 The other anecdotal counterpoint to Britain raised earlier – Russia – is harder to categorise using Levine's criteria. Prohibition was implemented by the Tsarist government in 1914 and retained for several years by Bolsheviks after the October Revolution. In the absence of a significant social movement campaigning for this measure, Schrad portrayed Russian prohibition as a top-down regulation. See: Schrad, *Political Power of Bad Ideas*.

76 Pittman, David J., 'International Overview: Social and Cultural Factors in Drinking Patterns, Pathological and Non-Pathological', 1967, viewed at www.api.or.at/akis/donauuni/pittman.pdf, p 3. Pittman actually suggested that France might be overly permissive, although consumption has fallen since he wrote this in the 1960s.

77 Osterberg, Esa L., 'Alcohol Tax Changes and the Use of Alcohol in Europe', *Drugs and Alcohol Review*, vol 30 (2), pp 124-129.

78 See: Blocker, Jack S., Fahey, David M. and Tyrell, Ian R., *Alcohol and Temperance in Modern History: An International Encyclopaedia*, Santa Barbara, CA: ABC-CLIO, 2003.

79 Reinarman, 'The Social Construction of an Alcohol Problem'.

80 Ibid, p 91.

81 Gusfield, *Contested Meanings*; Sulkunen, Pekka, *The Saturated Society: Governing Risk and Lifestyle in Consumer Culture*, London: Sage, 2009; Valverde, Mariana, *Diseases of the Will: Alcohol and the Dilemmas of Freedom*, Cambridge: Cambridge University Press, 1998.

82 Durkheim, Emile, *Suicide*, London: Routledge, 1970.

83 Corrigan, Phillip, and Sayer, Derek, *The Great Arch: English State Formation as Cultural Revolution*, London: Basil Blackwell, 1985, p 4.

84 Ruonavaara, Hannu, 'Moral Regulation: a Reformulation', *Sociological Theory*, 1997, vol 15 (3), pp 277-293.

85 Ibid.

86 Hunt, *Governing Morals*, p 1.

87 See: Hunt, *Governing Morals*; Ruonavaara, 'Moral Regulation'.

88 Ruonavaara, 'Moral Regulation'.

89 Foucault, Michel, *The Government of Self and Others*, Basingstoke, Palgrave, 2010, p 6; Hunt, *Governing Morals*, p 2.

90 Ben-Yehuda, Nachman, 'Moral Panics – 36 Years On', *British Journal of Criminology*, 2009, vol 49, pp 1-3; Jenkins, Philip, 'Failure to Launch: Why do

Some Social Issues Fail to Detonate Moral Panics?', *British Journal of Criminology*, 2009, vol 49, pp 35-47.

[91] Cohen, Stanley, *Folk Devils and Moral Panics*, London: MacGibbon and Kee, 1972, p 9.

[92] Gusfield, Joseph R., 'Status Anxiety and the Changing Ideologies of the American Temperance Movement', in Pittman, David J., and Snyder, Charles R. (eds) *Society, Culture and Drinking Patterns*, New York, NY: John Wiley and Sons, 1962.

[93] Borsay, 'Historical Parallels?'. Critcher has also examined this period with reference to moral panic theory: Critcher, Chas, 'Drunken Antics: The Gin Craze, Binge Drinking and Political Economy of Moral Regulation', in Hier, Sean (ed) *Moral Panics and Politics of Anxiety*, Abingdon: Routledge, 2011, pp 171-189.

[94] Thompson, E.P., *Whigs and Hunters*, Harmondswoth: Penguin, 1977, p 195.

[95] Hunt, *Governing Morals*, p 28.

[96] Cohen, *Folk Devils*, p 9.

[97] Rowbotham, Judith, and Stevenson, Kim, *Behaving Badly*, Aldershot: Ashgate, 2003.

[98] Greenaway, *Drink and British Politics*, p 91.

[99] Afternoon closure of licensed premises was abolished by the Licensing Act 1988 and the statutory prohibition on morning opening was scrapped by the Licensing Act 2003.

[100] Hier, Sean P., 'Thinking Beyond Moral Panic: Risk, Responsibility, and the Politics of Moralization', *Theoretical Criminology*, 2008, vol 12 (2), pp 173-190.

[101] Ibid, p 174.

[102] Critcher, Chas, 'Widening the Focus: Moral Panics as Moral Regulation', *British Journal of Criminology*, 2009, vol 49 (1), pp 17-34.

[103] See: Bhaskar, Roy, *A Realist Theory of Science*, Hemel Hempstead: Harvester, 1978.

[104] Hunt, *Governing Morals*, p 19.

[105] Ibid.

[106] Critcher, 'Widening the Focus', p 32.

[107] Cohen, *Folk Devils and Moral Panics*, p 9.

[108] Ruonavaara, 'Moral Regulation', p 282. It should be stressed that, although sharing a rejection of human agency with structuralism, Foucault was a post-structuralist. Structuralists, such as Althusser, downplay the extent to which individuals control their own destiny and highlight the omnipotence of external social structures. By contrast, post-structuralists argue that an individual's knowledge or understanding of the social forces that govern their destiny are also socially constructed.

[109] Corrigan and Sayer, *The Great Arch*, p 9.

[110] Elias, *Civilizing Process*, p 444.

[111] I have explored the conceptual issues presented here in more depth in the following book chapter: Yeomans, Henry, 'Theorising Alcohol in Public Discourse: Moral Panics or Moral Regulation?', in Petley, Julian, Critcher, Chas, Hughes, Jason, and Rohloff, Amanda (eds) *Moral Panics in the Contemporary World*, London: Bloomsbury, 2013. See also: Yeomans, Henry, 'What did the British Temperance Movement Accomplish? Attitudes to Alcohol, the Law and Moral Regulation', *Sociology*, 2011, vol 45 (1), pp 38-53.

[112] Ayres, Ian, and Braithwaite, John, *Responsive Regulation: Transcending the Deregulation Debate*, Oxford: Oxford University Press, 1992.

[113] Rose, Nikolas, and Miller, Peter, 'Political Power Beyond the State: Problematics of Government', *British Journal of Sociology*, 1992, vol 43 (2), p 175.

[114] Ruonavaara, 'Moral Regulation', p 290.

[115] Harcourt, Bernard E., 'The Collapse of the Harm Principle', *Journal of Criminal Law and Criminology*, 1999, vol 90 (1), pp 109-194.

[116] Mill, John Stuart, *On Liberty*, London: Penguin, 1985, p 72.

[117] Ibid, p 68.

[118] Hart, Herbert L.A., *Essays in Jurisprudence and Philosophy*, Oxford: Oxford University Press, 1983.

[119] Simmonds, Nigel E., *Central Issues on Jurisprudence*, London: Sweet and Maxwell, 1986.

[120] Ibid, p 79; Hart, *Essays in Jurisprudence and Philosophy*, p 54.

[121] Hart, *Essays in Jurisprudence and Philosophy*, p 64.

[122] Ibid, pp 64-70.

[123] See, for example: *Oxford Dictionaries*, 'Morality', http://oxforddictionaries.com/definition/english/morality?q=morality

[124] Lukes, Steven, *Emile Durkheim: His Life and Work*, London: Penguin, 1973, pp 410-430.

[125] See, for example: Sulkunen, *The Saturated Society*. Sulkunen defined morality primarily in relation to a shared social vision of 'the good life'.

[126] Lukes, *Emile Durkheim*; Donajgrodzki, A.P., 'Introduction', in Donajgrodzki, A.P. (ed) *Social Control in Nineteenth Century Britain*, London: Croon Helm, 1977.

[127] See: Sandel, Michael J., *Justice: What's the Right Thing to Do?*, London: Penguin, 2009; Smith, Alexander Thomas T., 'Fear and Loathing in Kansas City', *Anthropology Today*, 2010, vol 26 (4), pp 4-7.

[128] Hunt, *Governing Morals*, pp 7-8.

[129] Wiener, *Reconstructing the Criminal*, pp 3-4.

[130] Emsley, Clive, *The English Police*, London: Longman, 1991, p 5.

[131] Corrigan and Sayer, *The Great Arch*, p 14.

[132] Rose and Miller, 'Political Power Beyond the State', pp 190-191.

[133] This sample was Part 1 of the BL's digitisation project (as Part 2 was not available at the time research was conducted). Also, although Scottish and Irish

newspapers are contained within the BL's catalogue, they are not utilised unless they bear some specific relevance to events in England and Wales.

[134] Rowbotham, Judith, and Stevenson, Kim, 'Causing a Sensation: Media and Legal Representations of Bad Behaviour', in Rowbotham, Judith, and Stevenson, Kim (eds) *Behaving Badly*, Aldershot: Ashgate, 2003, pp 33-46.

[135] In documentary analysis, it is usual for sources to be studied for what they tell us about the social world and as features or constructs of that social world. See: Prior, Lindsay, 'Following in Foucault's Footsteps', in Silverman, David (ed) *Qualitative Research*, London: Sage Publications, 1997, pp 64-65.

[136] Bryman, Alan, *Social Research Methods*, Oxford: Oxford University Press, 2004, p 381; Matthews, Bob, and Ross, Liz, *Research Methods*, Harlow: Pearson, 2010, pp 278-279.

[137] Bingham, Adrian, *Family Newspapers? Sex, Private Lives and the British Popular Press, 1918–1978*, Oxford: Oxford University Press, 2009, p 11.

[138] I very deliberately say 'skewed towards' rather than 'determined by' dominant groups. There are two main reasons for this linguistic choice. First, I do not think that dominant interests are always homogenous and believe that it is important to recognise that diverse attitudes can often exist within social elites. Second, I have much sympathy for Stephen Turner's description of liberal democracy as 'government by discussion'. This is not a naive assertion of the importance of public opinion to government; rather, it is a recognition that, as parts of this chapter have already explained, consent and legitimacy are crucial considerations for liberal democratic governments. This encourages social elites to engage in public discourse, to persuade, to challenge, to motivate and perhaps occasionally to listen, rather than just to dominate through actual or threatened coercion. This form of public engagement means that public attitudes are not purely or simply those held by social elites and even elite attitudes expressed in public may have been adapted in order to better generate approval from a wider public. See: Turner, Stephen, *Liberal Democracy 3.0*, London: Sage Publications, 2003.

[139] See: Moss, Stella, '"A Grave Question": The Children Act and Public House Regulation, c.1908-1939', *Crimes and Misdemeanours*, 2009, vol 3 (2), pp 98-117; Valverde, *Diseases of the Will*.

[140] Those interested in the policing of drunkenness and the enforcement of licensing laws are directed to: Jennings, 'Policing Drunkenness'; Jennings, Paul, 'Policing Public Houses in Victorian England', *Law, Crime and History*, 2013, vol 3 (1), pp 52-75.

TWO

Temperance and teetotalism

Introduction

This book concerns the historical development of public attitudes and the regulation of alcohol. Within this broad remit, the last chapter noted the potential salience of the Victorian temperance movement to these issues and outlined the book's specific intentions to explore this further. How did this social movement relate to public attitudes to alcohol and the governance of drinking in England and Wales? This chapter will investigate this question through an examination of public discourse on alcohol and legal sources before and during the period in which the temperance movement emerged. Somewhere in the region of 500 newspaper and periodical sources have been considered and, additionally, a number of other sources are used, from David Wilkie's painting 'The Village Holiday' to *A History of Teetotalism in Devonshire* by the West Country temperance activist W. Hunt. These sources supplied a large quantity of evidence with which certain key issues are explored. What were the views of the first wave of temperance followers? Did these differ from 18th-century concerns about drinking? How did the temperance movement relate to the legal and ideological context of its period?

The emergence of the British temperance movement could feasibly be explained, using either moral panic theory or the rational, objectivist model of alcohol policy, as a straightforward response to a liberal legal stimulus. The first British temperance groups were formed in the late 1820s, before spreading across the country in the 1830s. The advent of temperance societies, therefore, coincided with a period of licensing reform, most notably engendered by the Beer Act 1830. This was a liberalising piece of legislation, which enabled householders to sell beer without the permission of the local licensing justice. This Act, in addition to the gradual replacement of domestic brewing with large-scale commercial brewing,[1] coincided with a surge in the numbers of premises nationwide selling beer and an accompanying increase in the number of arrests for drunkenness.[2] These trends were not unnoticed and, ultimately, the Beer Act 1830 fermented considerable unease about the drinking habits of the population. It was in this context of increased availability of alcohol and apparently diminishing social order that the early temperance movement flourished. So, was the growth of the movement attributable to increasing 'rational' concerns about 'real' social problems caused by drink? Or did, as moral panic theory might postulate, the British temperance movement tap into a reservoir of social anxiety stored up by a liberalising Act of Parliament or other social changes? Or was there, perhaps, more to it than either of these theoretical positions can encapsulate? Is it worth considering whether the British temperance movement was not a reaction, to either legislation or drinking habits, at all?

The 'second necessity of life'

Chapter One explained how beer and other forms of alcohol were socially ubiquitous substances that were viewed as largely unproblematic for much of British history. However, by the late 18th and early 19th centuries, these generally permissive attitudes towards drinking appeared increasingly inconsistent with the apparent pervasiveness of wider processes of moralisation. In 1787, William Wilberforce persuaded King George III to issue a Royal Proclamation, which called on local authorities to enforce existing laws that aimed to suppress vice and immorality. This new impetus towards moral reform was embodied in the actions of groups such as the Proclamation Society and the Society for the Suppression of Vice, which promoted much stricter personal codes of behaviour. Concerned with immorality broadly, these societies condemned, among other things, gaming, lewd plays, obscene publications, the breaking of the Sabbath and drunkenness.[3] While drunkenness was not their sole or paramount concern, the greater moralisation of everyday life promoted by such groups does seem at odds with the generally permissive, pre-modern attitudes to alcohol that were popular until well into the 19th century. This chapter aims to explore how new moral codes developed around alcohol and how they interacted with dominant attitudes, as expressed particularly through the law.

Classical virtues and Georgian excesses

Drinking was undoubtedly a major social, legal and political issue in the 18th century. Barr describes Georgian outrage about drinking habits and legal efforts to combat this problem behaviour as representing the beginnings of the temperance movement.[4] Is this accurate? What were the key features of public discourse on alcohol in the 18th century?

The problem of gin

The 'gin craze' or 'gin panics' occurred roughly from 1720 to 1750 and were largely centred on London. Gin was a relatively new drink to the British, having arrived with the Dutch King William III after the Glorious Revolution. Although brandy and whisky had been available previously, gin was the first alcoholic spirit consumed on a mass scale and its consumption appears to have increased dramatically from 1700 to 1750.[5] But historians frequently draw attention to additional or alternative reasons why gin became the subject of such frenzied attention during this period. Between 1632 and 1750, the population of London more than doubled[6] and this unprecedented growth is highlighted by Borsay as fostering social anxieties that came to be directed at gin.[7] Nicholls emphasises that in new, crowded urban spaces the sheer visibility of drunkenness among the lower classes prompted concern and outrage.[8] Both Sennett and Ehrenreich describe broader efforts to impose bourgeois notions of social order on all aspects of the behaviour of the new urban poor,[9] and Warner links this explicitly to drink by stating that 'the debate over gin was a debate over the nature of cities and the different sorts of people who inhabit them'.[10] In this context of rapid urbanisation, shifting demography and a bourgeois desire for social order, more usual concerns about drunkenness came to be articulated with an increased frequency and ferocity.

Gin-drinking thus became the focus of much public discourse. In 1710, *Athenian News* claimed that 'drunkenness is a vice epidemical among us'[11] and, in 1745, a letter in the *Universal Spectator* complained that 'those who drink only for the sake of Drunkenness ... have the peculiar felicity in this Island'.[12] A particular problem was identified in regards to female gin-drinking. Warner describes how, seeing as women drank and often sold the spirit, gin took on a feminine folk identity as 'Madame Geneva' or 'Mother Gin'.[13] This identity further fuelled alarm; one writer, after expressing dismay at reports that women, 'the weaker vessels', were out-drinking men, then asked: 'What words can prevail on Mankind, when such dreadful Appearances of Drunkenness can't?'.[14] This gendered preoccupation is apparent in, the most famous record of the 'gin panics', William Hogarth's 'Gin Lane'. Amid a grim carnival of brawling, sickness and death, Hogarth's aesthetic centrepiece is a woman who, too drunk to support it, has dropped her child head-first off some steps.[15] For many, gin and female drunkenness were huge, daunting social problems. A letter in the *Grub Street Journal* claimed that 'nothing but an omnipotent Agent can stem the torrent of Vice and Intemperance which rages thro' the land'.[16]

Contextualising responses to gin-drinking

Regardless of what the *Grub Street Journal* printed, 18th-century mortals drew on the old wisdom of temperance in an attempt to reduce gin-drinking. The influence of this concept is clearly apparent in 18th-century discourse; for example, after his death, Henry Hoare was described by *Covent Garden Journal* as 'an example of Temperance' and 'every good and aimiable [sic] Quality'.[17] But temperance was not just an admirable character trait; a volume advertised in the *London Evening Post*, of '16 discourses upon doctrines and duties more peculiarly Christian; and against the reigning Vanities of the Age', named temperance as one of several necessary Christian virtues.[18] This advertised text reflected the accepted theological importance of temperance. In the fourth and fifth centuries, drunkenness was attacked as a 'a work of the flesh' by Christian scholar Augustine of Hippo, and in the 13th century temperance was ranked as one of four cardinal virtues by Thomas Aquinas.[19] Prior to its codification as a Christian virtue, temperance had been considered highly valuable by the Classical civilisations of Greece and Rome. Moreover, the continued vitality of Classical temperance was apparent, for instance, in 1797 when the *Oracle and Public Advertiser* printed a list of quotes on the subject of drunkenness, which featured the likes of Hippocrates, Cicero and Zeno. Zeno's quote, emphasising the need for moderation and balance, captures Classical temperance well: 'A wise man will drink wine but will not suffer himself to be intoxicated by it.'[20] The Georgian writer Philotechnos's statement that the best kind of life is a 'simple, sober and modest Life; adorned with Temperance and Continence' reflects the 18th-century popularity of both Christian and Classical notions of temperance.[21]

Importantly, temperance was not just a virtue to be applied to drinking. In 1729, a letter in the *London Journal* defined intemperance as 'that Use of Meat and Drink, or whatever the natural Appetite invites to, which is pernicious to the Health and Vigour of any Person, in the Discharge of the Offices of Life'.[22] Moderation in eating was also seen as essential and *Lloyd's Evening Post* went as far as asserting that 'Intemperance in Eating is the grossest abuse of the gifts of Providence', it decays the body and impairs our 'nobler faculties'.[23] Additionally, 'an injudicious pursuit of sensual gratifications' would make a man 'a Fornicator' as well as 'a Glutton, or a Drunkard'.[24] A piece in *World* in 1756 claimed that to reform a 'luxurious person' one had to show him 'the deformity of intemperance and debauchery' and then instruct him to 'fast and pray, to sleep little, and to avoid the company of women'.

If these directions are followed, soon 'he will scarce bear to hear a female mentioned, and nauseate the very thought of a sumptuous entertainment'.[25] Heavy drinking was not, for the most part, the singular concern of those who moralised about personal behaviour. Eating and sexual behaviour were also areas of conduct in which it was necessary to apply the virtues of Classical and Christian temperance.

Drinking was just one aspect of behaviour in which moderation was required, and the alcoholic drink itself was not the primary problem. Prater explained: 'the Juice of the Grape, when administered from the Cup of Temperance, is an innocent, grateful and salutary Potion. 'Tis Excess only which adulterates it, and renders it a deadly Poison.'[26] Drinking was not, therefore, immoral in itself; concerns lay primarily with drunkenness and the kinds of actions it may occasion. As the *Universal Spectator* explained: 'Drunkenness is a Vice which seldom comes alone, but generally draws after it some other *Shameful Consequences*'.[27] Intemperance 'makes the Throne of Reason totter from its Basis',[28] meaning the drunken individual is 'prepared for the committing of every sin'.[29] For *E. Johnson's British Gazette*, drinking affects memory and imagination, and hence tends to disqualify wealthy drunkards from 'intellectual attainments' and leads poor drunkards into 'want and wretchedness'.[30] *Athenian News* was more specific about the sort of problems drunkenness leads to and divided them into 'inward Dangers', which cover various sicknesses, and 'outward Dangers' such as 'being engag'd in deceitful Bargains, firing of Houses, &c'.[31] Excess in drinking therefore, as with food and sex, was dangerous due to its capacity to produce a multitude of sinful behaviour.

The problem, therefore, was gin-drinking and the drunkenness it so readily produced. Hogarth contrasted 'Gin Lane' to another print of 'Beer Street'. 'Beer Street' is a more orderly and prosperous vision in which alcohol is enjoyed without the horrific consequences depicted in 'Gin Lane'. Borsay explains how, while gin was often seen as a French drink, beer was represented as patriotic; Hogarth depicted 'a weedy Frenchman being manhandled out of the street by a corpulent English artisan holding a jug brimming with beer'.[32] For Hogarth, therefore, the solution to the 'gin craze' lay in encouraging the consumption of beer instead of alcoholic spirits. It should be noted that beer consumption was not universally approved of. In 1758, the *London Chronicle* told the story of a Venetian who was 'greatly injured' by intemperance and so became abstemious, afterwards living to over 100 years of age.[33] Similarly, a piece in the *Public Advertiser* claimed that 'abstinence and sobriety do always fortify observers thereof against many evils'.[34] Praising the water-drinking Rechabites and other biblical ascetics, this article spoke of abstinence, alongside temperance, as a virtuous practice in regard to alcohol, food and exercise. While this piece presented abstinence as a moral positive, the continued association of drinking with food and other aspects of lifestyle suggests that the definition of the word may have been different from our modern understanding. Self-denial of food and 'a little gentle hunger', which that generates, are praised as beneficial, enjoyable experiences, but clearly abstinence from food cannot be permanent. As the author did not separate food and drink, this implies that permanent abstinence from alcohol was similarly unnecessary. Although permanent abstinence was occasionally seen to be efficacious, this was only as a personal remedy for the proven intemperate or as a short-term, Lent-like ritual, which, coupled with permanent temperance, would improve bodily and spiritual conditions.

So, alcohol per se was not commonly seen as immoral in the 18th century. Drunkenness, primarily caused by gin, was seen to be a huge problem with serious consequences. In public discourse, the remedies to this problem were abstinence from gin or all alcoholic spirits, short-term abstinence from all drink, or, most commonly, the virtuous exercise of temperance in regard to alcohol and all aspects of personal behaviour.

Legislation and reflection

There were a few groups, such as the Society for the Reformation of Manners and the Society for Promoting Christian Knowledge, which campaigned against gin-drinking. It should be noted that these groups were concerned not only with spirit-drinking, but also with a whole range of immoral behaviour.[35] Nevertheless, such groups did advocate greater restrictions on the gin trade and their demands were eventually, to some extent, addressed by legislation. For the first time, the Gin Act 1729 restricted the sale of gin to licensed premises in an effort to control the trade. The Gin Act 1736 went much further, increasing the duty on gin as well as raising the annual cost of a gin licence to £50. Warner and Ivis describe how, given that the fine for trading gin illegally was £10, many sellers preferred to take their chances and operate illicitly. So, rather than curbing gin consumption, the Gin Act 1736 spawned only disrespect for the law.[36] The Gin Act 1743 abandoned these counterproductive provisions and lowered the annual cost of a spirits licence, before the Gin Act 1751 fixed the fee at 40 shillings. The legislative frenzy, apparent in the quick succession of so many Gin Acts, reveals that a sense of anxiety prevailed until the 1751 legislation provided some alleviation. Nicholls describes how, by restricting spirits licences to premises that cost a minimum of £10 per year to rent, the Gin Act 1751 gentrified the gin trade by making it, to many, respectable. Some notion of social order was seen to be restored and the 'gin panics' petered out in the 1750s.

There are two important points to make here. First, although gin was a relatively new substance in Britain, it was constructed and regulated through existing frameworks. Sellers of beer and wine had required a licence granted by a local magistrate since the Alehouse Act 1552 and, in 1729, this control measure was extended to gin. Similarly, the imposition of duty on the sale of gin was consistent with procedures through which other alcoholic drinks were bought and sold. Through these frameworks, governments could employ high licence fees and inflated duties in an effort to manage gin consumption. This involved a higher level of government intervention than Georgian society was accustomed to; for example, the raising of the licence fee to £50 in 1736 amounted to a near prohibition of gin, but these interventions were based on established practices of governance. Government interventions were also based on older moral foundations. They were attempts to promote sobriety by discouraging excessive drinking generally, and gin-drinking particularly. The regular, moderate consumption of beer or wine was not problematic and, as in 'Beer Street', was acceptable or even commendable. The Gin Acts, therefore, are consistent with the dominance of Classical/Christian notions of temperance, which prized moderation and balance in worldly affairs.

The second noteworthy point is the apparent consistency of the 'gin craze' with moral panic theory (as discussed earlier). Demographic changes and societal transformations, also as discussed earlier, unsettled certain sections of society and gave rise to anxiety that came to be directed at the new drink, gin. Gin-drinkers, especially female drinkers, were identified as 'folk devils' and Hogarth and others 'manned the barricades' in order to loudly condemn these deviants. After a flurry of legislation, government actions eventually calmed tensions and restored a perception of social equilibrium with the Gin Act 1751. The selection of gin as a target for the release of anxiety does not appear to have been driven purely by a rational assessment of the harm it caused. Although spirits consumption rose from approximately 1700 to 1740, perceptions of alarming levels of drunkenness were not matched by prosecution levels, which Hunt found were fairly low in London in the early 18th century.[37] Warner's description of how, although tailing off somewhat in the immediate aftermath of the Gin Act 1751, spirits consumption actually began to rise again by the mid-1750s is more telling.[38] The widespread beliefs that, to borrow from the *Covent Garden Journal*, the Gin Act 1751 had 'very considerable [sic] lessened the pernicious Practice of Gin-drinking'[39] was not therefore entirely accurate. Perceptions of both the 'threat' posed by gin-drinking and its resolution were questionable as there appeared to be some distance between the measurable and perceived realities of the 'gin problem'. The 'gin panics', therefore, appeared as an exaggerated or disproportionate reaction, which resulted in an episode of mass opprobrium about a specific type of behaviour. As Borsay and Critcher have explored, the events of the 18th century can be readily explained using the concept of a 'moral panic'.[40]

As discussed in Chapter One, there appears some ontological distance between attitudes towards alcohol and actual drinking habits. The rise and fall of a specific social problem is not linked, in any straightforward way, to the objective or measurable occurrences of the problem behaviour. Nor do periods of heightened concern, which may be termed 'moral panics', necessitate new heuristic or legislative apparatuses. The period from 1720 to 1750 was an episode of public alarm about spirits drinking, but it did not witness the generation of new forms of conceptualising or regulating alcohol use. While outcry was loud, there was very limited organised campaigning for legal change or efforts to reform gin-drinkers. Despite Barr's claims, it is difficult to see the beginnings of an anti-alcohol social movement within this period.

The 'temperance reformation'

Shifting attitudes in the 1820s

Traditional notions of temperance continued to be apparent in the early 19th century. In 1814, the *Liverpool Mercury* published the story of Thomas Wood from Billericay who, being affected by 'frequent sickness of the stomach ... a constant thirst, a great lowness of spirits ... and fits of the gout', resolved to become more temperate.[41] As with earlier tales of sickness, Wood's curative regime involved moderating his consumption of meat and initially abstaining from alcohol also. However, Wood soon gave up the consumption of all liquids, including water, suggesting he was motivated more by asceticism generally than a specific problematisation of alcohol. Another personal story in *The Examiner* in 1827 recorded that: 'I was sensible from my earliest years, that nothing was so injurious to my health as indulgence in what are commonly termed pleasures'.[42] Despite the 'raillery and facetiousness' of his friends who criticised his lifestyle, the author lived 'sparingly and frugally', giving up wine altogether as it was deemed to be 'a poison to my constitution'.[43] Both sources display a slightly harder attitude towards alcohol and the latter, in particular, stresses the need for self-discipline in the face of pressure from others. But both sources include food or meat alongside intoxicating drinks as damaging substances. Intemperance still meant excess in any area of a broader spectrum of behaviour.

The focus on self-discipline in *The Examiner* piece is, perhaps, indicative of a wider valuation of this concept in the 1820s. In 1827, *The Times* published a poem by Mr Nicholson[44] entitled 'Genius and Intemperance':

> Oh! could I write that I myself could save
> From this one curse, this sure untimely grave,
> This endless want, that soon must stop my breath,
> These flaming draughts, which bring the surest death,
> Then should my Muse upon her wings advance,
> And Genius triumph o'er Intemperance.[45]

The poem describes how drinking is enjoyable at first and attractive to 'thousands of hopeful youths' as they begin to mix socially with friends. But, drinking is a 'bewitching sin', which eventually 'drowns all genius, wealth, and hope', leaving the drinkers as 'starving wretches'. Nicholson viewed intemperance as a serious, tragic problem: 'I could employ my pen for weeks, for years, Write on this subject, wet it with my tears.' The best defence against the corrosive effects of drink 'is well to know the moment to depart.... That I may know these ills, and stop in time, Is my last wish, as I end this rhyme'. The portrayal of drinking as essentially corrosive, the tragic depiction of the problem and the plea for self-discipline allude to a new seriousness in debates about alcohol. Interestingly, Nicholson's poem also associates temperance with the use of alcoholic drinks only, making no mention of food, sex or any other potentially de-moralising influence.

Other, more vivid illustrations of changing attitudes to drink were also produced in this decade. In 1826, *The Times* printed a damning report on America's drinking habits, which was originally published in the *New York Inquirer*. In this piece, the term 'intemperance' was again discussed only in reference to drunkenness, which was said to be increasing to 'a fearful extent' among young New Yorkers.[46] Drunkenness was said to be 'the besetting vice of our country', affecting not just the 'low and vulgar' but also the well heeled and educated. The piece echoes Nicholson: 'At first, the practice may be harmless' but it soon becomes 'a fixed and pernicious habit', which 'deluges the gaming-room and the brothel with their pestilent population'.[47] The idea that drunkenness leads to other temptations was not new, but other aspects of the article were novel. Drinking was seen as degrading, it was an 'indulgence' and related to 'sensualities'; these terms indicate an ascetic suspicion of pleasure congruous with the emerging influence of evangelicalism. Additionally, the piece demanded that drunkards be subjected to 'a broad and public stamp of moral reprobation'; 'Let them point out by name the many and memorable instances of degradation and ruin which have happened in this city'.[48] Drunkenness is thus singled out as a specific social threat and, through calls for the societal denunciation of intemperance, a need to thoroughly moralise this behaviour is identified. Warner links changes in American attitudes to alcohol during this period to the evangelical revival[49] and the coverage in the British press of drink stories in the United States (US) suggests a similar hardening of views may have been occurring on this side of this Atlantic also.

In a similar vein, the *Hull Packet* chose, in 1826, to print an extract by the famous jurist and 17th-century Puritan Sir Matthew Hale. Hale criticised the young man who 'in the full career of his vanities and pleasures' denies himself 'no pleasures, can drink, and roar, and debauch, and wear the newest fashions'.[50] This type of person thinks that devotion to God and the practices of religious duty are foolish until, that is, he becomes sick. Now that 'his glass is almost out, and but a few sands left in it' he realises his previous ways were 'perfect follies' and commits himself to religion, prayer and obedience to God.[51] 'Affliction is the school of wisdom' and so only through sickness does the intemperate man learn that 'intemperance, wasting of time, unlawful lust' are all sins.[52] The need for self-denial, selfless devotion to God and the association of intemperance with the sinful act of wasting time are all indicative of a puritanical approach to the topic of drinking. Despite the fact that Hale was concerned with the wider indulgences of vain youth and not just drinking, the fact that his ideas were again circulated in the 1820s implies that attitudes to alcohol were becoming more disapproving than in the 18th century.

Intensified disapproval of drinking was far from universal, however. Referring to its display in the National Gallery, the *Morning Chronicle* presented a vivid description of David Wilkie's painting 'The Village Holiday' (see Figure 2.1). The paper described the painting's 'innocent gaiety' and 'rural frolic and hilarity', scenes that evoke the *joie de vive* of Hogarth's 'Beer Street'.[53] It was also noted that 'the beginning, middle, and end of the enjoyment is drinking'.[54] But the article on Wilkie's painting was disapproving, stating that 'unhappily for rural morals, it is but too faithful a picture of country festivity'.[55] The portrayal of individual moral choices perhaps shows that the artist himself shared the *Morning Chronicle*'s concern. A woman is shown trying to lead her husband away from the festivities while 'he hesitates between the forcible tenderness of his wife, and the seduction of a full bottle'.[56] In a similar vein, in 1828 the same paper reported on the apparently hilarious court appearance of a 13- to 14-year-old boy who had smashed a shop window while drunk. It was reported that the boy explained that he had been drinking 'gin, and rum, and Meux' and this caused laughter. When the Lord Mayor asked if he meant Meux water, the boy replied, to even more laughter, 'God love you, no. Strong heavy wet. Everybody knows what it is'.[57] The amusement at the boy's behaviour felt by many of those present was not shared by the Lord Mayor, who referred to this case as 'the most deplorable instance of the increasing immorality of youthful persons he had ever beheld' and 'lamented the state that the vice of drinking had become more prevalent of late'.[58] While drinking was still viewed in a light-hearted way by some, others saw the problem as both serious and worsening.

Although older, more permissive attitudes to drink persisted, public discourse was certainly becoming more disapproving in the 1820s. Rather than being only one aspect of intemperance, alcohol was increasingly becoming a specific, serious problem in its own right. Hilton examines the rise of evangelicalism during this period, which he

Figure 2.1: 'The Village Holiday' by David Wilkie, 1809–11

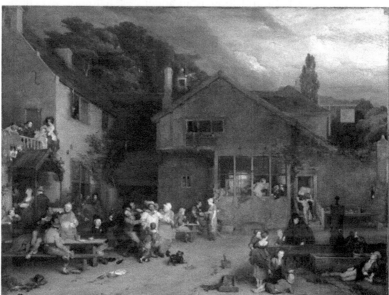

© Tate, London, 2013

defines as a belief that this world is an arena of moral trials, filled with depravity and temptation, and that the only possibility of redemption (enabled by Christ's atonement on the cross) is through individual conscience.[59] Hilton argues that this vision of the world spread outward from Non-conformist and Anglican churches and was connected to the eminence of personal agency and laissez-faire individualism within politics for much of the 19th century.[60] This broader ideological context appears reflected in the circulation of Puritan ideas from America or 17th-century Britain and their application to alcohol in this period. The British public would soon come to express their own views on alcohol in similar attitudinal terms to the *New York Inquirer* article and Hale but, in the 1820s, attitudes towards drinking were still hardening. The decade was a turning point in which, like the man in Wilkie's painting, public attitudes were torn between, on the one hand, a tendency to celebrate the festivities of the bottle and, on the other, an increasing belief that the trials of life could be passed by shunning the immorality of drinking.

Importing the temperance society in 1829

In one sense, events in 1829 represented merely the continuation of the hardening attitudes towards alcohol apparent in the preceding years. The *Morning Chronicle*, for example, recalled excerpts of a sermon by the evangelical Reverend Thomas Chalmers, who claimed that wine 'shall bite as a serpent and sting as an adder'.[61] Chalmers' serpentine depiction of this 'bacchanalian indulgence' shows echoes of puritanism and an intensification of moral disapproval. More interestingly, in 1829 the British press also reported extensively on the formation of temperance societies in the US. In August, the *Hull Packet* and *Morning Chronicle* both reported that 'the general prevalence of intemperate habits in the US have at length produced a re-action in the public feeling' and temperance societies were spreading across the US in order to 'put down that destructive practice of hard-drinking'.[62] Both papers reported the case of a Massachusetts judge and war veteran who, despite being initially reluctant to join his local society, soon resolved never 'to stand in the way of a measure so necessary for his country as the temperance reformation'.[63] The increasingly serious 'drinking problem' and what the Americans were doing about it were given extensive coverage in the British press.

Events in the US were an inspiration to men like John Edgar who, in mid-August, wrote to the *Belfast News-Letter* to call for the sanctification of the Sabbath. Primarily this was to be achieved through targeting 'the most flagrant and inveterate cause of profanation.... The sale and use of intoxicating liquors'.[64] Intemperance was described as 'the source of evils of incalculable magnitude', a threat to 'the temporal and eternal interests of individuals, families and communities' and disastrous for 'the moral and religious improvement of men'.[65] Moreover, this dire social problem was said to be 'widely spreading'.[66] Edgar was far from despair, however, and spoke glowingly of the successes of the US temperance societies and their labours to engender 'a change in public sentiment', 'a renovation of habits of the individuals, and the customs of the community'.[67] Inspired by this example of voluntary social action, Edgar ended with a call to arms: 'Up then and be doing, men of patriotism, men of piety; a tide of intemperance, rising every hour, is hurrying all moral and religious institutions before it, up and be doing, now, or weep when all is over, on the closed grave of your country's glory.'[68]

The efforts of Edgar and others soon resulted in the formation of the Cookstown Temperance Society, the first such organisation in Britain.[69] Although it should be remembered that Edgar only called for collective action against the use of alcoholic *spirits*, these events nevertheless represented an important development.

Moreover, Edgar was not alone in following the American example. In October 1829, John Dunlop gave a lecture in Glasgow claiming that American consumption of spirits had been greatly reduced by temperance societies and calling for the formation of more temperance societies.[70] Similar assessments of US temperance groups were reported in the *Hull Packet and Humber Mercury*, which claimed that in one part of the US, the campaigns had been so successful that 1,500 spirit vendors had given up the trade.[71] While publishing the sermons of American temperance pioneer Lyman Beecher, the *Leeds Mercury* echoed Dunlop and Edgar's calls for more societies.[72] There was a clear momentum to this trans-Atlantic movement and, by mid-1830, temperance mobilisation was apparent in London, Liverpool and across England and Wales.[73]

This mobilisation reflected how seriously the issue of drink was being taken. In January 1830, the Secretary to the New Ross Temperance Society stated his belief that 'a drunkard, though unfit to die, is entirely unfit to live'.[74] When the drunkard does die, the author went on to explain that: 'I would feel upon his death, as I would upon the death of the murderer dying on the scaffold – that he had paid the forfeit of his life to the offended justice of earth and of heaven.' By his own admission, the author looked upon drunkenness with 'a hatred and abhorrence quite peculiar'. But this was not out of step with the prevailing moral climate; attitudes were hardening and those who failed to mend their ways faced not only the worldly ruin of poverty and sickness, but also eternal ruin. In October 1830, the *North Wales Chronicle* related drinking to spontaneous human combustion. The apparent propensity of drunkards to burst into flames was not a new belief; in 1804, for example, the *Derby Mercury* printed Thomas Trotter's case notes from examples of the 'igneous quality of the Human Body, in People addicted to the use of Spirituous Liquors'.[75] But Trotter's detailed observations of the aftermath of such cases contrasted the alarming reports in the *North Wales Chronicle*. The paper related how, in his last minutes, the drunkard in question reported that 'he was suffering the torments of hell; that he was just upon its threshold, and should soon enter its dismal cavern; and in this frame of mind he gave up the ghost'.[76] The old connection of drinking to combustion was therefore reinterpreted; the burning quite literally became the drunkard's descent into hell and damnation represented his eternal recompense for a life of sinful intemperance. In the context of 'the temperance reformation', drinking was much more than just a matter of life and death.

Drunkenness and the consumption of spirits were viewed in increasingly stark terms as a social and moral evil. Moreover, given the coverage of American events, Edgar, Dunlop and others had an idea, based on voluntary association, of what could be done about this deadly, sinful social problem.

The teetotal turn

From relatively humble beginnings in the 1820s, the temperance movement grew into a huge and fascinating social phenomenon. While Georgian outrage about gin had remained largely confined to the south-east of England,[77] the temperance movement spread across the whole country. England's first temperance society was established in Bradford in Yorkshire, an area that, along with Lancashire, became in some respects the heartland of the movement.[78] Temperance was also particularly strong in Wales and Cornwall, the latter having had, as Harrison demonstrates, a higher membership of the British and Foreign Temperance Society per head of population than any other area of England or Wales.[79] Although its popularity and influence varied somewhat across the regions of Britain, the temperance movement was truly national in scope. The British Association for the Promotion of Temperance (BAPT – later the British Temperance League) and the British Teetotal Society (later the National Temperance League) were among the first nationally organised temperance groups,[80] although the UK Alliance, the Band of Hope and the Church of England Temperance Society (COETS) would later follow their lead. By the end of the century, the membership of temperance societies nationwide numbered in the millions.[81] This was a national social movement on a massive scale and so clearly distinct from any previous expression of anti-alcohol sentiments.

Interestingly, the temperance movement was probably weakest in London, the hub of the 'gin panics' in the preceding century.[82] Moreover, while concerns about gin-drinking had been expressed largely by London's social elites, from bishops and physicians to the Middlesex justices,[83] the temperance movement spanned a broader cross-section of British society. Karl Marx, a contemporary of the movement, criticised temperance strongly; he derided it as a 'bourgeois infection' constituted of those who wished for 'redressing social grievances in order to secure the continued existence of bourgeois society'.[84] Although clearly a polemical comment, the class composition of the temperance movement is significant. Shiman describes how the early temperance movement was dominated by the mid-echelons of society,[85] and Harrison explains how it thrived on middle-class benevolence or philanthropy as well as the aspirations of sections of the working class to appear respectable and 'civilised'.[86] This connection to working-class self-improvement explains the strong links of the temperance movement to the early labour movement, as well as other 'progressive' causes such as Chartism.[87] The fact that the temperance movement was radical, national (although stronger in provincial areas) and spanned the middle and working classes again suggests that it bore little relation to preceding anxieties about drink.

The temperance movement was also historically unprecedented due to its high level of organisation. The 'gin panics' were typified by outrage and alarm more than concerted action against drinking habits; but the temperance movement was coordinated at local, regional, national and even international levels. American orators, for example, were often involved in spreading the temperance gospel in Britain as well as Sweden, which received American and British temperance missionaries in the 1840s and 1850s.[88] On a local level, temperance groups were routinely involved in activities such as public meetings and the publication of campaign literature, such as the *Alliance News*. Later in the century certain groups became involved in more innovative means of targeting those most affected by drink; Shiman describes how the Salvation Army held prayer meetings outside London pubs, Miss Weston established temperance sailors' missions in Portsmouth, Devonport and Keyham, and the COETS established a 'Prison Gates

Mission' to help newly released prisoners lead a sober, law-abiding life.[89] In addition to their evangelical focus on new converts, temperance societies provided their members with fraternal support and a social life not centred on the local pub.[90] The level of organisation and the wide variety of tactics reveal that the temperance movement was a sophisticated and multifaceted campaign.

Perhaps most importantly, the temperance movement came to embody a whole new discourse on alcohol. In July 1832, the *Preston Chronicle* reported on a 'Temperance Tea Party' where guests were offered tea, coffee and cakes, and 'nothing was wanting to enliven the scene but a good band of music'.[91] It is not especially noteworthy that the party-goers were then addressed on 'the evils and dangers of inebriation'; but that they listened to a talk on 'the advantages and blessings of abstinence from intoxicating drinks' is remarkable. This tea party, and a subsequent field meeting attended by 2,000 people, constituted some of the early formative stages of abstinence-based temperance. One of the organisers of these gatherings was Joseph Livesey who, in 1832, began administering what are usually accepted as the first teetotal pledges. It is not clear whether teetotalism internationally sprang from Livesey's innovation or whether, as Cook suggests, it emerged simultaneously in parts of Britain and America.[92] But it is evident that the concept of the 'teetotal pledge' spread rapidly on both sides of the Atlantic. Livesey's BAPT and the London-based New British and Foreign Society for the Suppression of Intemperance were both established in 1835 to advance teetotalism[93] and, by 1840, even moderationist pioneer John Dunlop had joined the teetotal ranks.[94] This new temperance, based around total abstinence from alcoholic drinks, represented a clear break from the anti-drunkenness or anti-spirits discourses that had preceded it.

So, how did this discursive mutation, from moderation to abstinence, occur? The key concern is one of causal inevitability. A letter published in *The Times* in 1830 expressed the relationship of alcohol with a variety of nasty eventualities by asserting that 'the worst cases of murder, street robbery, housebreaking, seduction, and suicide, may all be traced to this horrid source'.[95] This is not a peculiar comment and, as has been discussed, alcohol had been associated with similar problems since earlier historical periods. But what distinguishes teetotallers from earlier parties concerned with the effects of drinking is that, to Livesey and his followers, moderate consumption of beer or wine was regarded as unavoidably connected to problems such as murder and robbery. A moderate drinking habit was conceived as a temporary state; it was, to borrow the words of W. Hunt, the first step on 'the highway to drunkenness'.[96] Hunt, a West Country teetotal activist, also used the metaphor of a whirlpool to describe how even moderate drinkers soon find that 'their giddy heads quickly sink in the deep waters of intemperance – perhaps to rise no more'.[97] Drinking was thus construed as a slippery slope, meaning that the negative potential consequences of alcohol use came to be viewed as the inevitable result of even modest consumption.

Alcohol thus went from being associated with a variety of immoral behaviour, to being conceived as immoral in itself. While intemperance had long been viewed as a sin, Cook describes how, given the inevitability of drinking leading to drunkenness, abstainers such as Dawson Burns came to view any consumption of alcohol as intemperate and therefore sinful.[98] In this moral climate, it became common to refer to drinking as 'a terrible evil'[99] of such magnitude that there is not 'anything to compare'.[100] Given this conceptualisation of drinking as a negative moral absolute, the previously advised remedies of moderation or abstinence from spirits were incapable of preventing drinkers from descending the slippery slope. In 1834, Livesey claimed that moderation was based on 'delusive notions' and produced 'baneful effects'.[101] In 1841, the *English Chartist Circular* went further; by claiming that 'the only true mode of killing drunkenness and the equally mischievous habits of "moderate" tippling is the adoption of Teetotal pledge', the publication asserted that moderation was morally tantamount to drunkenness.[102] As drinking rather than drunkenness was increasingly moralised, so abstinence and the teetotal pledge were constructed as the only viable means to escape the 'deep waters of intemperance'.

The idea of abstaining from alcohol was not entirely new. As aforementioned, reformed drunkards in the 18th century sometimes practised abstinence and, inspired by the water-drinking Rechabites from the Bible, abstinence within small ascetic religious groups was not unheard of. But Livesey's brand of teetotalism was not medically driven but, in his own words, based on the need to disseminate 'moral principles'.[103] Plus, and to borrow Weber's terminology, this was not the cloistered self-abasement of individual ascetics or isolated communities, but the everyday, 'worldly asceticism' of ordinary members of society.[104] In actuality, some of the topics explored in Weber's *Protestant Ethic* thesis resonate strongly with discourses of teetotalism. Weber proposes that the Calvinist belief in predestination shifts people's focus away from *achieving* a state of grace, which is the abiding concern of Lutheranism or Catholicism, and towards *proving* your own state of grace through such 'rational worldly activity' as working hard, saving money and controlling emotional or physical impulses.[105] Calvinism thus inflated the moral currency of thrift and self-control and, it is argued, supplied the ascetic Protestant spirit, which was instrumental in the growth of Western capitalism. Although Hilton describes how the centrality of predestination was somewhat diminished in 19th-century theology, he does argue that a related rationalistic world-view in addition to beliefs in the depravity of humankind and the virtue of self-denial were evident in a wider current of evangelical Protestantism.[106] It is therefore feasible that the ethical valuation of worldly asceticism necessary to sustain a commitment to an everyday routine of self-discipline, such as the teetotal pledge, resulted from the Calvinist-influenced aspects of evangelical Protestantism.

Ascetic values are apparent in much early teetotal discourse. Livesey argued that 'a working man, in health, with good food, can work better without ale than with it'.[107] As well as making more productive workers, Livesey believed that teetotallers were more ethically sound individuals, a point demonstrated by his description of 'the contentment, happiness and independence of a life of industry and sobriety'.[108] Hard work and abstinence from alcohol were thus crucial qualities of the model of the respectable working man promoted by Livesey and his followers. Just as Weber described how ascetic Protestantism demanded calculative rational actions from its adherents, so Livesey put forward his arguments in a decidedly rational fashion. In the early 1830s he forcefully argued that, as the brewing process extracted sugars and starch in order to produce alcohol, beer had far less nutrition than could otherwise be taken from the materials used to make it. It was also expensive; Livesey claimed that there was not more than one penny's worth of nutrition in a gallon of ale costing one shilling and four pence.[109] Appealing to the evangelical spirit of rationality, Livesey argued that money could and should be used to purchase more nutritious foodstuffs than beer. If alcohol costs money, disinhibits behaviour and reduces capacity for work (both when consuming and often the next morning), it becomes apparent why it was moral anathema to Calvinist-influenced, evangelical Protestants.

Given these ethical foundations, it is unsurprising that the temperance movement initially drew the majority of its support from more ascetic Protestant groups. Levine documents how abstinence-based temperance movements were popular in countries where Calvinist-influenced groups flourished,[110] and Gusfield describes how the US temperance movement drew support from the same denominations.[111] In Britain, Harrison describes how the early temperance movement included large numbers of Methodists, Baptists and Quakers;[112] a point that goes some way to explaining why temperance support was weaker in the more Anglican south-east of England than it was in Wales, Cornwall and the north of England where more ascetic forms of Protestantism were well established. This denominational explanation is not total, however, as it must be acknowledged that an evangelical faith in asceticism was apparent in the Anglican Church also; Hilton estimates that in 1850 one third of Anglicans were evangelical. Nevertheless, Hilton states that at the same point in time most Non-conformists were evangelical[113] and, indeed, as late as the mid-20th century, debates over Welsh licensing reforms were viewed through a denominational lens as a conflict of Church against Chapel.[114] Controversy over the reform of Welsh licensing reforms in the 1960s was seen to pit the 'puritanism' or 'Calvanism' [sic] of supporters of Sunday closing against the more permissive, pro-reform stance of a group characterised as Anglican.[115] There is, therefore, an enduring sense that the regional profile of the temperance movement owes something to the geographical character of more ascetic, evangelical forms of Protestantism.

The religious background of the temperance movement also helps to explain its qualitative character. Self-deprecatory commentaries were recurrent in temperance discourse. Although in 1745 the *Universal Spectator* compared British drinking habits unfavourably with those of the Spanish,[116] by the mid-19th century references to 'our national intemperance' were almost routine.[117] At a temperance meeting in 1872, Mr Heywood spoke of the shame that British drinking habits made him feel.[118] This comment evokes the total separation of the divine sphere from the sin and depravity of the earthly realms that Hilton sees as characteristic of 19th-century evangelicalism.[119] E.P. Thompson quotes the Methodist preacher Jabez Bunting's claim that 'the dust of self-abasement is our place before God'; a point that renders guilt, shame and self-repulsion, as expressed by Heywood and others, as the only emotions suitable to human beings.[120] Given the apparent preponderance of depravity, it might be expected that concerned onlookers would have despaired. But, in keeping with the work ethic that Weber identifies, Harrison highlights an evangelical commitment to the notion of 'the struggle', which inspired their zealous temperance campaigning. He quotes temperance supporter Sir Wilfrid Lawson saying 'we live in a world full of sin, of wrong, and of injustice, and if we are not to struggle, the sooner we are out of this world the better'.[121] Similarly, Richard Passmore Edwards reminded people 'that to him that knoweth to do good, and doeth it not, to him it is sin'.[122] Faced with the overwhelming sin and immorality, it was therefore imperative for good Protestants to struggle against it with all the devotion and self-discipline they applied to other worldly labours.

Confronted by evil and convinced of the rewards of hard work, the only option for temperance believers was therefore to fight – and 'fight' is very much how many advocates understood their cause:

> Hail Livesey! still onward – the cause is divine,
> Thy zeal over warm – in this war thou dost shine,
> As Preston exulting can tell.
> There Temp'rance hath flourished; the banner is there
> Triumphant displayed; and the glorious war
> Makes patriots bosoms so swell....
>
> To battle with these; may the task still be mine,
> They struggle for freedom, for virtue divine –
> The Temperance watchword is 'On!'[123]

The 'battle', repeatedly referred to by Edward Morris, in this piece from 1834, was the battle to convert drinkers to teetotalism and thus reform the behaviour of the population. Imbued with this evangelical spirit, the temperance movement set about promoting the teetotal pledge in Victorian society. It was not enough, therefore, for Livesey and others to simply abstain from drink themselves or seek separation from the immoral sections of the population. The hard-working, worldly Protestant was compelled to eradicate any evil they perceived, even if the evil lay in the behaviour of other people. The temperance movement thus traverses the divide between what Foucault calls the 'government of self' and the 'government of others'.[124]

This divide, following Hunt, is precisely where moral regulation projects are usually situated. The temperance movement fits the mould of a moral regulation project in other ways too, including its denunciation of a certain type of behaviour and the promotion of an alternative, teetotal lifestyle. It is apparent that this was not the worried reaction of social elites, but a movement predominantly instigated by the middle class and focused on the working class. It thus corresponds to Hunt's typical campaign 'from below' or 'from the middle'.[125] Hunt lists other requisites of a moral regulation project,[126] all of which were fulfilled by the temperance campaign: a target (drinkers), agency (societies), tactics (promotion of the pledge), discourse (abstinence based) and a political context (the Beer Act). Harrison is, therefore, right that the temperance movement was more organised than any previous instances in which anti-alcohol sentiment became popular; but it also possessed:

- broader national support;
- refined tactics;
- more evangelical members;
- a heightened belief in the need for radical behavioural reform;
- a clearer, more distinct discourse than any previous outburst of alarm directed at alcohol.

The reaction of Hogarth and his Georgian contemporaries to gin consumption is not an equivalent as it was limited in organisation, confined in geographical and social spread, restricted in target (to spirits-drinking) and reliant on older frameworks for understanding and regulating the problem behaviour. The temperance movement, therefore, was different from what had come before. It is a classic example of a moral regulation project (as defined by Hunt) and quite distinct from any historical antecedents.

The Beer Act 1830

So, what part did the Beer Act 1830 play in the temperance reformation? Since the Alehouse Act 1552, sellers of intoxicating drinks required a licence granted by a local magistrate and, from 1808 onwards, sellers of beer had further required an excise licence in order to ply their trade.[127] The Estcourt Act 1828 began to loosen some restrictions; it scrapped certain 18th-century statutory provisions, including the requirement for licence applicants to provide character references and recognisance or surety of £10 against disorder on their premises.[128] The Beer Act 1830, however, vastly accelerated this liberalising trend by enabling people to sell beer, ale or cider without magisterial permission, requiring only that beer-sellers possess an excise licence (which was obtainable upon the payment of a fixed fee). The legislation was partially motivated by free trade logic. At the time, persistent references were made to the need to tackle monopolies, which breweries had reportedly established in particular areas.[129] It was not believed that the existing system was equipped to tackle this problem; there was a degree of hostility to the 'arbitrary and injurious power' of local magistrates.[130] The concentration of licensing power in the hands of magistrates led to widespread fears of corruption and Anderson argues that, in light of this, the Beer Act 1830 should be understood as enacting a desire to replace the murky procedures of magisterial discretion with a more transparent, rule-based system.[131] The Act would, therefore, simultaneously strike a blow against commercial monopolies and for rational governance.

There were also other potential motives behind the Beer Act 1830. Nicholls notes that Wellington's government was facing a General Election and increasing the availability of beer may have been seen as a vote winner.[132] Whether electioneering was a motivation or not, the reform was certainly advocated with reference to free trade ideas as well as older, 18th-century conceptions of the drink problem. Consistent with the views of their Georgian predecessors as well as their temperance contemporaries, many people continued to view alcoholic spirits as the real problem. During parliamentary debates of the legislation in 1830, the Member of Parliament (MP) for Shrewsbury, Mr Slaney, argued that 'all disorder and immorality consequent on tippling arose from the drinking of spirits, and not from the drinking of beer'.[133] As in Hogarth's day, beer was still commonly perceived in a morally neutral or positive light; a letter in *The Times* expressed the view that beer was a normal commodity and so asked why its sale 'should not be as free as the sale of bread and cheese, or bacon?'[134] Legislative attempts to liberalise the trade in beer were therefore positioned as attempts to reduce the consumption of alcoholic spirits. As Slaney described, the debate was largely concerned with 'a healthful nutricious [sic] beverage and demoralising and destructive spirituous liquors'.[135]

However, the belief that beer consumption was harmless was not universal. The MP for Reading, Mr Monck, argued that the existence of a licensing system showed that common law pronounced 'public houses to be public nuisances',[136] which 'ought not to be erected in low, retired, and improper situations'.[137] Monck believed that the Beer Bill threatened this state of affairs by carrying 'the principle of competition to a new and indefinite extent'.[138] Sir T. Gooch gave some support to Mr Monck, stating that 'he was a friend to free trade in beer, but he thought the magistrates ought to have some control over the licences'.[139] Reservations were not restricted to Parliament; the *Hampshire Telegraph* reported on a public meeting in Newport at which it was agreed that the indiscriminate sale of beer would 'be productive of serious evil to the morality and good order of society'.[140] During 1830 a number of anti-Beer Bill petitions were presented to Parliament. Although many petitions came from licensed victuallers, who feared that the freeing up of the beer trade would threaten their livelihoods,[141] a petition from the vicar and church wardens of Isleworth expressed non-pecuniary worries about the 'most ruinous effects' the Bill may have.[142] Although Monck and those at the Newport meeting are not reported as raising objections to moderate use and properly regulated sale of beer, they did highlight the potential problems that beer may produce.

Many people soon came to agree with the vicar of Isleworth's concerns, mainly as the Beer Act was frequently seen as worsening the very problem it sought to solve. After this legislation came into effect, there was a large increase in the number of premises selling beer[143] and significant decreases in the price of their product.[144] This was not unexpected, but it was also apparent that the consumption of spirits was not significantly reduced[145] and that arrests for drunkenness were rising.[146] The fears of the moralist 'who trembles lest our streets should become too narrow for a staggering population' appeared to have been realised.[147] In Parliament in 1839, Mr Pakington referred to 'the evils which had resulted from the beer act of 1830'.[148] In the same year, a group of Watford magistrates petitioned Parliament calling for a clampdown on beerhouses, describing them as those 'schools of vice' that have 'corrupted' and 'seduced' young people into 'riotous debauchery'.[149] It became commonplace to echo these sentiments by referring to 'the evils of the Beer Act', a phrase that featured in the *Newcastle Courant* in 1850,[150] *The Era* in 1857, and was used by prohibitionist Dawson Burns as late as 1908.[151] The Beer Act 1830 thus provided a focus for critical social commentaries for some years to come, and, for many people, its very name became synonymous with legislative failure and moral bankruptcy.

Nowhere was criticism of the Act stronger than in the ranks of the prohibitionist UK Alliance. Harrison reports that in the 1860s the Alliance, Britain's largest temperance society, had three principal aims:

- the restoration of beer shops to magistrates' control;
- opposition to Gladstone's attempts to open up the wine trade;
- opposition to the free licensing policy of the Liverpool magistrates.[152]

All of the UK Alliance's aims relate to either the Beer Act 1830 or the related free trade model of alcohol governance. Interestingly, advocates of free trade were not disheartened by the Beer Act 1830's apparent lack of success and blamed these eventualities on a surfeit of regulations. A letter in *The Times* in 1860 claimed that the statute failed because beerhouses could not compete equally with public houses, which could stay open for longer hours and sell wine and spirits as well as beer.[153] This letter was prompted by Gladstone's contemporaneous attempts to liberalise the wine trade by reducing duties and encouraging imports. Gladstone, like free traders before him, was motivated by the idea that competition would improve the quality and price of drinks, and so in turn reduce the dangers of adulteration and provide an alternative to spirit-drinking.[154] This mixture of free trade and anti-spirit/pro-beer ideas thus formed a potent and lasting cocktail. Also, the historical legacy of the Beer Act 1830 clearly structured debates about alcohol for several decades.

It must be remembered that attitudes to drink were hardening several years before the Beer Bill was first debated in Parliament. But, from 1830 onwards, these changing attitudes were increasingly expressed in reference to the Beer Act 1830. The Act did not engender a fundamentally novel discourse of anti-alcohol sentiment. It did, however, create a discursive arena in which the potentially negative effects of beer-drinking and the need for proper regulation were stressed. Both the traditional idea of beer as healthy and harmless, and the conception of spirits as somehow different and more malevolent, were challenged. As a piece in the *Derby Mercury* argued, beer was not just a nutritious beverage but potentially a 'moral poison' also.[155] By the time legislative amendments were debated in Parliament in 1839, Mr Warburton was able to make a case that beer is an intoxicating drink and should be subjected to the exact same regulations as wine or gin.[156]

Reflections

The Beer Act 1830 did not, therefore, instigate the increasing problematisation of alcohol, but it did contribute to a much wider acceptance that beer, as well as spirits, can produce social problems. It is tempting to say that this legislation was, therefore, a prerequisite for the emergence of teetotalism. However, it must be remembered that groups such as the Society for the Suppression of Vice demonstrated that aspects of social life were becoming increasingly moralised anyway. Moreover, this chapter has shown that attitudes to alcohol were already in the process of becoming harder as more puritanical or evangelical beliefs were increasingly applied to drink, and that teetotalism emerged almost simultaneously on both sides of the Atlantic. The Beer Act 1830 structured debate and perhaps accelerated the problematisation of all alcoholic drinks; but, based on this analysis, it appears only as a local contributing factor within a bigger, cross-national attitudinal shift. This conclusion means that neither moral panic theory, which applies to short-term reactions to social issues that are deemed irrational, nor the rational model, which refers to logical or defensible responses to identifiable social problems, are suitable heuristic frameworks. The temperance movement was more than simply a reaction to a legislative reform and changing drinking habits. The campaign's emergence from the 1820s onwards embodied some fundamental transformations in understandings of alcohol, a reformation of public attitudes and the beginning of a new and distinct project to morally regulate the use of alcohol.

The genesis of the temperance movement and its problematisation of all forms of drinking represented, therefore, the start of a new chapter in Britain's relationship with alcohol. Indeed, the very concept of 'temperance', the virtue used to morally regulate consumption, came to be redefined in this period. Victorian usage of the term 'temperance' came to refer almost exclusively to drinking habits and largely to teetotalism, rather than the word's more literal meanings of restraint, moderation or balance. This linguistic change was emblematic of a national attitudinal remaking. The results of this remaking will be explored in the subsequent chapters.

Notes

[1] Burnett, *Liquid Pleasures*, pp 111-140.

[2] Wilson, *Alcohol and the Nation*, pp 99-101; Harrison, *Drink and the Victorians*, pp 64-86.

[3] For further information on these groups, see: Roberts, *Making English Morals*.

[4] Barr, *Drink*, pp 288-289. Nicholls, similarly, highlights some similarities by saying the 18th-century gin campaigners articulated the same concerns for religious piety, reason and desire to work as Victorian temperance activists and 17th-century Puritans (Nicholls, *Politics of Drink*, p 44).

[5] Nicholls, *Politics of Alcohol*, pp 34-37. Although it should be noted that Nicholls points out the difficulty in historically assessing the level per capita gin consumption.

[6] Sennett, Richard, *The Fall of Public Man*, Cambridge: Cambridge University Press, 1974, pp 50-53.

[7] Borsay, 'Historic Parallels?'.

[8] Nicholls, *Politics of Alcohol*, pp 36-37. As well as the increased visibility of drinking in urban environments, it is feasible that the greater anonymity of city life removed some of the stigma associated with drunkenness and thus facilitated heavier consumption. But, as discussed in Chapter One, an objective increase in drunkenness resulting from urban anonymity would not provide sufficient explanation of how this objective trend relates to understandings and regulation of alcohol.

[9] Sennett, *Fall of Public Man*, pp 48-49; Ehrenreich, Barbara, *Dancing in the Street*, London: Granta, 2007, pp 105-180.

[10] Warner, *Craze*, p x.

[11] 'The Drunken Post', *Athenian News or Dunton's Oracle*, 23 May 1710.

[12] Anonymus, 'From My Own Chambers', *Universal Spectator and Weekly Journal*, 21 September 1745.

[13] Warner, *Craze*, pp 62–63.

[14] 'The Drunken Post', *Athenian News or Dunton's Oracle*, 23 May 1710.

[15] See: Borsay, 'Historic Parallels?'.

[16] 'Proposals', *Grub Street Journal*, 1 April 1736.

[17] 'Modern History: Abridged. Saturday', *Covent Garden Journal*, 10 March 1752.

[18] 'This Day Was Published ...', *London Evening Post*, 18 June 1754.

[19] Cook, *Alcohol, Addiction and Christian Ethics*, pp 52–66.

[20] 'Original Remarks of Eminent Persons on Temperance', *Oracle and Public Advertiser*, 20 March 1797.

[21] Philotechnos, 'To the Printer of the *Middlewich Journal*', *Schofield's Middlewich Journal or Cheshire Advertiser*, 10 May 1757.

[22] 'Private Vices, no Publick Benefits: To the Editor of the London Journal', *London Journal*, 14 June 1729.

[23] 'Remainder of the Extracts and Tracts on the Choice of Company, and Other Subjects', *Lloyd's Evening Post and British Chronicle*, 21 December 1761.

[24] 'Venienti Occurite Morbo', *Prater*, 18 September 1756.

[25] Academicus, 'To Mr Fitz-Adam', *World*, 18 March 1756. Although this piece is focused on the male 'luxurious person', it should be noted that female drunkenness was a particularly acute public concern in the 18th century, especially during the 'gin panics'.

[26] 'Venienti Occurite Morbo', *Prater*, 18 September 1756.

[27] Anonymus, 'From My Own Chambers', *Universal Spectator and Weekly Journal*, 21 September 1745.

[28] 'Venienti Occurite Morbo', *Prater*, 18 September 1756.

[29] 'For the Sunday Monitor: The Consequences of Actions are to be Considered', *E. Johnson's British Gazette and Sunday Monitor*, 18 March 1798.

[30] Ibid.

[31] 'The Drunken Post', *Athenian News or Dunton's Oracle*, 23 May 1710.

[32] Borsay, 'Historic Parallels?'.

[33] 'Postscript: To the Editor of the *London Chronicle*', *London Chronicle*, 10 August 1758.

[34] Setaymot, 'To the Printer of the Public Advertiser', *Public Advertiser*, 18 July 1789.

[35] Critcher, 'Drunken Antics'.

[36] Warner, Jessica, and Ivis, Frank, '"Damn You, You Informing Bitch": *Vox Populi* and the Unmaking of the Gin Act 1736', *Journal of Social History*, 1999, vol 33, p 4.

[37] Hunt, *Governing Morals*, pp 36–38.

[38] Warner, *Craze*, pp 206–208; Warner et al, 'Can Legislation Prevent Debauchery?'. See also: Nicholls, *Politics of Alcohol*, pp 47–48.

[39] 'Modern History: Abridged. Saturday', *Covent Garden Journal*, 10 March 1752.

[40] Borsay, 'Historic Parallels'; Critcher, 'Drunken Antics'.

[41] 'Miscellaneous Extracts: Extraordinary Instance of Extreme Temperance', *Liverpool Mercury*, 4 February 1814.

[42] 'Newspaper Chat: A Temperate Man', *The Examiner*, 29 July 1827.

[43] Ibid.

[44] As far as I can tell, this refers to John Nicholson, a Yorkshire poet who lived from 1790 to 1843. He reportedly drowned when, after visiting several public houses, he attempted to cross the River Aire near Shipley, West Yorkshire. See: 'John Nicholson', *Oxford Dictionary of National Biography*, www.oxforddnb.com/view/printable/20140

[45] 'The Yorkshire Poet', *The Times*, 1 December 1827.

[46] 'Drunkards in New York', *The Times*, 16 October 1826.

[47] Ibid.

[48] Ibid.

[49] Warner, Jessica, 'Temperance, Alcohol and the American Evangelical: A Reassessment', *Addiction*, 2009, vol 104 (7), pp 1075-1084.

[50] 'Sir Matthew Hale's Counsels of a Father', *Hull Packet and Original Weekly Commercial, Literary and General Advertiser*, 14 February 1826.

[51] Ibid.

[52] Ibid.

[53] 'The National (Angerstein) Gallery', *Morning Chronicle*, 8 December 1824.

[54] Ibid.

[55] Ibid.

[56] Ibid.

[57] 'Police', *Morning Chronicle*, 18 December 1828.

[58] Ibid.

[59] Hilton, Boyd, *The Age of Atonement*, Oxford: Clarendon Press, 1988, p 8.

[60] Ibid.

[61] 'The Reverend Thomas Chalmers D.D.', *Morning Chronicle*, 17 April 1829.

[62] 'Miscellaneous Intelligence', *Hull Packet and Humber Mercury*, 11 August 1829; 'News', *Morning Chronicle*, 5 August 1829.

[63] Ibid.

[64] Edgar, John, 'To the Editor of the News-Letter', *Belfast News-Letter*, 14 August 1829.

[65] Ibid.

[66] Ibid.

[67] Ibid.

[68] Ibid.

69 'Cookstown Temperance Society', *Belfast News-Letter*, 23 October 1829.

70 'Temperance Societies', *Newcastle Courant*, 10 October 1829.

71 'Foreign Intelligence', *Hull Packet and Humber Mercury*, 1 December 1829.

72 'Latest Intelligence', *Leeds Mercury*, 23 January 1830.

73 'Miscellaneous Intelligence', *Hull Packet and Humber Mercury*, 16 February 1830; 'Temperance Society', *Liverpool Mercury*, 23 July 1830.

74 Carr, Reverend G.W., 'Temperance Societies', *Morning Chronicle*, 6 January 1830.

75 'Morning Address – Animal Combustion', *Derby Mercury*, 15 November 1804.

76 'Drunkenness – Spontaneous Combustion', *North Wales Chronicle*, 21 October 1830.

77 Warner, *Craze*.

78 See: Harrison, *Drink and the Victorians*, pp 109, 140.

79 Ibid, p 109.

80 Shiman, *Crusade Against Drink*, p 58.

81 Shiman reports that, at the turn of the 20th century, the Band of Hope alone had three million members (Shiman, *Crusade Against Drink*, p 154).

82 Warner, *Craze*, p x.

83 See: Nicholls, *Politics of Alcohol*, pp 34-50.

84 Harrison, *Drink and the Victorians*, p 395.

85 Shiman, *Crusade Against Drink*, p 4.

86 Harrison, *Drink and the Victorians*, pp 24-26.

87 Ibid.

88 Eriksen, Sidsel, 'Drunken Danes and Sober Swedes? Religious revivalism and the temperance movements as keys to Danish and Swedish folk cultures', in Strath, Bo (ed) *Language and the Construction of Class Identities*, Gothenburg: Gothenburg University Press, 1989, pp 55-94.

89 See: Shiman, *Crusade Against Drink*, pp 104-105, 130-133.

90 Shiman, *Crusade Against Drink*.

91 'Temperance Tea Party', *Preston Chronicle*, 14 July 1832.

92 Cook, *Alcohol, Addiction and Christian Ethics*, pp 81-82.

93 Harrison, *Drink and the Victorians*, pp 139-142.

94 Ibid.

95 Homo, 'Abuse of Spirituous Liquor', *The Times*, 4 January 1830.

96 Hunt, W., *History of Teetotalism in Devonshire*, UK: Western Temperance Advocate Office, 1841, p 14.

97 Ibid.

98 Cook, *Alcohol, Addiction and Christian Ethics*, pp 94-104.

99 'Annual Tea Meeting of the Fisher-Gate Chapel Band of Hope', *Preston Guardian*, 26 October 1872.

100 'Conference on the Reform of Temperance in the Corn Exchange', *Preston Guardian*, 16 November 1872.

101 'Lecture on Temperance', *Preston Chronicle*, 8 March 1834.

102 'Temperance Record', *English Chartist Circular* (1841-1844).

103 'Lecture on Temperance', *Preston Chronicle*, 8 March 1834.

104 Weber, Max, *The Protestant Ethic and the Spirit of Capitalism*, London: Unwin, 1965.

105 Ibid, pp 98-103, 126-127.

106 Hilton, *Age of Atonement*, pp 8-9.

107 'Lecture on Temperance', *Preston Chronicle*, 8 March 1834.

108 'Temperance Tea Party', *Preston Chronicle*, 14 July 1832.

109 'Lecture on Temperance', *Preston Chronicle*, 8 March 1834.

110 Levine, 'Temperance Cultures'.

111 Gusfield, 'Status Conflicts'.

112 Harrison, *Drink and the Victorians*, pp 179-184.

113 Hilton, *Age of Atonement*, p 26. It is also worth iterating that Methodism began as a movement within the Church of England and did not separate from the established church until the 1790s, after Wesley's death.

114 'Dangers of Disunity', *The Guardian*, 24 February 1961.

115 'Right to Drink in Welsh Clubs', *The Times*, 22 March 1961.

116 'From My Own Chambers', *Universal Spectator and Weekly Journal*, 5 October 1745.

117 'Permissive Bill Meeting in Leeds', *Leeds Mercury*, 12 December 1872.

118 'United Kingdom Alliance, Preston Auxiliary', *Preston Guardian*, 17 September 1870.

119 Hilton, *Age of Atonement*. It is useful to note that Weber sees this faith in depravity, which has been theologically demonstrated by Eve's 'original sin' and the crucifixion of Jesus at the hands of humankind, as originating from Calvinism. But whether or not he is correct, it is hard to disagree with Hilton that, by the 19th century, a preoccupation with depravity was a characteristic of broader forms of evangelical Protestantism. See: Weber, *Protestant Ethic*, pp 102-103.

120 Thompson, *Making of the English Working Class*, p 400.

121 Harrison, *Drink and the Victorians*, p 377.

122 'Temperance Conference at Portsea', *Hampshire Telegraph and Sussex Chronicle*, 4 September 1872.

123 Morris, Edward, 'The British Banner of Temperance', *Preston Chronicle*, 15 November 1834.

124 Foucault, *Government of Self and Others*.

[125] Ibid, pp 1-2.

[126] Ibid, p 28.

[127] See: Jennings, Paul, 'Liquor Licensing and the Local Historian: Inns and Alehouses 1753-1828', *The Local Historian*, 2010, vol 40 (2), pp 136-150.

[128] Ibid.

[129] For example, see: Probus, 'Sale of Beer Bill: To the Editor of *The Times*', *The Times*, 21 June 1830.

[130] Mr Western MP, 'Sale of Beer Bill', *Morning Chronicle*, 22 May 1830.

[131] Anderson, Stuart, 'Discretion and the Rule of Law: The Licensing of Drink in England, c.1817–40', *Journal of Legal History*, 2002, vol 23 (1), pp 45-59.

[132] Nicholls, *Politics of Drink*, p 91.

[133] 'Sale of Beer Bill', *Hull Packet and Humber Mercury*, 25 May 1830.

[134] Probus, 'Sale of Beer Bill: To the Editor of *The Times*', *The Times*, 21 June 1830.

[135] 'Sale of Beer Bill', *Morning Chronicle*, 22 May 1830.

[136] 'Sale of Beer Bill', *Hull Packet and Humber Mercury*, 25 May 1830.

[137] 'Sale of Beer Bill', *Morning Chronicle*, 22 May 1830.

[138] 'Sale of Beer Bill', *Hull Packet and Humber Mercury*, 25 May 1830.

[139] Ibid.

[140] 'To the Printer of the *Hampshire Telegraph*', *Hampshire Telegraph and Sussex Chronicle*, 26 April 1830.

[141] See: 'Imperial Parliament', *Morning Chronicle*, 27 April 1830.

[142] 'House of Commons', *Jackson's Oxford Journal*, 8 May 1830.

[143] Harrison, *Drink and the Victorians*, pp 64-86.

[144] 'Postscript', *Bristol Mercury*, 28 June 1830; 'London', *Hampshire Telegraph and Sussex Chronicle*, 4 October 1830.

[145] Harrison, *Drink and the Victorians*, pp 81-86.

[146] Wilson, *Alcohol and the Nation*, pp 99-101.

[147] 'The New Beer Bill', *Hampshire Telegraph and Sussex Chronicle*, 25 October 1830.

[148] 'The Parliament', *The Examiner*, 24 March 1839.

[149] 'Repeal of the Beer Act', *The Era*, 3 February 1839.

[150] 'The Lords' Committee on the Beer Act', *Newcastle Courant*, 21 June 1850.

[151] Burns, Dawson, 'The Licensing Bill', *The Times*, 1 May 1908.

[152] Harrison, *Drink and the Victorians*, p 348.

[153] A Thirsty Soul, 'The Brewer's Monopoly', *The Times*, 16 February 1860.

[154] See: Harrison, *Drink and the Victorians*, pp 248-250.

[155] 'The Beer Bill', *Derby Mercury*, 14 July 1830.

[156] 'The New Beer Act', *The Operative*, 24 March 1839.

THREE

Balancing acts or spirited measures?

Introduction

Academics studying the British temperance movement tend to regard it as having had little effect. Warner asserts that 'the most salient feature of the British temperance movement is how little it was able to accomplish'[1] and Nicholls' history of the drink question seems to position the temperance movement as something that rose up before falling down, leaving little meaningful imprint on society.[2] More popularly, Ian Hislop's recent BBC series, *Age of the Do-Gooders*, portrayed the Victorian temperance movement as a curious phenomenon that, despite the apparently continuing relevance of its message, sunk without a trace.[3] But is this negative assessment of impact accurate? Did this well-supported, highly organised and discursively novel social movement really effect no changes in the way British people relate to alcohol?

Building on the argument in the previous chapter that the emergence of the British temperance movement represented the start of a potent and distinct movement to morally regulate the use of alcohol, this chapter begins an assessment of the impact of this project. The particular utility of the moral regulation approach is that it enables a concentration on the attitudes towards alcohol that are discernible in public discourse as well as forms of regulation, legal or otherwise, that affect people's behaviour. Hence, this chapter focuses on the legal impacts of the temperance movement as well as the subtler attitudinal changes it may have engendered. These attitudinal changes are investigated primarily through the study of newspaper sources and, for this chapter alone, approximately 350 articles have been analysed. Drawing on these sources, this chapter focuses on the more immediate effects of temperance campaigning in the Victorian period. Subsequent chapters examine public attitudes in the 20th and 21st centuries and so give some consideration to its longer-term significance.

'A new moralising subtext'

The massive social and economic upheavals of the 19th century were accompanied by the expansion of government into new areas of social life. Many previously untouched spheres of social life, from working practices to education, became increasingly subject to government regulation. Moreover, as Emsley highlights, 19th-century laws tended increasingly to be countrywide rather than local; problems and solutions began to be conceived on a national level.[4] The Education Act 1870, for example, signalled a commitment to the nationwide provision of education by establishing local boards to build and manage schools. Similarly, the Habitual Criminals Act 1869 established a system for centrally recording crime and the Prison Act 1877 transferred control of prisons from local authorities to central government. It is not entirely surprising, therefore, that from the mid-1860s onwards the sale and consumption of alcohol was subject to new, national legislation. Wiener has also described how around the middle of the 19th century, the whole spectrum of law was characterised by 'a new moralizing subtext, a hardly questioned acceptance of the importance of strengthening the self-discipline, foresight, and reasonableness of the public and of the suitability of law as a medium for expressing and furthering these values'.[5] Given this description, nor is it surprising that the sort of theoretical concerns that occupy this book, with their focus on moral discourse, should find a convenient subject in alcohol regulation during this period.

In light of the apparent shift towards more government intervention and greater moralisation, the task in hand then becomes to discern whether changes in the regulation of alcohol from the mid-1860s onwards can be explained solely by this generalised governmental transformation, or whether more specific attention to the discursive configuration of alcohol regulation is required. As useful as Wiener and Emsley are, it is reasonable to consider whether their broad histories of the legal system during this period are sufficient for understanding particular changes in the regulation of alcohol and the role that the temperance movement may (or may not) have played in their creation.

The split personality of Victorian temperance

Chapter Two examined how the early British temperance movement was rapidly converted to a doctrine of total abstinence from alcohol, which was embodied in the teetotal pledge. The first groups of abstinence-inspired campaigners, such as Joseph Livesey's BAPT, are often referred to as 'moral suasionists' due to their preference for persuasive tactics. Livesey described their activities as based on 'kindly Christian-like teaching and admonition … visiting the back slums, holding temperance meetings everywhere, and circulating sound information and temperance tracts and publications'.[6] But BAPT and other groups were not only concerned with new initiates; for those already pledged, temperance societies sought to aid continued abstinence. Shiman describes how the societies provided their members, many of whom had recently migrated into cities from rural areas, with a social life not centred on the local pub, and later in the century some provided the kind of financial services associated with friendly societies, such as sick pay and death payments.[7] Moral suasionists possessed social and financial incentives that might encourage individuals to take the teetotal pledge and stick to it.

More importantly, suasionists used a potent moral discourse to promote their cause. Harrison examines how between 1830 and 1870 the temperance movement promoted a model of the respectable, sober working man and its popularity 'flourished on the genuine desire for respectability and self-reliance which prevailed within the working class'.[8] Much of this longed-for respectability could be found in the routine of individual self-denial engendered by the pledge. Livesey spoke in 1873 of the 'extraordinary results' of 'earnest self-denying labours'[9] and William Harcourt MP espoused the value of denying one's self 'indulgences' in drinking and fostering 'voluntary self-control'.[10] Even Lord Stanley, no teetaller himself, equated the pledge with resistance of temptation and the 'conferment of moral strength'.[11] In all three cases, a behavioural routine of self-discipline and self-control was associated with moral or psychological benefits as well as social respectability. In the Victorian period, campaign groups would sometimes commission special envelope designs so that those sending, receiving and handling post would see their message. In 1851, a London temperance group produced an envelope that starkly depicted the chaotic depravities of Hogarth's 'Gin Lane' on one side and an idyllic family scene of Victorian sobriety, social order and restrained prosperity on the other (see Figure 3.1). The caption 'Intemperance: Bane of Society' encircles a cup from which a snake is emerging. Conquering the serpentine temptation of drink through teetotalism therefore developed and exhibited an enviable level of personal character, ethical backbone and social respectability.

But from the 1850s onwards, questions began to be asked about the efficacy of the teetotal pledge and moral suasionism in general as a means to produce total societal abstinence. In a famous exchange

Figure 3.1: Envelope issued by The Temperance Society, 1851

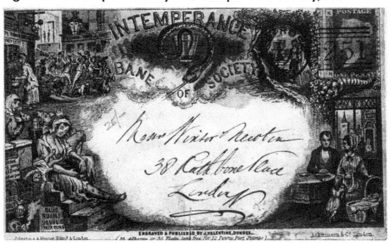

© Royal Mail Group 2012, courtesy of The British Postal Museum & Archive (www.postalheritage.org.uk)

of views with Lord Stanley in 1856, lawyer Samuel Pope did not refute that achieving collective abstinence through self-control was hypothetically desirable, but asked: 'how are the people to reach that state – how to acquire that habit in the midst of the sad and sorrowful circumstances which surround them?'.[12] This negative assessment of the social environment was mixed with scepticism over the general moral fortitude of the population; in 1872, *The Times* declared that 'there never was a time when the hard-working but thriftless and improvident Englishman was not notorious for want of self-control'.[13] In 1873, Dawson Burns echoed these points when he mockingly asked Livesey: 'Had all the residents of Preston who have signed kept their pledge, what would have been the temperance condition of Preston to-day?'.[14] Many people would never take the pledge in the first place and, as Burns highlighted, there was no guarantee that those who did would stick to it. Voluntary acts of self-denial may have been admirable but, given people's social circumstances, could not be widely replicated and so were deemed incapable of producing the 'temperance reformation' that was envisaged. As Pope argued, 'moral force is not enough for the world as it is',[15] meaning that moral suasionism's faith in the pledge and the self-reforming power of the individual was fanciful.

Motivated, in the words of the *Newcastle Courant*, by years of 'disheartening failure through moral suasion',[16] Pope and Burns became prominent advocates of a new method for achieving collective abstinence: prohibition. Prohibitionists shifted the focus of temperance discourse away from the moral defects of the individual drinker, which could not be altered, and towards external, social factors that, they argued, held far greater potency as means through which behaviour could be altered. They were not alone in reaching this conclusion; in the mid-19th century Friedrich Engels blamed the social system of industrial capitalism, rather than the individual, for drunken excesses.[17] But for prohibitionists, the primary external factor that fostered intemperance was not a socioeconomic system but a legal one; they targeted, in Pope's words, the 'legalized system of temptation'[18] that governed the drinks trade. Inspired by the implementation of prohibition in the US state of Maine, the UK Alliance was established in 1853 to campaign for a similar legal intervention on this side of the Atlantic. Its membership numbers and finances swelled rapidly; Brown reports that the Alliance's revenue, in 1881 alone, was more than six times higher than the National Liberal Federation's.[19] The UK Alliance soon became Britain's largest temperance society and a formidable campaigning force. The idea, that if individuals could not or would not regulate their own behaviour then the state must employ the law to do it for them, was a powerful and popular one.

The replacement of a persuasive focus on nurturing individual voluntary change with a more paternalistic and utopian faith in the capacity of the law to reform society, is significant. Incumbent within this change was the creation of new discursive targets at which the moral regulation campaigners could take aim. It was no use targeting individual citizens to tackle what Burns called 'temptation under sanction of law';[20] clearly those propagating or perpetuating this legal arrangement must be confronted. Hence, the UK Alliance was heavily involved in lobbying Parliament, sponsoring Private Members' Bills and supporting the electoral campaigns of prospective MPs who supported the cause. In this sense, the UK Alliance waged a largely top-down campaign, which stood in stark contrast to the bottom-up, conversion-seeking activities of moral suasionists. Additionally, in prohibitionist discourse a new folk-devil was formed in the shape of the landlord or brewer. In a lecture in Preston in 1872, Mr Fothergill said that the current legal system allowed 'the rich brewer to tempt the poor sinners to their ruin'.[21] He went on to speak of the injustice of a magistrate punishing 'a victim of the liquor seller, and allowing the seller to go free'.[22] Sir Wilfrid Lawson MP claimed that the Alliance was fighting 'a system which inflicts as large and as wide-spread human misery as ever resulted from negro slavery',[23] and so publicans and brewers were constructed as morally tantamount to slave traders; they kept the drunkard 'in chains'[24] and sought to profit from his misery. There were clear discursive and tactical differences between prohibitionists and moral suasionists.

Nevertheless, there were discursive congruencies between the two strands of the temperance movement. The *Leeds Mercury* quoted Alliance member Reverend C. Garrett describing how drinking was an insult to God that resulted in 'misery and eternal death',[25] clearly showing that prohibitionists shared the problematisation of all forms of alcohol, which had been advanced by teetotal suasionists in the 1830s. The temperance belief in 'the struggle' or 'battle' was, if anything, intensified by prohibitionists. Drink was a negative moral absolute and, for people such as Mr Heywood, every aspect of life became a 'protest against this evil'.[26] Heywood described how 'the question of temperance was one of more progress and triumph of the gospel, and all others sank into insignificance with it'.[27] At a public meeting in Bradford, Reverend Garrett was reported to passionately proclaim that: 'The Alliance was simply the vanguard of the army that was marching on....The Alliance had prepared a battering ram to bring down the drinks traffic, the Good Templars had come forward to work it, and the building would fall amidst a rejoicing world'.[28] The Good Templars were a fraternal temperance society often painted as the shock troops of prohibitionism; according to another Bradford speaker, they 'neither took nor gave quarter'.[29] The persistent employment of the terminology of warfare belies something about how prohibitionists saw their campaign; this was a holy crusade, both good and righteous, which would lead to huge and radical social improvements.

Despite this aggressively utopian language, the UK Alliance's main demand was not the full enactment of prohibition but some form of local veto over the liquor traffic. A local veto would allow areas of the country to 'go dry' if this measure was supported by a majority (of usually two thirds) in a local referendum, and its preference to the full prohibition of Maine Law was used by Warner as evidence of the British temperance movement's either realism or lack of ambition.[30] However, it should be pointed out that, among the membership of prohibitionist groups, there was little doubt that the local veto would result in full national prohibition. They fervently believed that, in the words of J.H. Raper, the drinks industry was forced 'upon the community against the will of the community',[31] and, to quote Wilfrid Lawson, the attendant evils of 'pauperism, crime and drunkenness' were also 'inflicted upon them'.[32] People were imprisoned by cruel, manipulative publicans who used their inability to resist the temptation of drink to keep them in chains. But, given the opportunity, the population would vote overwhelmingly to free themselves from this slavery by 'going dry'. Addressing the obstacle of the parliamentary majority opposed to the local veto, Lawson confidently stated that 'before the breath of an aroused and enlightened public opinion that great majority would melt away like snow upon the mountain side'.[33] This unwavering faith was driven by the simple belief that God was on their side and so the Alliance was, in Reverend Garrett's words, 'sure to succeed'.[34] Drinking was sinful and 'No sin against God ... could succeed'.[35] Given this genuine conviction in the popularity of their cause and the inevitability of its success, relying on the local veto to banish the drinks trade appears utopian rather than pessimistic or realistic.

By the early 1860s, moral suasionism appeared in decline and the confident, strident campaigning of the prohibitionist UK Alliance took over the reformist momentum.[36] This was not a harmonious shift within the moral regulation movement; moral suasionists and prohibitionists frequently argued vociferously. In July 1873, the *Preston Guardian* featured a lively exchange of letters between Joseph Livesey and Dawson Burns, with the former forcefully rejecting the Alliance view that 'the people are unwilling slaves to the traffic, oppressed and yearning for "power" to be delivered'.[37] Livesey argued that the 'citizens of this country have a right, if they wish, to drink intoxicating liquors' and that, for the most part, people exercised this right.[38] To presume that these very same people should be allowed to decide the shape of the licensing system was dismissed as folly. In response, Burns criticised Livesey's view that, because so many people regularly succumb to the 'terrible temptation' of drink, the facility to legally remove this temptation should not exist.[39] Burns could not understand how someone may believe that the sale of liquor results in evil yet not wish to eradicate the sale of it. The exchange also touched upon the suitability of magistrates to make licensing decisions[40] and the effectiveness of various American policies.[41] But, despite their shared concern about drink, there was little consensus between the two; whether the temptation could and should be removed or people could and should be taught to resist it, remained an irreconcilable issue.

The problematisation of alcohol therefore produced two distinct variants of temperance: one preferring internal, voluntary solutions and the other seeking external, legally coercive measures. In 1873, Livesey signed off with a pointed attack on the Alliance, which was accused of 'busying themselves with politics'[42] while the teetotal cause lost ground. In 1887, Livesey's son, Howard, made a similar attack on prohibitionism for allegedly rendering the whole temperance campaign inert by diverting attention towards an unachievable legislative goal.[43] Howard Livesey's lament, for the replacement of the 'preaching of the gospel of abstinence'[44] with aggressively seeking legal compulsion to abstinence, inferred that moral suasionist campaigning had, for the most part, expired. If this position is coupled with the ultimate failure of the ascendant prohibitionist movement to achieve its primary legal demand, it is possible to understand Warner's claim that the British temperance movement accomplished very little.

Legal impacts of the temperance movement

Warner's classification of the British temperance movement as a failure seems based primarily on the lack of prohibition legislation enacted by Westminster. Comparison with the US, where prohibitionist temperance dominated and was successful to the extent that the trade in alcohol was outlawed (temporarily from 1919 to 1933), seems to heighten this perception of lack of accomplishments. A retrospective search for a British equivalent of the American 18th Amendment, which introduced prohibition, will always conclude in the negative. But does this mean that the British temperance movement accomplished nothing?

The birth of the modern licensing system

First, it must be acknowledged that Parliament voted many times on whether introducing some form of local veto, the principal demand of British prohibitionists, was desirable. In 1864, Alliance member and Liberal MP Sir Wilfrid Lawson introduced the Permissive Bill to Parliament as a Private Members' Bill. The Bill proposed that, with a two thirds majority in a poll, ratepayers would be able to veto the granting of licences in their local area and it was repeatedly re-introduced to Parliament up until the mid-1880s. Despite being rejected by Parliament at every opportunity, prohibitive measures did seem to be slowly gaining acceptance; the National Liberal Federation endorsed the local option in 1891 and it formed part of the Liberal Party's 1892 electoral platform. Having won the General Election, the Chancellor of the Exchequer, William Harcourt MP, introduced a Local Veto Bill in 1893. Harcourt was a convert to the cause, having vigorously opposed licensing restrictions in the 1870s, and was convinced of the need for local parishes to have the legal facility to ban the granting of licences if this was approved by referendum. With heavy opposition from the drinks trade, Harcourt's Bill was defeated in 1893. In 1895, a slightly softer Local Option Bill was debated, which would have allowed people to vote for a reduction in the number of licensed premises in their areas as well as being able to vote simply for the continuation or cancellation of all licences. The Bill had full government backing this time but the administration collapsed and was defeated at the 1895 General Election before the measures could be voted on.[45] Defeats aside, the very fact that Victorian Parliaments regularly debated the Alliance's demand for some form of local control of the drinks trade indicates a degree of impact. Its measures may have been rejected, but prohibitionists exhibited some potency in terms of setting the public and political agenda of the day.

Not all local veto-style legislation was unsuccessful. The Temperance (Scotland) Act 1913 was implemented after the First World War. Effectively, this statute enacted the UK Alliance's main aim by setting up local polls in Scottish areas on the future of the drinks trade, the results of which would dictate local licensing policy. Warner's dismissal of this Act as the sum total of six decades of prohibitionist campaigning is unfair for two reasons.[46] First, the derisory tone fails to acknowledge that, as described earlier, advocates of the local veto fully expected it to produce uniformly dry parishes. Second, while the local veto was never extended south of the border, other temperance demands were met. Sunday closing of public houses was implemented in Scotland by the Licensing (Scotland) Act 1853 and Wales eventually followed suit with the passage of the Welsh Sunday Closing Act 1881.[47] This Act survived until 1961 when it was replaced by local veto-style legislation allowing for the enforcement of local Sunday closing in Wales if it was approved by referendum. Sunday opening hours in England were limited by statutes in the mid-1850s[48] but, despite the House of Commons approving a Bill for Sunday closing in England in 1889, prohibition on the Sabbath day was never enacted.[49] Even where it was implemented, Sunday closing may seem a pallid measure when compared with the goal of total sobriety. But Sunday closing was a key demand for some temperance societies; the Central Association for Stopping the Sale of Liquor on Sundays, which was linked to the UK Alliance,[50] was established to further precisely this end. Measures such as Sunday closing and the local veto in Scotland demonstrate that the temperance movement did achieve *some* of its legislative goals.

In addition to these legal measures, there were other notable changes to the governance of alcohol in the Victorian period. The Liberal government's controversial 1871 proposal to cap the number of licences granted in any given area was rejected by Parliament, but other reforms were already under way. The free-trade approach to drink, ushered in by the Beer Act 1830 and apparent in Gladstone's reduction of import duties on wine in the 1860s, was eroded from the mid-1860s onwards.

The Wine and Beerhouse Act 1869 tightened licensing by requiring all retailers of intoxicating liquors to be of 'good character'. More importantly, this Act also required all persons selling beer, ale or cider to be in possession of a licence granted by a local magistrate, and so replaced the more laissez-faire system of the Beer Act, which required only that sellers obtain an excise licence. Section 3 of the Licensing Act 1872 reaffirmed this governmental shift, stating that 'no person shall sell or expose for sale by retail any intoxicating liquor without being duly licensed to sell the same'. The maximum penalty for the first breach of this rule was a hefty £50 fine or imprisonment with hard labour for up to one month, and rose exponentially with subsequent offences. The restoration of magisterial control and the reasonably harsh sanctions attached to illicit trading illustrate the re-absorption of licensing into the legal system.

During the 1860s and 1870s, liberal rules on public house opening times were also replaced with more restricted hours. While the opening times of beerhouses had been regulated since they were created in 1830, there were no statutory restrictions on pub opening, except on Sundays, until the mid-1860s. The Public House Closing Acts 1864 and 1865 implemented compulsory closure between 1am and 4am on weekdays, and enforced a closing time of midnight on Saturdays. The Licensing Act 1872 tightened these regulations by not allowing any pubs to open between midnight and 5am. Depending on the decision of the licensing justices and to some extent the size of the town or city in which premises were located, pubs would begin trading at some point between 5am and 7am, remain open all day before ceasing trading at 10pm, 11pm or midnight. In London, the presumption was that pubs would open from 5am until midnight, whereas the Act specified that normal hours in the rest of the country would extend from 6am until 11pm. Sunday hours were also shortened to 12:30–2:30pm and 6–10pm although, if the licensing justices approved, the London Sunday hours, of 1–3pm and 6–11pm, could be observed elsewhere.[51] These new stricter rules demonstrate that time was called on the previously more lax system of alcohol governance.

The Licensing Act 1872 markedly increased both the scale and scope of alcohol regulation. It created the first national, statutory age qualification to British alcohol regulations by banning pubs from selling spirits to the under-16s.[52] Statutory age restrictions on the purchase of alcohol were tightened in 1886 and 1901, before the legal age for purchase was fixed at 18 by the Licensing Act 1961 (for both on-licence and off-licence sales). Section 35 of the 1872 Act also increased the powers of the police to regulate drinking by stating that, for the first time, 'a constable may at all times enter on any licensed premises'.[53] Significantly, offences of simple drunkenness in 'any highway or public place' and drunkenness with aggravation, where a person behaved in a 'riotous or disorderly fashion', were also created by Section 12. Although the penalties incurred have been modified, Section 12 of the Licensing Act 1872 still forms the basis of the modern offences of 'drunkenness in a public place' and 'drunk and disorderly'. Drunkenness with aggravation was additionally used to police drink-driving for some time as it applied to persons who, as Section 12 specified, are drunk while in charge of a 'carriage, horse, cattle or steam engine'. Legislation relating to alcohol and age, public drunkenness and drink-driving, which will be discussed in more depth in Chapter Six, proliferated massively from the mid-20th century onwards. Suffice to say here, that the Licensing Act 1872 appears strangely prescient. Through criminalising aspects of drunkenness and increasing police powers to discipline sellers and consumers, this statute established significant and enduring frameworks through which the use of alcohol has been governed.

Given the reinstatement of magistrates' control, the restriction of opening hours, new drunkenness offences, the first age-based prohibition and increased police powers, licensing legislation produced between 1864 and 1872 embodied a new and much more restrictive model of regulating the sale and consumption of alcohol. Moreover, legal frameworks that sought to limit alcohol supply, restrict opportunities for consumption and criminalise its excessive use were all legislative efforts in keeping with the problematisation of alcohol. This sea change in governmental attitudes, which saw the abandonment of the laissez-faire and free trade inspired the Beer Act 1830 model, demonstrates an apparent acceptance of the temperance belief that all forms of alcohol, including beer, were essentially problematic and needed regulating. The discourse of the temperance movement legitimated a higher level of state intervention in the drinks trade and, by 1872, the law reflected this.

A wishy washy tyranny

Temperance discourse may have legitimated greater legal regulation, but how was this shift represented in public discourse more generally? By far the most common representation of the Licensing Act 1872 was as a balancing act. Temperance groups calling for prohibition, as well as drinks industry representatives who insisted on the maintenance of their commercial freedoms, were both heavily active in lobbying and protesting at this point in time. To both the *North Wales Chronicle* and *The Examiner* the government was therefore negotiating a course between 'the Scylla of "the trade" and the Charybdis of the alliance'.[54] Similarly, for (pre-conversion) Harcourt the situation was reminiscent of the 'unfortunate person I have read of, who found himself between a tiger and a crocodile, both ready to snap him up'.[55] Stuck between 'two flat contradictions',[56] the government's response was dismissed as a 'patched-up compromise',[57] a 'useless compromise',[58] and a 'milk and water, wishy washy compromise which will really effect little good'.[59] Even those such as Donald Dalrymple MP, who saw the Act as valuable, believed that it was only a temporary settlement.[60] The overriding characterisation of the Licensing Act 1872 was, therefore, as a compromise between trade and temperance, or, as one newspaper asserted, between 'Good Templars and Good Tipplers'.[61]

Despite the characterisation of the Act as timidly expedient, it did provoke extensive and sometimes furious debate. Geographic variations in opening hours attracted some comment; in regard to tying opening hours to the size of settlement, the *North Wales Chronicle* suggested that there were more 'seductions' and 'exciting allurements' in towns and cities where hours were being less severely curtailed.[62] The newspaper rhetorically asked: have 'drunkenness, immorality and crime [been] found to be in inverse ratio to the density of population?'[63] The differing hours that applied to London pubs were referred to as an injustice by some provincial commentators,[64] although London newspaper *The Era* responded by arguing that these reforms had been prompted by the representatives of northern towns who 'have presented us with terrible pictures of depravity prevailing in their imaginations among their constituents'.[65] MP for Leeds, Edward Baines, is cited as one of these representatives who engineered a situation where, through uniform (although uneven) shortening of opening hours, the government was effectively 'visiting the sins of the "Tykes" on the heads of the cockneys'.[66] Uneven opening hours in different areas of the country was clearly a sensitive prospect.

More pertinent than geographical issues, however, was the accusation that the Licensing Act was a 'flagrant piece of class legislation'.[67] This claim was based on the premise that wealthy people, who could afford private wine cellars and membership of private clubs (to which the statutory closing times did not apply), would not be affected by the new rules. Although *The Times* protested that the drinking habits of rich men did not result in 'breaches of the Queen's peace',[68] *Lloyd's Weekly Newspaper* branded the Act as a 'tyranny' on 'the public who have no wine-cellars'.[69] A letter in the *Derby Mercury* derided the reforms as 'a disgrace to any civilised community',[70] while *Reynolds's Daily Newspaper* described the Liberal Party's actions towards ordinary people as equivalent to 'flagellating them with scorpions'.[71] *Lloyd's Weekly Newspaper* said that the reforms were 'uncompromising; dictated by Puritanic and unreasoning spirit', which, nevertheless, reasoned it to be efficacious to leave 'gentlemen to tipple ... as they choose'.[72] These commentators were motivated by a class-conscious conviction that the rule of law was not being properly applied; as one newspaper asserted, the law *should* affect Pall Mall as much as Whitechapel.[73] Towards the end of the year, angry exasperation prompted *The Era* to mockingly report that Henry Bruce and Lord Kimberley, the architects of the Licensing Act, planned to close music halls at 8pm, outlaw smoking and make whistling in the street illegal. The punch-line read: 'The above regulations will be applicable only to members of working and middle classes who cannot afford to become members of clubs.'[74]

As well as geography and social class, the Act was accused of undermining traditional rights of consumption. The *Daily News* struggled with the idea, inherent in the licensing restrictions, that beer must be viewed as problematic; 'It was supposed to be the thing which enabled us to fight the French and grow fat and live long'.[75] Beer was not viewed by all as possessing quite the patriotic bombast that the *Daily News* attributed it; although many others saw it as a normal part of everyday life. A letter to the *Birmingham Daily Post* from James Penner pointed out that 'great numbers of people regard beer as a necessity' and so enforcing the closure of pubs at certain times of day amounted to a 'dietary curfew'.[76] Lord Stanley supported this characterisation of alcoholic drinks when he described prohibition as 'a rule of diet'.[77] It follows from these neutral, even positive assessments of beer, that many people still regarded the adulteration of beer as the 'real evil' responsible for drunkenness and other problems, not the beer itself.[78] At a public meeting, reported by the *Leeds Mercury*, when Reverend Flood claimed that 60,000 deaths per year were caused by drinking, someone in the crowd shouted 'adulteration!', to imply that good beer was not responsible.[79] Presumably these persons supported the new penalties on the adulteration of beer, contained within the new Act, but rejected its other provisions as unnecessary. Regardless, the persistence of older, positive views of beer demonstrates that the teetotal turn in attitudes to alcohol, which problematised all intoxicating drinks, had been far from universal.

The broader implication of this contestation over the character of beer was revealed by *The Times*, when it stated that 'Parliament is, in fact, going far beyond its proper scope in attempting to restrict the people in their private consumption of an article of diet'.[80] Compulsory closing times, along with greater powers for police and courts to discipline drinkers, were frequently seen as a 'meddlesome and mischievous'[81] interference with the everyday lives of ordinary people who, for the most part, 'drink when they want, and leave off when they don't'.[82] Alderman Brinsley saw the Licensing Act 1872 as an 'unjust and un-English interference with the requirements of working men';[83] *The Era* saw these new restrictions as 'paternal' and 'oppressive';[84] and (pre-conversion) Harcourt equated them with the actions of a 'grand-maternal Government which ties nightcaps on a grown-up nation by Act of Parliament'.[85] The *Ipswich Journal* attempted some historical perspective, claiming that in former days Englishmen would rather 'preserve the liberty he enjoyed, even though it occasionally extended to the liberty to do wrong'.[86] Whether they were normal dietary articles or aids to national security, many people struggled to swallow the problematisation of alcoholic drinks and hence found the new, more interventionist laws entirely unpalatable.

Apparent in Brinsley's reference to 'un-English' measures, aspects of public discourse located the Licensing Act 1872 within a longer-term patriotic narrative. The *Ipswich Journal* claimed that 'Englishmen have not been so tyrannically treated, since the days of the Norman Kings, as they are being treated by this Act'.[87] Similarly, Penner's letter in the *Birmingham Daily Post* reminded the reader that 'once upon a time the Norman oppressor decreed that every Saxon should, at the sound of a bell rung in the evening, extinguish his light and cover his fire' before asking 'are we coming back to legislation like that?'[88] These comments evoke what Christopher Hill calls 'the Norman Yoke', a populist creation myth of the English constitution in which essential freedoms were stolen by the Norman conquerors before being partially wrested back from King John in the Magna Carta.[89] In light of this, Penner's question cannot be taken lightly; the liberty to consume alcoholic beverages free from state interference was central to many people's conception of traditional English constitutional freedoms. The Bishop of Peterborough most aptly captured this relationship, existing in the public mindset, of the drink politics of 1870s to English history: 'Better is a nation of free drunkards than a nation of teetotal slaves.'[90]

This powerful sense that traditional, hard-won liberties were being lost made the implementation of aspects of the Licensing Act 1872 difficult. When, in August 1872, drink-sellers had to cease their business at earlier hours there were widespread instances of social disorder. The press reported rioting in Hull, Stalybridge,[91] Taunton, Leicester[92] and Oxford, and in the last of these, teetotallers reportedly had their windows broken.[93] A widely -reported incident in Exeter saw working-class men gather angrily outside a gentleman's club (which was still serving) after the pubs they had been drinking in had shut at 11pm.[94] As well as those seemingly above the new rules, those enforcing them also came in for criticism too. The *Manchester Times* reported on a Salford magistrate who convicted and fined a man for the new offence of being drunk in a public place, despite the fact that the man had been in his own home.[95] A police officer had pursued the man's cohabitant, who had been observed to be drunk on licensed premises, back to the address before arresting both of them. This rather (il)liberal interpretation of what exactly a 'public place' was led to the magistrate being mockingly described, by the *Bristol Mercury*, as a 'teetotal solon'.[96] Greater vitriol was reserved for the so-called Vigilance Committees, which many temperance groups established to monitor pubs' compliance with the new trading hours. *The Examiner* was particularly scathing, describing the Vigilance Committees as both 'a little comical' for taking the functions of amateur policemen upon themselves, as well as 'monstrous' due to their 'obtrusively obnoxious' practices.[97] The feeling that important liberties were being infringed upon, by law enforcers as well as law-makers, was a salient one.

Evidently, the ability to consume intoxicating beverages as and when one chose cut right to the heart of personal liberty for many people. The furore surrounding the Licensing Act 1872 was partly characterised by debate over whether alcohol in general or beer specifically was as thoroughly problematic as temperance supporters and increasingly politicians supposed. But, equally, there was fierce conflict over the basic capacity and legitimacy of the law in its aspirations to regulate this type of individual behaviour; can and should people be made sober by Act of Parliament? The repeated accusations of class rule, geographical injustice, Norman tyranny and maternal government, not to mention actual unruly protest at the new closing times, suggest that many people believed that the Act aligned the state to a more interventionist position on the issue of drinking. The Licensing Act 1872 may have been a compromise and a weaker version of the previous year's Bill, but, nevertheless, contemporary reactions suggest it remained an important and controversial rewriting of alcohol regulations.

A 'popular awakening'?

The temperance movement may have created an environment that, although still partially hostile, was more favourable to greater state intervention than previously. But, to what extent did the temperance movement force this intervention? First, a balancing act requires the existence of two opposing forces. Hence, the overwhelming characterisation of these legal reforms as a compromise can be understood partly as a widespread recognition that the temperance movement was involved in instigating them. Legal frameworks that seek to limit alcohol supply, restrict opportunities for consumption and criminalise its excessive use are all legislative efforts in keeping with the problematisation of alcohol. These qualitative affinities are no accident; Harrison highlights that the movement reached its campaigning peak in this period and increasingly influenced the governing Liberal Party. Harrison also points out that the Licensing Act 1872 closely followed the Reform Act 1867, which, he argues, weakened the power of vested drinks trade interests by expanding the franchise.[98] Perhaps more importantly, electoral reforms also meant that large swathes of the (male) middle class, the bedrock of the social movement, were now enfranchised. Given the level of temperance campaigning and enfranchisement, positing a causal connection of temperance to licensing reform is not unreasonable.

Contemporary commentaries tended to corroborate this connection. Just as the Vigilance Committees were attacked for their role in enforcing the Act, so the temperance movement more broadly was criticised for its role in producing this legislation. The *Ipswich Journal* wrote that Henry Bruce, the Home Secretary and chief architect of the Licensing Act, had been 'got at' by teetotallers.[99] Similarly, at a public meeting in Liskeard, E. Horsman MP claimed that Bruce had been persuaded to agree with both Permissive Bill campaigners and prominent brewer Mr Bass.[100] Such descriptions were unflattering for Bruce, depicted as weak-willed and easily co-opted, but they were no more complimentary about the temperance movement. For their alleged part in sullying the minds of MPs, temperance supporters were described as, at best, 'well-intentioned zealots' and, at worst, intolerant fanatics[101] and 'lantern-jawed friends of coercion'.[102] For a social movement that prided itself on its struggles for rational social progress and moral advancement, such words were no doubt unwelcome, but, in a sense, they again paid tribute to the influence the movement was believed to possess.

However, it must be pointed out that the provisions of the 1872 statute were far from ideal for the temperance movement. Harrison describes how, although the temperance movement created much of the momentum towards licensing reform in this period, it did not enthusiastically embrace the legislation.[103] The suasionist National Union for the Suppression of Intemperance gave the Act some support[104] and the UK Alliance treated it as a 'sign of progress'[105] or a step in the right direction.[106] As these quotes show, support was rather cautious; temperance groups were not entirely convinced by the legislation and tended to regard it, as the majority of others did, as a compromise. But within public discourse, both temperance and non-temperance voices were more assured of the role of the movement in instigating the reforms. At an Alliance meeting, delegates spoke of 'a popular awakening to the evils of the liquor traffic', which their campaigning had contributed to;[107] Band of Hope members believed that the Licensing Act 1872 'partially embodied' temperance principles;[108] and *The Times* wrote that without an agitation against the drinking habits of the lower classes there would have been no licensing reform at all.[109] In terms of the problems it caused and the regulation that was needed, it seems that the temperance movement shifted the goal-posts of the drink debate so far that, to even play in the same game, the government had to concede some ground. Even if the Licensing Act 1872 fell short, therefore, of the sort of measures that many temperance supporters desired, it is partly testament to their influence that there were any such measures at all.

Reflecting on legal changes

The temperance movement, therefore, had two significant effects on the regulation of alcohol: the partial or full realisation of some of its campaigning goals and, through its role in preparing the attitudinal ground and forcing the political agenda, the replacement of the minimal intervention-type approach to drink with a more restrictive model of governance. So, to an extent, Warner's conclusion can be challenged by a closer, more relative appreciation of legal and historical developments. Can the sociological insights provided by moral regulation theory shed further light on the issue?

Attitudinal or heuristic impacts of the temperance movement

The legal impact of the temperance movement as a whole has been examined. This section examines the public discourse surrounding the licensing reforms of the early 1870s in an effort to understand the qualitative character of the new system of regulation that the temperance movement helped to instigate. Do these legal frameworks owe more to prohibitionism or moral suasionism? And is the impact of either sufficient to refute Warner's judgement that the British temperance movement achieved very little?

'... to the spirits of just men more perfect'

Home Secretary Henry Bruce was the chief parliamentary backer of the Licensing Act 1872. Wiener presents Bruce as in agreement with Gladstone's description of the model citizen as possessing 'self-command, self-control, respect for order, patience under suffering, confidence in the law, regard for superiors'.[110] Gladstone made this remark as a description of those suitable for suffrage, but Wiener depicts Bruce as broadening its applicability to other areas of social life. He believed strongly in the use of prisons as correctional facilities and was also interested in reformatory schools for juvenile offenders. Interestingly, the biblical quotation inscribed on the Bruce family cemetery plot evokes this moral mission of social improvement; it reads: 'To God the Judge of all and to the spirits of just men more perfect'.[111] The crucial issue relating to alcohol was how to make the spirits of men more perfect. Although *The Era* described Bruce as committed to diminishing drunkenness,[112] he opposed prohibitory solutions in Parliament as well as Donald Dalrymple's 1870 proposal to give doctors the power to indefinitely detain habitual inebriates.[113] The explanation seems to lie in Bruce's enduring faith in self-command and self-control; he stated that he had 'no faith in any remedy for intemperance but the improved intelligence and morality of the people'.[114] For Bruce, individuals were agents of behavioural self-reform rather than products of a deterministic social environment.

This faith in the responsible, self-improving citizen was not necessarily incompatible with the laissez-faire restrictions of the Beer Act 1830; the behaviour of responsible citizens might not need regulated by the state. But, by the late 1860s and early 1870s, drinking and drunkenness were discussed in increasingly heightened moral tones. For example, *The Times*, which was generally opposed to the temperance movement and licensing restrictions, complained of the nuisance and scandal of 'our national drunkenness'.[115] In a similar vein, Bruce was quoted by a group of prohibitionists as saying that intemperance in Britain is 'a blot in their social system and a disgrace to their civilisation'.[116] The *Hampshire Telegraph* claimed that 'England has always been a drunken nation'[117] and the *Birmingham Daily Post* reported that 'the French think we are a nation of drunkards'.[118] The heightened alarm in these statements and their pejorative judgements on British drinking habits evoke both the self-denigration of temperance discourse (identified in

Chapter Two) and, more fundamentally, the temperance movement's belief that all alcoholic drinks are in essence problematic. Public and political discourse was decreasingly hospitable to the old idea that beer was a dietary essential and only adulterated beer and spirits produced social problems. As 'our national drunkenness' was seen to result from beer as much as gin, so it was deemed necessary for the Wine and Beerhouse Act 1869 and the Licensing Act 1872 to bring the regulation of beer, ale and cider back into line with the more proscriptive treatment of alcoholic spirits. With the problem treated increasingly seriously, the self-control of the responsible citizen did not supply sufficient regulation.

But the government was keen to ensure that this expansion of regulation would not be seen to constitute an excessive intervention. There was a pervasive public belief during this period that individuals could not and should not be made sober by force of law. The normative and practical aspects of this position often overlapped or coincided. That said, the practical inefficacy of state-enforced sobriety was often highlighted in discussions of the effects of (prohibitionist) Maine law,[119] and the political or constitutional dangers inherent in such a project were articulated as liberal warnings of the possibility that a powerful or popular group (in this case teetotallers) may be able to force their will onto the disempowered or numerically weaker in society.[120] Lord Kimberley, the key promoter of the Licensing Act in the House of Lords, thus argued that people cannot be compelled by law to abstain from alcohol[121] and *The Times* supported this position by claiming that 'no moral work was ever achieved without personal agencies' and 'an appeal to the free will ... of our race'.[122] The intensifying view of all alcoholic drinks as problematic meant that adhering to the doctrine of minimal government was not feasible, but overly stringent legal measures, such as prohibition, were also rejected. To the government and *The Times* at least, state intervention was no worthy substitute for self-improvement.

People could not be coerced into sobriety any more than they could be left to govern themselves. Nevertheless, there was a discernible belief in this period that the state could practically and legitimately use the law to limit the temptations of drink. In Parliament, Bruce complained that: 'At present, at most hours of the day, men and women are invited by illuminated Publichouses to spend a few pence on a dram of Liquor. The society and attractions of the House invite them linger, and they are tempted to consume far more than is good for them.'[123]

Bringing such premises under magistrates' control, giving the police the power to enter them and reducing their hours of trade would, it was believed, reduce the 'temptation to drink in excess'.[124] In a speech prior to the Preston by-election in 1872, Liberal candidate Mr German claimed that although people could not be made sober by Act of Parliament it was possible to limit temptation and so make drunkenness more difficult. German went on to support earlier pub closing times by arguing that 'the hour between 11 and 12 was a time of temptation, when very often the seeds of bad habits grew'.[125] Reducing rather than removing the temptation of drink was deemed by the government and its supporters to be a tolerable restriction on personal liberties.

The creation of legal frameworks amenable to behavioural change is relevant to earlier discussion of the causation of drink problems. It was noted that debates within the temperance movement pitted moral suasionists, arguing that intemperance resulted from individual moral failings, against prohibitionists, who believed that the (legal) environment was largely responsible. In a sense, restrictions on the drinks industry engendered by the Licensing Act 1872 implicitly attributed some causal importance to the external environment. But in terms of solving the problem of 'our national drunkenness', the dominant position reflected a belief that the individual should be the primary unit of social change. During an 1872 meeting on the subject of licensing reform, Mr Straight MP spoke of 'the great bulk of the nation' for whom 'freedom of action' was a crucial consideration.[126] Equally, *The Times* asserted that 'we shall not be able to check, or even much diminish, the continual stream of besotted votaries to the gin palace; at least, not by law';[127] external stimuli could not effect the sort of moral improvements needed. These arguments, and the form of governance they supported, were demonstrable of the belief that individuals were not constituted purely by their environments but were actively engaged in processes of self-formation. As in moral suasionism, behavioural reform was therefore achieved by fostering ethical self-reformation.

So, the reforms of the mid-1860s and early 1870s, culminating in the Licensing Act 1872, established a system whereby drink was governed through restriction and encouragement. Contained within these frameworks was an inherent problematisation of all alcoholic drinks, a heightened belief in the gravity of the drink problem, a valuation of persuasive above coercive tactics, and corresponding efforts to reduce rather than remove the temptation of drink (in order to help the self-improving citizen). Given this characterisation, the post-1872 system of alcohol governance begins to appear as distinctly suasionist in flavour.[128]

Moral obligations and behavioural choices

The fostering of behavioural change did not end with the legal regulation of the temptation of drink. Arguing that people cannot be forced to adopt more moderate drinking habits, Lord Kimberley spoke of the need to persuade individuals to govern their own behaviour.[129] To an extent, the exhortations to self-improvement and the condemnations of drunkenness that were apparent in Bruce's rhetoric, as well as public and political discourse more generally, constitute a form of official persuasion. Similarly, Harcourt's commendation of self-denial,[130] which was strongly reinforced by temperance advocates,[131] may be seen as a stimulus towards behavioural change. Other politicians were more specific in their advice: Charles Turner MP asked workmen 'to discourage intemperance by giving the cold-shoulder to any of their fellow-workmen who were addicted to drinking heavily'[132] and Lord Kimberley reiterated that people cannot be forced into sobriety before urging teetotallers to 'persevere in spreading the rules of temperance as far as they can'.[133] It should be stressed that this governmental project to persuade and encourage within restrictive legal frameworks cannot be equated with the liberal notion of free choice. It is significant that even legally permitted forms of drinking could be morally censured. To elaborate, Bruce left individuals with the legal freedom, within certain administrative and behavioural parameters, to drink as much as they wanted; but by stating that drunkenness is 'a disgrace to their civilisation', he left no doubt about the officially designated moral parameters in which this freedom was constructed.

The construction of behavioural choices about drinking with reference to officially encouraged and morally censured forms of behaviour was not restricted to political discourse. Echoing The Temperance Society's envelope of the 1850s, an *F. Allen & Sons' Cocoa Chocolate and Confectionery* advert produced in the 1880s featured illustrations connecting the avoidance of drink to general wellbeing (see Figure 3.2). The image 'Intemperance & Poverty' shows a slouched man, clutching a bottle, in a bare room with a shabbily dressed, miserable-looking family. This picture is juxtaposed with another of the same family entitled 'Temperance & Prosperity'. In the second picture, they appear cheerful and well dressed, and are sat at a table in a well-furnished room, enjoying (what presumably is) cocoa chocolate and cakes. The implication is clear: the choice of hot chocolate above alcoholic drinks leads to a wealthier, healthier and happier life for oneself and one's family. These examples of political rhetoric and advertising demonstrate that the moral construction of choices about alcohol had ceased to be purely the business of temperance societies. From the 1870s onwards, more numerous and diffuse social agents were involved in the transposing of binary behavioural categories onto choices about drinking.

Figure 3.2: F. Allen & Sons' Cocoa Chocolate and Confectionery Works London, circa 1880

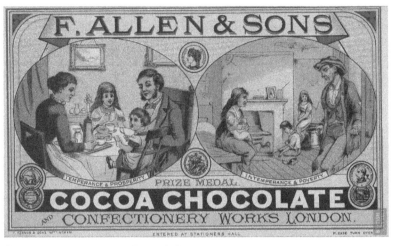

© The British Library Board (Evan. 6343)

So, individuals may have been superficially presented with a behavioural choice, but in moral terms there was no doubt about which type of conduct they should and should not choose. Instead of a legal regime that precludes the possibility of deviance, the Licensing Act 1872 is better understood as a regulatory framework allowing for a series of behavioural choices that are constructed in moral terms as either approved or condemned, right or wrong, or good or evil. Interestingly, 'the wrong choice' about alcohol, which leads to drunkenness, continues to be legally defined in a fashion not unbecoming of the moral suasionist temperance movement. *Neale v RMJE* [1984] decreed that the offences of drunkenness created by Section 12 of the Licensing Act 1872 refer to persons who have taken intoxicating liquor to the extent that 'steady self-control' is affected.[134] Subsequent cases, such as *R v Tagg* [2001] and *Carroll v DPP* [2009], have applied the same definition of drunkenness and so the legal eminence of self-control is discernible.[135] The fact that offences contained within the 1872 legislation are still employed shows some legal impact; but the affinity of the dominant legal interpretation of drunkenness with the notion of individual self-control, so evident in Victorian political and suasionist temperance discourse, indicates the deeper qualitative impact that the temperance movement had over the way alcohol is viewed and regulated in this country.

But, can regulatory licensing reform really be connected to the project to morally regulate alcohol? In some ways, these licensing reforms appear diminutive next to the demands of prohibitionists, whose desire for the state to legally restructure social life can appear as a firmer conviction in the need to ethically reform people's behaviour. However, Ruonavaara[136] has sought to distance moral regulation from Corrigan and Sayer's[137] conception of a top-down governmental action and incorporated concerns for self-formation and self-governance of identity and conduct into the concept (as discussed in Chapter One). Ruonavaara thus recognises an enhanced role for non-state actors and persuasive tactics. From this perspective, the official promotion of the temperance movement's model of the sober, respectable working man is an ethical subjectivity that aims to engender, but not force, behavioural change. If a person comes to see himself as disrespectable and immoral due to his drinking, he may be persuaded to change his behaviour. Teetotal suasionist Joseph Livesey argued that alcohol regulation should restrain and not force, citing high duties and licensing controls as examples of legitimate legal restraint.[138] But within these restraints, 'people are fit to be made better, and they can be made better',[139] or, to use the terminology of Bruce's epitaph, made 'more perfect'. The establishment of restrictive, non-prohibitive, legal frameworks around alcohol can thus be seen as an attempt to encourage behavioural reformation. Following Ruonavaara, this project is consistent with the characteristics of moral regulation.

The problematisation of all alcohol, the normative saturation of behavioural discourse and the focus on ethical self-formation all testify to the salience of moral regulation within the model of alcohol governance established by the Licensing Act 1872. Moral regulation must be construed, therefore, as something broader than just legal regulation. Akin to the legal moralist Lord Devlin (who is discussed further in Chapter Five), prohibitionists seemed to conflate legal regulation and moral regulation, believing that without the former the latter could not be realised. To suasionists, however, legal regulation was never the sum total of their aims. Their focus on self-denial and self-control indicate that there was a practical and moral currency invested in personal or extra-legal regulations. In 1841, temperance campaigner W. Hunt argued that 'every Christian professor is laid under a *moral obligation* … to abstain for his own benefit as well as the benefit of others'.[140] The significance of this quotation is that for suasionists, unlike prohibitionists, a moral obligation takes precedence over a legal obligation. Governance of the drinking habits of the population does not, therefore, end at the boundaries of legal imperatives but extends to broader areas where regulation is constituted largely by moral compulsion. Choices are delineated by legal parameters of permissible and indictable conduct; but within the space afforded by these parameters, the persuasive faculties of moral discourse construct individual behavioural decisions.

Reflecting on attitudinal/heuristic changes

It is therefore possible to reappraise the impact of the temperance movement. Ruonavaara's distinction of coercive and persuasive tactics focuses attention on the division in the temperance movement between the externally driven, coercive social change sought by prohibitionism and the behavioural self-reformation promoted by moral suasionists. It is the latter type of moral regulation that is most pervasive; the system of governance established by the early 1870s appears as an active, moderately interventionist promotion of individual behavioural change by the state. The Licensing Act 1872 in particular sought to aid total sobriety by establishing legal rules more amenable to improving the 'intelligence and morality' of the population. Given that this statute constituted a significant break with the Beer Act's model of alcohol governance, it is defensible to assert that the British temperance movement, particularly its suasionist strand, does possess some enduring social legacy.

The legacy of the temperance movement

The idea, propagated by Warner and others, that the British temperance movement achieved very little has been challenged in three main ways. First, a more relative appreciation of legal changes has flagged up the importance of measures such as Welsh Sunday closing and the Scottish local veto. Second, the role of the temperance movement in legitimating and instigating licensing reform in the early 1870s must be acknowledged as a form of impact, especially given that the resulting measures controversially and permanently ended the more relaxed regulatory system of the Beer Act. Third, the role of the temperance movement in colouring dominant public attitudes is revealed by the manifold interpretive affinities between temperance ideas and the qualitative character of the system of governance used to regulate alcohol. It is likely that both strands of the temperance movement contributed towards the first two impacts, but moral suasionism was noticeably more important in producing the third. Prohibitionism has thus been shown as something of a distraction that encourages academics to focus on the achievement (or non-achievement) of absolute campaigning goals. This search for a defining temperance victory, a British 18th Amendment, is erroneous. In Britain, the temperance movement placed greater emphasis on individual behavioural solutions, rather than collective legal coercion, and achieved more incremental legal measures. The legal and attitudinal or heuristic impacts of the temperance movement have therefore been attributed to moral suasionism more than prohibitionism.

Causally speaking, there are three layers of association that connect these legal and attitudinal/heuristic changes to the British temperance movement. First, there is a geographical or international association that suggests that the character of national temperance movements corresponds, to some extent, to the historical legal regime that governed alcohol use. Prohibition was enacted in the US where the prohibitionist strand of temperance dominated; but in Britain, where the character of temperance remained split, a system of legal restrictions and moral compulsion was established. Second, there is a chronological association of licensing reform with a period of heightened campaigning activity, which further suggests temperance influence. Of course, government in general was changing anyway during this period (as discussed earlier), becoming moralised, increasingly national and more interventionist. But the particular configuration of this post-1872 model of alcohol governance, based around the facilitation and encouragement of individual self-reform, demonstrates that it was, to some degree, infused with suasionist spirit. The problematisation of all forms of alcoholic drinks, recognisable within the new licensing laws, was a discursive feature common to both main types of Victorian temperance. But the increasing concentration on the personal obligation to refrain, as well as the focus on the facilitation of behavioural change through the dual use of legal restrictions and the normative construction of behavioural choices, reveals tangible affinities with the beliefs and tactics of moral suasionists. Crucially, it is these interpretive affinities that help separate more general changes in governance during the period from the discernible historical impacts of temperance campaigns. The qualitative dimension thus adds ontological substance to the connection of changing regulatory frameworks to parts of the temperance movement.

The governmental frameworks established in 1872, based around legal restriction and moral compulsion, consist of more than the simple balancing of competing interests. Indeed, they show that the influence of the British temperance movement has been subtler and more complex than its American counterpart, yet not necessarily lesser in magnitude. Building on the conceptual discussion in Chapter One, this argument is based on the premise that regulation is not reducible only to legal regulation and may entail 'softer' compulsion towards self-reform as well as coercive attempts to alter behaviour. To assess the success of the temperance movement, it is necessary to look beyond narrow assessments of legal change and consider also the changing qualitative character of the law over time. Without this interpretive appreciation of the normative foundations beneath debates about drink, Warner's conclusion would likely have been more agreeable.[141]

Notes

[1] Warner, Jessica, 'Are you a Closet Fabian? Licensing Schemes Then and Now', *Addiction*, 2006, vol 101, pp 909-910.

[2] Nicholls, *Politics of Drink*.

[3] Hislop, Ian, 'Sinful Sex and Demon Drink', 2010, episode 3 of series *The Age of the Do-Gooders*, BBC2, first screened 13 December 2010.

[4] Emsley, Clive, *Crime and Society in England, 1750–1900*, Harlow: Longman, 1994, pp 11-12.

[5] Wiener, *Reconstructing the Criminal*, p 83.

[6] Livesey, Joseph, 'The Alliance and the Permissive Bill', *Preston Guardian*, 26 July 1873.

[7] See: Shiman, *Crusade Against Drink*.

[8] Harrison, *Drink and the Victorians*, p 367.

[9] Livesey, Joseph, 'Dawson Burns and the Permissive Bill', *Preston Guardian*, 26 July 1873.

[10] 'Mr Cardwell and Mr Harcourt', *The Times*, 31 December 1872. Harcourt would later perform something of a U-turn and become a fervent supporter of prohibition.

[11] Lord Stanley, 'Reasons Against Attempting the Total Suppression of the Liquor Traffic', *The Times*, 2 October 1856.

[12] Pope, Samuel, 'Reply by the Honorary Secretary', *The Times*, 2 October 1856.

[13] 'That Portion of the British Public ...', *The Times*, 9 August 1872.

[14] Burns, Dawson, 'The Permissive Bill Movement', *Preston Guardian*, 19 July 1873.

[15] Pope, Samuel, 'Reply by the Honorary Secretary', *The Times*, 2 October 1856.

[16] 'The Newcastle Teetotallers and the Licensing Act', *Newcastle Courant*, 8 November 1872.

[17] In *The Conditions of the Working Class in England*, Friedrich Engels blamed industrial capitalism for the drunken excesses of Victorian workers, as they are 'deprived of all enjoyments except that of sexual indulgence and drunkenness, are worked every day to the point of complete exhaustion of their mental and physical energies, and are thus spurred on to the maddest excess in the only two enjoyments at their command'. See: Engels, Friedrich, *The Condition of the Working Class in England*, New York, NY: University of New York Press, 1993, p 109.

[18] Pope, Samuel, 'Reply by the Honorary Secretary', *The Times*, 2 October 1856.

[19] Brown, James B., 'The Temperance Career of Joseph Chamberlain, 1870-1877: A Study in Political Frustration', *Albion*, 1972, vol 4 (1), p 30.

[20] Burns, Dawson, 'The Permissive Bill Question', *Preston Guardian*, 23 August 1873.

[21] 'Second Lecture by the Teetotal Nutcracker', *Preston Guardian*, 20 April 1872.

[22] Ibid.

[23] 'Permissive Bill Meeting', *Liverpool Mercury*, 24 May 1873.

[24] 'Second Lecture by the Teetotal Nutcracker', *Preston Guardian*, 20 April 1872.

[25] 'Bradford Auxiliary of the United Kingdom Alliance', *Leeds Mercury*, 19 October 1872.

[26] 'United Kingdom Alliance, Preston Auxiliary', *Preston Guardian*, 17 September 1870.

[27] Ibid.

[28] 'Bradford Auxiliary of the United Kingdom Alliance', *Leeds Mercury*, 19 October 1872.

[29] Ibid.

[30] Warner, 'Are you a Closet Fabian?'.

[31] 'Bradford Auxiliary of the United Kingdom Alliance', *Leeds Mercury*, 19 October 1872.

[32] 'Permissive Bill Meeting in Leeds', *Leeds Mercury*, 12 December 1872.

[33] 'Permissive Bill Meeting', *Liverpool Mercury*, 24 May 1873.

[34] 'Bradford Auxiliary of the United Kingdom Alliance', *Leeds Mercury*, 19 October 1872.

[35] Ibid.

[36] For much examination of the competing fortunes of different temperance strands, see: Harrison, *Drink and the Victorians*.

[37] Livesey, Joseph, 'The Alliance and the Permissive Bill', *Preston Guardian*, 19 July 1873.

[38] Ibid.

[39] Burns, Dawson, 'Dawson Burns and the Permissive Bill', *Preston Guardian*, 26 July 1873.

[40] Ibid.

[41] Livesey, Joseph, 'The Alliance and the Permissive Bill', *Preston Guardian*, 23 August 1873.

[42] Ibid.

[43] Livesey, Howard, 'The Futile Policy of Prohibition', *The Times*, 8 January 1887.

[44] Ibid.

[45] For more details on the 1890s, see: Nicholls, *Politics of Alcohol*.

[46] Warner, Jessica, Riviere, Janine, and Carson, Jenny, 'On Wit, Irony, and Living with Imperfection', *American Journal of Public Health*, 2008, vol 98 (5), pp 814–822.

[47] Interestingly, this was the first piece of legislation since the 16th-century union of England and Wales to apply to one country and not the other.

[48] The Sale of Liquor on Sunday Act 1854 restricted Sunday opening in England and Wales to only four hours. This unpopular measure, which provoked rioting, was revisited by Parliament in 1855, which saw fit to allow pubs to open from 1–3pm and 5–11pm – enacted through the Sale of Liquor on Sunday Act 1855.

[49] The exception to this is the county of Monmouthshire, to which the provisions of the Welsh Sunday Closing Act 1881 were applied in 1921, although, historically, there has been some contention over whether Monmouthshire is rightly part of England or Wales.

[50] Harrison, *Drink and the Victorians*, pp 257-258.

[51] That said, magistrates could also force pubs to close at 9pm on Sunday if they chose to. Also, exemptions to these restricted trading hours applied where the customers were 'bona fide travellers' or the premises was a refreshment room in a railway station. Further extension of trading hours could also be granted to public houses in the vicinity of theatres or markets.

[52] Section 42 of the Metropolitan Police Act 1839 banned the sale of spirits to the under-16s for consumption on the licensed premises. This statute, however, only applied to the metropolitan district of London.

[53] It should be noted that these powers were temporarily removed by the Licensing Act 1874.

[54] 'The Government Licensing Bill', *North Wales Chronicle*, 15 June 1872; 'The Licensing Act and Playgoers', *The Examiner*, 7 December 1872

[55] 'Public Meeting in Oxford', *The Times*, 31 December 1872.

[56] 'That portion of the British public ...', *The Times*, 9 August 1872.

[57] 'The Session', *North Wales Chronicle*, 17 August 1872.

[58] 'The Licensing Question', *Derby Mercury*, 24 April 1872.

[59] 'Ministerial Shortcomings and Backslidings', *Reynolds's Daily Newspaper*, 14 July 1872.

[60] 'Temperance Conference at Portsea', *Hampshire Telegraph and Sussex Chronicle*, 4 September 1872.

[61] 'Bridgwater', *Bristol Mercury*, 2 November 1872.

[62] 'The Government Licensing Bill', *North Wales Chronicle*, 18 May 1872.

[63] Ibid.

[64] See: 'The Licensing Act – Town Hall Meeting', *Birmingham Daily Post*, 12 September 1872.

[65] 'To Licensed Victuallers: The Licensing Question', *The Era*, 11 August 1872.

[66] Ibid.

[67] 'The Licensing Act – Town Hall Meeting', *Birmingham Daily Post*, 12 September 1872.

[68] 'That portion of the British public ...', *The Times*, 9 August 1872.

[69] 'Health and Happiness Bills', *Lloyd's Weekly Newspaper*, 21 July 1872.

[70] Observer, 'Mr M.A. Bass and the Licensing Bill: To the Editor of the Derby Mercury', *Derby Mercury*, 27 November 1872.

[71] 'The New Licensing Law', *Reynolds's Daily Newspaper*, 25 August 1872.

[72] 'The Operation of the Licensing Act', *Lloyd's Weekly Newspaper*, 29 September 1872.

[73] 'The New Licensing Law', *Reynolds's Daily Newspaper*, 25 August 1872.

[74] 'Looming in the Future', *The Era*, 10 November 1872.

[75] 'London – Monday, Jan. 15', *Daily News*, 15 January 1872.

[76] Penner, James, 'The Government Licensing Bill: To the Editor of the Daily Post', *Birmingham Daily Post*, 29 June 1872.

[77] 'Lord Derby on Education and Diet', *Pall Mall Gazette*, 10 January 1872.

[78] 'The Sale of Liquor Bill', *Pall Mall Gazette*, 17 April 1872.

[79] 'The Government Licensing Bill. Town's Meeting in Leeds', *Leeds Mercury*, 4 July 1872.

[80] 'The Licensing Bill was appointed for ...', *The Times*, 7 August 1872.

[81] 'The Working Men and the Licensing Act', *Ipswich Journal*, 17 December 1872.

[82] Penner, James, 'The Government Licensing Bill: To the Editor of the *Daily Post*', *Birmingham Daily Post*, 29 June 1872.

[83] 'The Licensing Act – Town Hall Meeting', *Birmingham Daily Post*, 12 September 1872.

[84] 'To Licensed Victuallers: The New Licensing Act', *The Era*, 25 August 1872.

[85] 'Public Meeting in Oxford', *The Times*, 31 December 1872.

[86] 'The Session and its Lesson', *Ipswich Journal*, 3 August 1872.

[87] 'Current Topics', *Ipswich Journal*, 8 October 1872. The reference to 'Englishmen' here may not be entirely incidental; a letter in the *Pall Mall Gazette* equated licensing restrictions with womanly fussing over men's behaviour. See: *Pall Mall Gazette*, 9 August 1872.

[88] Penner, James, 'The Government Licensing Bill: To the Editor of the *Daily Post*', *Birmingham Daily Post*, 29 June 1872.

[89] Hill, Christopher, *Puritanism and Revolution*, London: Panther, 1968.

[90] 'Shall we Submit?', *Reynolds's Daily Newspaper*, 22 September 1872.

[91] 'To Licensed Victuallers: The Licensing Act', *The Era*, 10 November 1872.

[92] 'The Licensing Act', *Jackson's Oxford Journal*, 31 August 1872.

[93] 'To Licensed Victuallers: The New Licensing Act', *The Era*, 20 October 1872.

[94] 'Public Houses and Clubs', *The Examiner*, 24 August 1872.

[95] 'The Right to Get Drunk at Home', *Manchester Times*, 7 September 1872.

[96] 'The New Licensing Act', *Bristol Mercury*, 7 September 1872.

[97] 'The Good Templars', *The Examiner*, 31 August 1872.

[98] Harrison, *Drink and the Victorians*, pp 259-270.

[99] 'Current Topics', *Ipswich Journal*, 16 July 1872.

[100] 'Parliament Out of Session', *The Times*, 19 January 1872.

[101] 'To Licensed Victuallers: The Licensing Act', *The Era*, 6 October 1872.

[102] 'The Teetotallers in Leeds', *The Era*, 25 August 1872.

[103] Harrison, *Drink and the Victorians*.

[104] 'Suppression of Intemperance', *The Times*, 13 July 1872.

[105] 'To Licensed Victuallers: The New Licensing Act', *The Era*, 20 October 1872.

[106] 'The United Kingdom Alliance', *Daily News*, 16 October 1872.

[107] 'The United Kingdom Alliance...', *The Times*, 17 October 1872.

[108] 'Annual Tea Meeting of the Fisher-Gate Chapel Band of Hope', *Preston Guardian*, 26 October 1872.

[109] 'The London Newspapers will be Read To-day...', *The Times*, 17 April 1872.

[110] Wiener, *Reconstructing the Criminal*, pp 144-150.

[111] 'Henry Bruce, 1st Baron of Aberdare', henry-bruce-1st-baron-aberdare.co.tv

[112] 'To Licensed Victuallers: The Licensing Question', *The Era*, 11 August 1872.

[113] Wiener, *Restructuring the Criminal*, p 297.

[114] Harrison, *Drink and the Victorians*, p 263.

[115] 'That portion of the British public...', *The Times*, 9 August 1872.

[116] 'The Licensing Act', *Hampshire Telegraph and Sussex Chronicle*, 17 April 1872.

[117] 'Portsmouth, Saturday, May 11', *Hampshire Telegraph and Sussex Chronicle*, 11 May 1872.

[118] 'Independent Order of Good Templars', *Birmingham Daily Post*, 10 September 1872.

[119] 'The Government Licensing Bill', *Leeds Mercury*, 17 April 1872.

[120] 'The Working Men and the Licensing Act', *Ipswich Journal*, 17 December 1872.

[121] 'The Government Licensing Bill', *Leeds Mercury*, 17 April 1872.

[122] 'That portion of the British public ...', *The Times*, 9 August 1872.

[123] 'The Licensing Bill was appointed for ...', *The Times*, 7 August 1872.

[124] Ibid.

[125] 'Preston Election', *Preston Guardian*, 7 September 1872.

[126] 'The Government Licensing Bill', *The Times*, 2 July 1872.

[127] 'That Portion of the British Public ...', *The Times*, 9 August 1872.

[128] That is not to say, necessarily, that Bruce and others were converts to the suasionist cause; rather that when the government's faith in self-reform met an agenda for licensing reform and a problematisation of alcohol, both of which had been advanced by the dual strands of the temperance movement, the results were far closer to suasionism than prohibitionism.

[129] 'News of the Day', *Birmingham Daily Post*, 13 May 1872.

[130] 'Public Meeting in Oxford', *The Times*, 31 December 1872.

[131] See: Livesey, Joseph, 'The Alliance and Permissive Bill', *Preston Guardian*, 26 July 1873.

[132] 'Conservatism in Lancashire', *Reynolds's Daily Newspaper*, 8 September 1872.

[133] 'News of the Day', *Birmingham Daily Post*, 13 May 1872.

[134] *Neale v RMJE* [1984] Crim LR 485.

[135] *Carroll v DPP* [2009] EWHC 554; *R v Tagg* [2001] EWCA Crim 1230. These cases dealt with distinct, separate issues and are cited here purely to illustrate and provide some support for the contention that the definition of drunkenness as loss of 'steady self-control' is now legally well established.

[136] Ruonavaara, 'Moral Regulation'.

[137] Corrigan and Sayer, *The Great Arch*.

[138] Livesey, Joseph, 'The Alliance and the Permissive Bill', *Preston Guardian*, 19 July 1873.

[139] Livesey, Joseph, 'The Alliance and the Permissive Bill', *Preston Guardian*, 26 July 1873.

[140] Hunt, *History of Teetotalism in Devonshire*, p 33.

[141] Some of the arguments pursued here are also covered in the journal article: Yeomans, Henry, 'What did the British Temperance Movement Accomplish? Attitudes to Alcohol, the Law and Moral Regulation', *Sociology*, 2011, vol 45 (1), pp 38-53.

FOUR

The apogee of the temperance movement

Introduction

The previous chapter identified certain frameworks of moral compulsion that, in addition to purely legal measures, governed the consumption of alcohol under a system established primarily the Licensing Act 1872. This chapter applies the same concern for extra-legal, normative forms of regulation to the period 1914–21. Harrison and Shiman describe how temperance societies were in decline by the turn of the 20th century; memberships were falling and influence was waning.[1] Congruously, historians studying drink during the First World War tend to overlook the issue of public attitudes or morality and their historical precedents.[2] The temperance movement is thus largely removed from studies of drink debates during the First World War and the consensus opinion is captured by Greenaway's argument that '[t]he outbreak of war in 1914 transformed the whole issue of liquor control ... now it was primarily redefined in terms of national efficiency'.[3] Greenaway's discussion focuses largely on the rise to dominance of the secular issues of industrial productivity and military discipline. Older moral positions on drink were regarded as of limited relevance; 20th-century drink debates were largely seen as rational and secular.

But were these 'rational' concerns for national efficiency really the primary drivers of public discourse on alcohol from 1914 to 1921? Had the British temperance movement and the moral regulation project it initiated ceased to be a significant feature of public attitudes towards alcohol? Interestingly, Greenaway describes drink debates during the First World War as a 'moral panic'.[4] On the one hand, this is entirely fitting; a new or redefined social problem, which Greenaway identifies, is the typical subject matter of moral panic theory. In Cohen's classic theoretical formulation, moral panics are short-term, temporary phenomena, which rise up 'every now and then'[5] before submerging again as some form of equilibrium is reached or restored. In this classic episodic approach, each panic appears, essentially, as an independent event with little or no causal relation to preceding or succeeding historical events. On the other hand (and as described in Chapter One), this classic approach has been criticised; Critcher defines moral panics as high points within established currents of moral regulation[6] and Hier presents them as manifestations of volatility within longer-term processes of moralisation.[7] Following Critcher and Hier, whether a 'rational' response or an irrational moral panic, drink debates in any period must be positioned within historical processes of moral regulation.

This chapter therefore examines whether the consideration of the drink problem from 1914 to 1921 as a largely independent historical entity is feasible. Over 400 newspaper sources from 1914 to 1921, in addition to legal materials and temperance sources, are used to investigate the important issues relating to public attitudes and regulation. To what extent was this an episode in which the discourse relating to the retail and consumption of alcohol was fundamentally redefined by the issue of national efficiency? Do ongoing discursive trends that originated in earlier historical periods shed any light on public discourse and regulation of alcohol during this period? Given the starkly differing contexts of war and peace, this chapter aims to fulfil this brief by examining wartime and the post-war years separately before reflecting on developments across the whole period from 1914 to 1921.

Drink as a national problem

Between 1872 and 1914, British society and public attitudes changed in several significant ways. From the second half of the 19th century onwards, there was a growing interest in the capacity of external social forces to shape individual lives. The emerging labour movement, as well as researchers such as Charles Booth and Joseph Rowntree, promoted a less personal and more structural or environmental focus on social problems such as urban poverty and crime. Wiener describes how, for many, these new social outlooks were daunting and led to individuals feeling dwarfed by their natural and social environments.[8] Given this recognition of environmental influences, it became decreasingly acceptable and even possible to blame, as the original teetotallers had done, individual personal failings for social problems. Wiener identifies that, in issues of social reform, harm reduction began to take precedence over moral culpability.[9] Just as problems became, in this sense, de-personalised or collectivised, governmental solutions became increasingly interventionist. From the rise of compulsory education to the creation of court-appointed probation officers, the role that state activity played in everyday lives was greatly enhanced around the turn of the 20th century. The individual, in possession of self-command and self-control, was no longer the centre of the heuristic universe; both causes and solutions of social problems were conceived in increasingly environmental or collectivist ways.

Wiener elaborates on these changes, describing how early Victorian 'fears of a dam-busting anarchy began to be replaced by opposite fears of a disabled society of ineffectual, devitalized and over-controlled individuals moulded by environmental and biological forces beyond their control'.[10] Turn-of-the-century discourse was thus typified, especially in the wake of Britain's defeat in the Boer War, by a pessimistic obsession with national efficiency and racial degeneration. The effects of these broader changes can be related to alterations in the governance of alcohol. The Inebriates Act 1898 increased the power of the state over some of these flawed, ineffectual citizens by allowing courts to order that, if they were deemed to be habitual drunkards, offenders could be confined to an inebriate reformatory. This new therapeutic or welfarist tone was complemented by an increased use of taxation to govern the consumption of alcohol, as evidenced particularly in David Lloyd George's 1910 Budget.[11] While habitual inebriates legislation embodied a focus on a certain group within the population, so tax increases conceivably showed an attempt to reduce consumption at a population-wide level and thus alleviate problems of a weak, inefficient nation. Instead of concentrating on morally defective individuals, the shift towards more social and environmental understandings of how individuals were constituted led to the concentration of regulation on both problem populations and the population at large.

Temperance discourse was certainly not insulated from the growth of this increasingly collective or demographically inspired conception of the nation. At a teetotal meeting in early 1914, Mrs Lloyd George named alcohol as one of the 'great evils which were paralysing our national resources everywhere'[12] and, in a piece on new treatment programmes for habitual drunkards, the *Daily Express* referred to alcohol as 'a great national evil'.[13] This collective ownership of the drink problem corresponded to an enhanced concentration on the wellbeing of children: at a meeting of the Women's Total Abstinence Union, John Newton declared his desire 'to protect the child life of the nation against the contamination of the public-house bar'.[14] Newton articulated the threat to children, the future of the nation, in the medical language of contamination rather than the moral rhetoric of temptation; responsibility for the drink problem was thus located outside of the individual. Valverde identifies an opposition between free will and determinism within understandings of the causes and cures these conditions. It is not the case, Valverde argues, that determinism necessarily took total precedence over free will in this period;[15] but it is reasonable to suppose that, given the inflated importance attributed to contamination, demography and the nation, the heuristic scales tipped slightly towards the determinism of external constitution.

By early 1914, the heuristic landscape of public discourse had already shifted since the 1870s and war would soon bring further changes. This chapter examines public attitudes and efforts to regulate alcohol from 1914 to 1921 and considers whether war altered the contours of the 'drink problem' in England and Wales. Following the conclusions of the previous two chapters, it specifically investigates whether either suasionist or prohibitionist ideas still held much governmental sway and analyses how the regulatory regime they helped shape, instituted by the Licensing Act 1872, fared during war and the subsequent peace.

Responses to war

In the summer of 1914, the outbreak of war created a new geopolitical arena in which issues of governance were played out. Many existing policies and political principles had to be fundamentally re-evaluated in the context of total war and alcohol was by no means exempt. The growing acceptability of more collectivist and interventionist approaches to social problems had been apparent pre-war and was drastically intensified during the war years. From compulsory conscription to requisitioning, previously sacrosanct rights to liberty and property were fundamentally challenged. The relationship between the individual and the state changed (at least temporarily) and the previously unthinkable became increasingly thinkable or indeed actual. Given this new form of wartime governance, in addition to its commitment to the socially curative power of radical legal intervention, prohibitionism became highly plausible once more. This section examines the enigma of why the temperance movement's primary legal demand was not enacted during the First World War and how, in its absence, alcohol use was governed in England and Wales.

The enigma of British alcohol policy, 1914–18

To many, war intensified the need for tighter restrictions. Leif Jones MP stated that '[i]f drink was a national danger in peace times it was such tenfold in war'.[16] Jones argued that national survival hinged on the combat readiness of large swathes of the young male population and others, such as H.H. Croydon, extended this argument to the 'productive classes', whose drinking endangered the war effort by incurring 'terrible wastage and loss'.[17] Drink 'robbed the soldier of his efficiency'[18] and worker of his or her commitment to hard labour. Alcohol was regarded as a threat to both military discipline and industrial productivity and so it became seen as a serious threat to the nation. In February 1915, Chancellor of the Exchequer David Lloyd George declared that 'drink is doing us more damage in the war than all the German submarines put together'.[19] One month later, he famously proclaimed that 'we are fighting three foes, Germany, Austria and Drink: and as far as I can see the greatest of these deadly foes is Drink'.[20] So, given this opprobrium, why did the British government not enact prohibition?

The demands of war produced tough restrictions on the drinks trade in many countries. Belgium, Canada (with the exception of the province of Quebec), Romania and Russia were among 10 countries that adopted prohibition as a wartime measure. After the First World War, prohibition remained a viable legal option; a number of countries, including Finland, Iceland and Norway, upheld its implementation for several years.[21] Most notably, in 1919 the US amended its constitution in order to make the trade in alcohol illegal. The symbolic significance of this emerging world superpower enacting prohibition is worth noting; to many, this type of legislation represented the future.[22] That said, prohibition was not the only wartime drink measure and some countries focused instead on specific drinks that were seen to be especially problematic; France, for example, outlawed absinthe. In addition, Sweden strengthened its existing system of municipal ownership of the drinks industry and introduced an alcohol rationing regime. In the 1910s, the outbreak of war saw strict legal regulation of alcohol become a feasible action in many countries during wartime and beyond. Britain's failure to implement prohibition, rationing or any other radical measures certainly appears curious.

The peculiar comparative situation becomes doubly strange if Britain's temperance history is considered. Many of the countries that implemented prohibition during wartime, such as Canada, Finland and the US, had experienced large-scale abstinence-based temperance movements in the 19th century similar to Britain's. Interestingly, despite the decline in temperance mobilisation in the early 20th century, pre-war temperance sympathies had not dissipated entirely in Britain and proved resurgent during wartime. This was particularly evident in the formation of the Strength of Britain Movement (SOB) in 1916, a prohibitionist group, whose advocates argued that '[t]he use of alcohol lessens the fighting value of men in all ranks and impairs their thinking power and the speed and soundness of their judgement'.[23] The SOB's message, that sobriety and hard work were needed to maximise national efficiency, was popular. At a meeting of the 'free churches', Mr Parr claimed that 'during the war, patriotism demands prohibition'[24] and, towards the end of the war, the National Liberal Federation came out in favour of full local control of the liquor traffic.[25] There was a tangible sense that, for the sake of winning the war, strict measures such as prohibition may have to be swallowed by a generally reluctant populace. This new wave of patriotic prohibitionism, in addition to pre-war temperance sympathies, suggests that strong legislative action against drink would have commanded reasonable support.

The issue of how to deal with alcohol during the war was complicated by the increased popularity of other radical ideas, particularly the idea that the state should purchase the drinks industry and run it as an ongoing concern. Such proposals were inspired by the Swedish 'Gothenberg Model' of municipal ownership of the drinks trade and had been championed in Britain in the 1870s and 1880s by Joseph Chamberlain.[26] The basic logic to such proposals was that salaried management of public houses by state-appointed persons would free pub managers from the need to generate profit by encouraging excessive drinking. War gave this cause new urgency; the *Manchester Guardian* lent its support to the nationalisation of the drinks trade due to the worry that 'our national vice' may become 'our national undoing'.[27] A newspaper editorial argued that, although it is more visible in wartime, private vice always impacts upon the state and so state intervention is legitimate. The *Manchester Guardian* went on to claim that state ownership was preferable as it 'would for the first time make it possible to legislate other than by mere prohibition on the vice of drinking'.[28] Support for these radical interventions was evident in public discourse about alcohol before, during and after the war.

It should be stressed that prohibition and nationalisation were still contentious proposals. Nationalisation was derided by representatives of the drinks trade as 'the rankest Socialism ever invented'[29] and, as the *Daily Express* explained, many temperance supporters were equally hostile to these proposals as they did not want the state to make a profit 'in partnership with the devil'.[30] The *Daily Express* also attacked prohibition, evoking the Bishop of Peterborough's rhetoric from an earlier age by arguing that 'it is a free England for which our sons are giving their lives'.[31] Union leader Ben Tillet rejected the broader terms of this debate by arguing that there was nothing within the drinking habits of the working man that required radical reform; Tillet cited the millions of working-class men fighting abroad as evidence that this 'was a class to be honoured and not degraded'.[32] But Tillet's critique represented a minority opinion. The *Daily Express* reported that temperance supporter Reverend Mottram was deeply suspicious of any state purchase of the immoral drinks trade but would accept such an action if it would help the war effort.[33] Also *The Times*, for so long a bastion of free trade resistance to state interventions in the economy, came out in favour of the prohibition of alcoholic spirits in order 'to deepen the national efficiency for the purpose of the war'.[34] Moreover, *The Times* accepted that 'if further restrictions on the sale of liquor ... will help us to this end, let the Government impose them without delay'.[35] Public discourse was overwhelmingly characterised by an acceptance that compromises and sacrifices were necessary and justified in order to win the war.

In addition to the international context and public support for stricter drink laws, the links of the temperance movement to the Liberal Party render the lack of radical reform curious. The Liberals grew closer to temperance groups in the 1870s, although some blamed these associations for electoral losses. In the wake of the unpopular Licensing Bill 1871 and the Licensing Act 1872, the Liberals lost the 1874 General Election heavily. Gladstone blamed the defeat on a reaction to these restrictive reforms, declaring that 'we have been borne down in a torrent of gin and beer'.[36] Given Gladstone's views, it would have been understandable if the Liberal Party had shied away from formulating strict alcohol measures in the aftermath of 1874. But, nevertheless, it continued to maintain links with the temperance movement and, after once again forming a government in the 1890s, tried unsuccessfully to implement a variant of the (prohibitionist) local option. Not dissuaded, the Liberals included a limit on the number of licensed premises per head of population in the Licensing Bill 1908, although these proposals were rejected by the Conservative-dominated House of Lords.[37] The Liberals did not, therefore, distance themselves from temperance measures post-1874 and actually retained an active interest in strict drink laws up until the outbreak of war. Lloyd George, who served as Chancellor and then Prime Minister during the war, is an important figure. He came from a Welsh Methodist background and had expressed support for the temperance cause and nationalisation.[38] The position of Lloyd George and others meant that, in the words of historian Green, the Cabinet had never been so 'self-consciously abstemious'.[39] Radical interventions therefore commanded sympathy or support at the highest political levels.

The British government's refrain from implementing radical alcohol policies during the First World War is not just a curious riddle given the spread of collectivism and the erosion of traditional liberties engendered by war. This central riddle is wrapped in the mystery of the comparative international situation and Britain's temperance history, as well as being concealed within the enigma of public and high-level political support for radical interventions at the time. So if strict measures such as prohibition and nationalisation were avoided, what exactly did the government do?

What was the government's response?

Some aspects of the governmental response were entirely predictable. One such unremarkable measure was the increase in levels of taxation levied on the trade in alcoholic drinks. By the 20th century, it was well established that taxation could be used to either discourage consumption or raise government revenue; the Gin Act 1736 raised the excise duty on gin in an effort to discourage consumption and Lloyd George's 1910 Budget also contained considerable tax rises for both brewer and pub licences.[40] Slightly more novel was the decision, enforced by the Central Control Board (CCB), which oversaw most British alcohol policy during the First World War,[41] to limit the strength of alcoholic spirits available for public purchase.[42] Such a measure, not entirely dissimilar to France's banning of absinthe, had never been enacted before, albeit the Gin Act 1736 did inflate the cost of a licence to such an extent that it amounted to a prohibition of gin.[43] Moreover, various licensing initiatives, from the Beer Act 1830 to Gladstone's liberalisation of the wine trade in the 1860s, were at least partially motivated by an attempt to wean people off spirits by promoting the trade in weaker alcoholic drinks. Increased taxation and restrictions on the strength of spirits did not, therefore, amount to any radical new departure in alcohol policy.

The same point can be made in respect of one of the key planks of the wartime alcohol policy: restricted hours of sale. During the war, the CCB restricted public houses to opening from midday to 2:30pm and 6:30pm to 9:30pm.[44] The implementation of morning and afternoon closure was novel, but the idea of restricted hours of sale was not new to the drinks industry. As described in previous chapters, statutory closing times were established in the Victorian period; beerhouses had operated within set hours since their creation in the 1830s and public houses were restricted from mid-1860s onwards. It is now relatively common to hear it said that closing times were first introduced in Britain during the First World War, but they were actually significantly older. Wartime opening hours were stringently reduced but, as with taxation, this was the tightening of an existing regulation rather than the creation of a new one.

Some of the government's measures had less historic precedents. On the outbreak of war, the 'treating' of soldiers and sailors to drink immediately became a public issue.[45] In September 1914, H.H. Croydon, of the COETS, wrote to *The Times* imploring people to refrain from this popular custom.[46] This call was echoed by both the Minister of War Lord Kitchener and his sister, Mrs Frances Parker, who asked people not to 'treat' servicemen in the interests of their 'efficiency and wellbeing'.[47] While initially the justification for such concerns about treating referred to the need to reduce the consumption of alcohol by servicemen in order to maximise military effectiveness, the terms of the debate quickly encompassed the drinking habits of the civilian population also. In late 1914, a letter in *The Times* from E.F. Chapman asked: 'Do we, as a nation, realize that temperance is necessary to efficiency in war? Can we understand that it must be adopted by our civilian population as well as by our sailors and soldiers as a national habit?'.[48] There was a certain rational logic at work here, as the continued productivity and wealth of a nation becomes particularly important during wartime. Thus, under the auspices of the CCB, treating was banned in 1915. Attracting much comment at the time, this was an unusual measure, historically speaking.[49] But if it is compared with some of the measures, such as prohibition or nationalisation, contemplated at the time, it hardly appears radical.

The concentration on maximising the productive capabilities of the civilian population was also behind one truly radical policy pursued by the wartime administration. In certain areas the CCB did enact a type of localised nationalisation of the drinks industry. In 1916, the state began purchasing pubs in Enfield Lock, Cromarty Firth and, on a huge scale, Carlisle and its environs. These areas were selected because they were home to large munitions factories and so the sobriety of the local population, many of whom worked in these factories, was seen to have a strategic importance for the war effort. In these localities, the CCB replaced the private profit motive with a system of 'disinterested management' and, freed from the pursuit of financial gain, salaried managers began making a number of improvements to pubs. Improvements affected the physical condition and decor of many premises, as well as the provision of food and soft drinks.[50] Pubs were often operated as works canteens, in the hope that the provision of food would mean workers would not opt for a 'liquid lunch'. But this was also an attempt to change the culture of the pub, to make it more comfortable, more respectable and more family friendly. According to a post-war letter in *The Times*, these efforts were successful in creating something 'like the Continental restaurant ... where a better moral atmosphere may reinforce a healthy public opinion and create self-respect'.[51] The nationalisation of the drinks industry as an effort to promote sobriety and productivity was, therefore, a radical measure; but it was pursued in only a handful of areas.

Prior to the First World War, Britain already had reasonably restrictive drink laws. It was established practice for British governments to regulate who may sell alcohol, when and (through taxation) at what price; the governmental response to the First World War instigated no paradigmatic shift away from these legal frameworks. The legal response was therefore moderate; it was a mixture of tightening existing restrictions, implementing a new but hardly radical ban on 'treating' and undertaking a radical yet small-scale scheme of nationalisation. But were these moderate legal measures the sum total of ways in which sobriety was promoted in Britain during the war?

'England expects every man to do his duty'

An examination of public discourse during the First World War provides some fascinating new perspectives on this issue. Press coverage in the early years of the First World War reveals that voluntary, as well as legal, action was demanded. As with treating, these demands were initially directed at servicemen. Robert B. Batty wrote in the *Manchester Guardian* that 'the greatest enemy to military efficiency has been insobriety, and its greatest support abstinence'.[52] Batty cited the Russo-Japanese War as evidence, claiming that the humiliating Russian defeat was due to the drunkenness of many of its officers. In another letter to the *Manchester Guardian*, one S.M. Mitra echoed Batty's concerns and called for military clubs, whose clientele were officers, to stop selling alcoholic drinks. It was seen to be unfair to expect the rank-and-file to abstain from alcohol unless their superiors were prepared to observe the same form of teetotal conduct. Mitra explained that 'an example set by a military club would go a great way towards making Tommy a teetotaller and would be an object lesson to Germany'.[53] There appears, therefore, to have been a strong belief that teetotal soldiers were markedly more effective soldiers. Batty's quotation of the late Field Marshall Lord Roberts encapsulates this point: 'Give me a teetotal army,' he said, 'and I will lead it anywhere.'[54]

'Tommy the Teetotaller' was promoted as an aspirational behavioural ideal partly through imploring Britons to follow the example of their allies. Legislative restrictions on alcohol in France and even 'Barbarous

Russia'[55] had set a 'glorious example',[56] imbued with the 'spirit of sacrifice'.[57] While Britain's allies were viewed as respectable and sober, her German enemies were constructed as beer-drinking savages to be reviled. H.H. Croydon (COETS) contrasted good sober soldiery, as apparently typified by the British campaigns in Egypt, with the alleged drunken savagery of German soldiers. He explained that 'the trail of the German troops is marked, as innumerable witnesses testify, by myriads of empty bottles', and went on to claim that 'in some measure, the horrors of the German atrocities have had their origin in intemperance'.[58] This was not an isolated point: in 1915, John Rae of the National Temperance League connected beer-drinking with the 'animal and uncivilised habits' of German soldiers in Belgium.[59] Furthermore, a cartoon by Sidney Strube in the *Daily Express* in May 1915 depicted Kaiser Wilhelm II and Admiral Tirpitz celebrating the death of women and children onboard the Lusitania by drinking beer.[60] The First World War was not just Britain versus Germany; it was teetotalism versus drink, civilisation versus savagery.

The current of national self-denigration that had been prominent in Victorian discourse on alcohol was thus revised as the boundaries of national respectability and civilisation were redrawn along the lines of wartime alliances. Faith in our national depravity did not, however, subside and is evident within the heightened valuation of the evangelical notion of the struggle during the war. Previous chapters have described how temperance activists had long viewed their campaign as a battle against evil. In 1872, for example, Mr Hayle of Bury applied Admiral Nelson's famous statement of patriotic obligation – 'England expects every man to do his duty'[61] – to the war against drink. But the shared language of war and the temperance movement was not a mere rhetorical convenience; following Croydon and Rae's descriptions of German soldiers, it is clear that, for many people, the First World War represented a very literal rendering of this older conflict between good and evil. The *Manchester Guardian* reported on a 'very temperate man'[62] who promoted sobriety by urging a group of Scottish miners to view the national crisis as sportsmen. He explained that 'We needed every ounce of energy to be thrown in this struggle … and asked them to think that the first thing a trainer did when they put themselves in his hands to train for any great athletic event was to cut off all kinds of alcohol.'[63] To many people, the war was a physical, geopolitical manifestation of the moral and existential struggle against drink that they had long perceived themselves as fighting.

As the appeal to the Scottish miners shows, the strict behavioural standards initially demanded from the military were soon demanded of civilians also. In the early months of the war, the behaviour of British women became a significant issue as the focus shifted from 'the temptations put before not only our soldier's wives but our soldiers in the making'.[64] Given their importance as wives and mothers, the repeated allegation that women were succumbing to the temptation of alcohol, and drunkenness was thus increasing, was particularly scandalous.[65] Acute worry about 'women's duty and honour during this time of war' led Gertrude S. Gow and others to establish a 'League of Honour'.[66] The League aimed to combat the 'abnormal excitement' that had apparently gripped women and girls through the promotion of 'prayer, purity and temperance'.[67] Importantly, the League did not lobby for legal reforms but instead, in a thoroughly moral suasionist fashion, operated through 'mutual help, encouragement, and spiritual influence', which was provided by parish branches of this national group.[68] One of the League's chief 'weapons' was a pledge of total abstinence from alcohol for the duration of the war and, in an indirect way, the teetotalism of its female members would help men as 'the manhood of our country is raised or lowered by the influence of its womanhood'.[69] Drawing on teetotal moral suasionism, the League promoted female teetotalism through voluntary means.

Calls for the voluntary promotion of sobriety were not restricted to women as the pledge campaign also targeted male civilians. A letter in *The Times* one week after Mrs Gow's asked: 'can we understand that it [abstinence] must be adopted by our civilian population as well as by our sailors and soldiers as a national habit?'.[70] But this pledge campaign really started to gather momentum when prominent establishment figures began to endorse it. In November 1914, it was reported that a conference presided over by the Archbishop of Canterbury had endorsed a general pledge of abstinence for the duration of the war.[71] Many senior Anglican clergy soon began to echo this call; the Bishop of Durham,[72] the Bishop of London[73] and the Archbishop of York[74] were vocal in their support for this measure. A group of 22 Birmingham magistrates were reported as having taken the pledge[75] and, most notably, King George V and later Lord Kitchener forbade the consumption of alcohol in all their households. The *Daily Express* was particularly inspired by the King's example and repeatedly called for MPs to take similar steps.[76] Although MPs did not go as far the King, when they resolved to apply the same restricted opening hours to Parliament's bars as were applied elsewhere in the country the *Express* saluted this measure as a 'self-denying ordinance' and a 'great sacrifice'.[77] The highest echelons of British society thus traded voluntary acts of self-denial for a potent patriotic currency.

The Church of England was the main protagonist in the pledge campaign. Chapter Two summarised Hilton's research on how evangelical ideas permeated Anglican attitudes and wider political beliefs in the 19th century.[78] Its actions during the First World War suggest that many in the Church of England at that time were motivated by (originally) evangelical perceptions of the pervasiveness of sin and depravity as well as the importance of developing individual conscience. The Church thus sent pledge cards, adorned with patriotic colours, to churches and large workplaces. The cards featured quotes from members of the clergy as well as the text of the wartime pledge itself: 'I follow the King's lead, and promise to abstain from all intoxicating liquors during the war'.[79] Leaflets and 'chum cards', which could be given to friends, were distributed and many churches organised special 'Pledge Sundays' to further the campaign. Whether due to grassroots campaigning or public endorsements by national leaders, the pledge campaign gained ground fast and was apparently very effective. Both the *Daily Express* and *The Times* reported that workers were steering clear of pubs.[80] In late 1914, F. Milne claimed that 'greater self-control, along with greater self-denial, is expected of every citizen in the land'.[81] By April 1915, Milne's wish appeared to have been, partially at least, fulfilled.[82]

The 'official' rationale for the pledge campaign, as with treating and teetotalism within the military, was about civilians doing their utmost to help the war effort. Partly this was evident through a number of demands for the amount of cereal crops used in brewing to be reduced and diverted, instead, towards increasing national food production.[83] But expenditure was a much more prominent public argument in favour of the pledge. The Bishop of London highlighted that £160 million was spent annually on drink, money that could be either spent on paying off the war loan or used to provide relief to Serbia or Armenia.[84] The precise mechanics of this proposal, however, were unclear. First, there was the issue of how it was imagined these personal savings would contribute towards the national war effort: would tax, voluntary donations or something else be used? Second, expenditure on drink, unlike the Bishop of London's vague ideas, did make a direct contribution to the nation's coffers due to the high level of duty paid on alcoholic drinks. Industry groups were quick to emphasise this point; an advert in the *Daily Express* stressed alcohol's many advantages, including that it is 'a Revenue Producer' and therefore, in an ironic twist, 'part of the Strength of Britain'.[85] As well as the financial wellbeing of the British state, there were also complaints over falling revenues from wine-exporting allies. A Frenchman wrote to *The Times* in 1915 pleading with the British not to stop purchasing French wine as this would be 'another blow to the few remaining trades of France'.[86] There seemed a genuine risk that collective teetotalism would deprive both the British government and some of Britain's allies of much-needed revenue. The 'rational' arguments in favour of the wartime pledge were far from watertight.

Legal or governmental actions did not, therefore, constitute the totality of ways in which drink was governed during the war. This examination of public discourse has highlighted that the pledge campaign embodied a powerful movement of voluntary, persuasive action that targeted all members of society. But, although reduced drinking may feasibly have contributed to improved industrial productivity or military discipline, many of the arguments used to justify the wartime pledge simply do not stand up to scrutiny. Why must those not fighting or working in munitions factories abstain from alcohol? And why, for that matter, abstinence rather than moderation anyway?

'An indefinitely mighty force': the pledge and providentialism

Regardless of the dubious economic rationale of the pledge, there was a sense that self-denial in itself, as enshrined within the pledge, would bring benefits. Mrs Parker claimed that if civilians as well as soldiers abstained 'then the men who have rallied to the colours would be linked to their wives, parents and families at home by a bond which would be for good of all'.[87] A newspaper letter in 1915 struck a similar note, arguing that 'the civilian should feel the sacrifice just as much as the soldier, the rich man just as the poor'.[88] The Bishop of London outlined how many people were asking: 'is there no sacrifice that I can make, which will at least cost me something, which may help shorten the war for them and save some of their lives?'.[89] The 'them' to which the Bishop referred were 'our gallant comrades' who, 'up to their waists in cold and muddy water, day by day and night by night', risk their lives to guard 'their country's honour' and the 'freedom of the world'. Given this patriotic military altruism, it was seen to be essential that civilians 'make some definite sacrifice to show that the country is to some extent worthy of its defenders'.[90] For many, the civilian pledge was about creating a metaphysical bond of solidarity through mutual sacrifice and, to some degree, enforcing a notional parity in suffering between soldiers and civilians. But the Bishop of London's comments also demonstrate a preoccupation with moral worthiness; the pledge campaign was, in some ways, about the nation showing itself to be deserving of its armed forces and worthy of the ultimate victory it was striving for.

Concerns with solidarity, shared suffering and national worthiness show that there was a potent moral dimension to debates about the wartime pledge, meaning that the campaign looks less like a purely secular and rational means to boost efficiency. But as with efficiency, it was widely believed that the discernible moral, even spiritual, elements involved in the pledge would help the war effort. As the Bishop of Durham explained: 'Given a nation virtuous, sober, God-fearing, those combatants will feel an indefinitely mighty force behind them and will be lifted even higher than before in courage and in the moral goodness which is of the soul of the highest forms of valour.'[91]

The civilian pledge was therefore connected to providentialism; if we do good, God will reward us. It was not, so far as the sources examined for this chapter show, explicitly justified as an attempt to curry divine favour. But the pledge was certainly a commitment to virtue and goodness that, it was widely believed, would help avoid total destruction. Hunt identifies providentialism as a prominent strand in moral regulation projects from the 18th century onwards.[92] It featured in Victorian temperance adherents' vision of a struggle against evil but was more vividly apparent in the pledge debates of the First World War, as the fiery end that temperance campaigners had long feared appeared genuinely at hand. Teetotalism, even just a crash course, was seen as a necessary collective defence.

The civilian pledge, as a boost to 'moral goodness', had its roots in the moral regulation project of the temperance movement. The 'worldly asceticism'[93] of the teetotal pledge, pioneered by Joseph Livesey in the 1830s, was visible in the routine of everyday discipline and self-control demanded of soldiers and civilians. Victorian teetotalism was partly about thrift, labour and material self-betterment. But it was also about moral self-improvement; alcohol was viewed as a corrupting influence, an absolute evil that was detrimental to both the drinker's earthly existence and, more importantly, their ultimate prospects for salvation. The temperance movement failed to achieve the total collective sobriety it aimed for, but some of its arguments did seem to become standard ideological currency. It was common, during the First World War, to see the pledge referred to as 'voluntary self-sacrifice'[94] or a 'heroic act of self-denial'.[95] Even when explaining his decision not to take the pledge, Lord Hugh Cecil acknowledged that 'all self-denial is admirable'.[96] Teetotalism specifically and self-denial generally were seen as positive moral actions, likely to providentially improve one's, or one's country's, prospects for salvation.[97]

Summary: 1914–18

The tradition of promoting voluntary teetotalism was clearly alive and well in Britain in this period. Originally connected to evangelical beliefs, the tradition was now evident in society more broadly. Moreover, such acts of self-denial as the teetotal pledge had become invested with a providential, national currency that forced routines of sobriety, as engendered by more interventionist government responses, could not match. The pledge campaign, coupled with legal restrictions, formed a governmental effort to lift the nation from alcoholic depravity, to purify it and thus propel it to victory. In a different social and moral climate, prohibition or nationalisation may have been seen as essential; but in Britain behavioural governance did not end at the limits of the law.[98] The pledge campaign was, therefore, an extra-legal supplement to the moderate legal response to alcohol during the war.[99]

Post-war: what now?

The context of war intensified the techniques of both legal restriction and moral compulsion used to regulate alcohol consumption. This section investigates the extent to which the heightened atmosphere of self-denial, self-sacrifice and providentialism continued to influence the governance of alcohol in the years following the First World War. How did the law and public discourse change with the outbreak of peace?

To CCB or not to CCB?

In the wake of the First World War, the CCB was frequently praised for having provided 'consistent and an intelligible' alcohol policy.[100] Measures such as restricted hours and the provision of workers' canteens had reportedly done 'much to diminish the temptation to drink'.[101] Beer consumption was down[102] and convictions for drunkenness, even among women who were tempted by drink in their husband's absence, had also decreased.[103] Of course, these statistical trends were no doubt influenced by the fact that so many young men were stationed abroad, meaning their drinking occurred outside of the remit of either excise figures or police statistics. Nevertheless, there was a tangible sense that there had been an 'extraordinary change' in national alcohol consumption across the 1910s.[104] In a letter to *The Times*, Beatrice Picton-Turbervill claimed that 'Great Britain is becoming a sober country by a process of natural development', which wartime restrictions had accelerated.[105] The questions that now came to occupy public discourse on alcohol therefore related to whether or not the CCB had a future: should the CCB and its apparently successful regulatory provisions be retained in peacetime?

First, it is necessary to emphasise that the two orthodox poles of the drink debate continued to exist. A letter in *The Times* in 1919 captured the traditional, anti-regulation position well, arguing that '[a] more wholesome and heartening drink was never made than good English beer'.[106] Evoking Harcourt's 1872 criticism of maternal government, the letter went on to claim that Englishmen 'want beer, and I do not see why we should be treated like children by sour persons who sit all day in an armchair'.[107] In a similar vein, the *Daily Express* consistently argued that the retention of wartime restrictions during peacetime was a form of tyranny; in February 1921 the paper stated that the British people 'gave up their rights because they were told that the concession was necessary to beat the Germans. Now they feel that they have been tricked'.[108] This position, mixing patriotism with libertarianism, was countered by the continuing campaigns of prohibitionist temperance. Although the SOB movement petered out post war, the Alliance remained active and its campaign was boosted in 1919 by the visit of American prohibitionist 'Pussyfoot' Johnson; 'Pussyfoot', incidentally, briefly became a pejorative synonym for a temperance supporter. Significantly, buoyed by contact with the original 'Pussyfoot' who had been part of a successful prohibition campaign, and encouraged by the looming local veto polls in Scotland,[109] the prohibitionist movement continued to push for an intensification of the CCB's wartime restrictions on drink in England and particularly Wales, where a Local Veto Bill was eventually debated (and rejected) in 1924. The ongoing presence of traditional patriotic and prohibitionist standpoints shows the similarity of post-war alcohol debates to pre-war and Victorian discourse.

Second, the new prominence of the topic of state purchase or nationalisation within public discourse differentiates 1918–21 from the pre-war period. The experiments with direct state control of the drinks trade were reviewed favourably. In the Carlisle district, the number of licensed premises was reduced from 200 to 128 and the number of breweries shrank from four to two. This considerable diminution of the size of the trade was accompanied by refurbishment and improvement of the remaining premises, particularly in regards to the increased provision of food. The results, reportedly, were improved 'physical welfare of factory workers', greater efficiency and reduction in convictions for drunkenness.[110] *The Times* saw fit to describe the Liquor Control Board as 'the most successful of all the administrative bodies set up in the war'.[111] The Labour Party, rapidly emerging as a serious electoral force, was particularly keen to promote the Carlisle model as an ongoing example of how the state could solve social problems. J.J. Mallon described the Labour position as holding that the drinks trade 'ought not to be left uncontrolled in the hands of persons who must live by it and may therefore be tempted to develop it at the cost of the well-being of community'.[112] Prior to 1914, pubs were characterised as 'brutalising' arenas of 'pre-war slavery'; they therefore needed to be reformed 'if the vision of a better world to live in is to be realised'.[113] The Labour Party was therefore among those who wanted localised aspects of the CCB's wartime regulations rolled out nationwide.

While not everyone endorsed the CCB's activities with quite the enthusiasm of Mallon and his Labour colleagues, there was a general acceptance that some wartime restrictions would be retained. The Archbishop of Canterbury spoke positively of the 'general sobriety that has so far characterized the period of the armistice' and warned against 'premature or unwise relaxation of the safeguards now in force'.[114] This recognition was not restricted to Anglican temperance sympathisers. *The Times* stated that:

> No one, for instance, is likely to contend that the abuse of liquor is a good thing, nor would anyone seriously maintain that indiscriminate temptation to excess should be allowed if can be avoided without excessive restriction on the supply of stimulants to those who can make proper use of them.[115]

The Times thus recommended that the 'middle way' that the CCB had found between the two extremes should be the basis of post-war alcohol policy. More remarkably, even the representatives of the drinks industry accepted that there would be no return to pre-war ways. In 1919 and 1921, trade-sponsored licensing Bills were debated in Parliament; interestingly, both Bills would have enforced closure of public houses at midnight and neither sought to permit more than 12 hours of pub opening time per day. As Labour's Arthur Greenwood pointed out, 'Even brewers ... agreed that there could not be a return to the *status quo*'.[116]

Be it shortened opening hours, increased provision of food or disinterested management, there was a general consensus that at least some of the CCB's wartime restrictions should remain in place. After the parliamentary failure of the two brewer's Bills, the onus fell on the Liberal government to provide a peacetime settlement for the ongoing issue of drink regulation.

The Licensing Act 1921

It should be emphasised that there had been changes in alcohol regulations since the armistice was signed. In 1919, the CCB extended evening opening hours slightly, increased beer production and lifted the ban on treating.[117] Other restrictions remained in place and so, regardless of opinions on the level of regulation that was desirable, a more permanent settlement to the drink question was required. A licensing committee, which included those affiliated to both the drinks trade and the temperance movement, was convened in 1921. Shortly after the committee's recommendations, the government published a Licensing Bill. The Bill passed through Parliament in summer 1921 and was enacted later that year.

The Licensing Act 1921 was an interesting piece of legislation. It was liberalising in the sense that it scrapped the wartime limitation on the strength of alcoholic drinks, but constricting in its clampdown on the serving of large measures ('the long pull') and its prohibition of the purchasing of drinks on credit ('the slate'). The Act also abolished the CCB yet left the state management of the drinks trade in the Carlisle area intact (where it endured until the 1970s). In most areas, the new Licensing Act's greatest significance lay in the hours during which it allowed for licensed premises to open for business. There was a shift in legal approach from specifying hours during which premises must remain closed (which had been the case with the Licensing Act 1872), to prescribing hours during which trade was permitted. In the majority of the country, these new permitted hours allowed pubs to open for a total of eight hours from 11.30am to 3pm and 5.30pm to 10pm or 10.30pm, if the licensing justices approved. In London, permitted hours totalled nine as licensed premises could open until 11pm; but, again, this required the approval of local magistrates. While more relaxed than during wartime, the retention of morning and afternoon closure meant that new opening hours were more stringently controlled than they had been in the pre-war system.

In 1872, private clubs had controversially remained unregulated in respect of their trading hours. But, interestingly, these new opening hours were to apply to private clubs as well as public houses. Similarly, the exemption from statutory closing times granted for the '*bona fide* traveller' by the Licensing Act 1872 was also scrapped; the Attorney-General Sir Gordon Hewart's joke that '[a] *bona fide* traveller was someone who took a *bona fide* walk to get a *bona fide* drink' implied that the law had been abused and ridiculed.[118] However, exemptions were retained for late meals, or so-called 'theatre suppers', which premises were able to serve. This meant that customers ordering a meal in a hotel or restaurant could purchase an alcoholic drink to go with it up to one hour after the usual time; although, again, this extension required magisterial approval. Other exemptions included the non-applicability of permitted Sunday trading hours of 12.30–2.30pm and 6.30–9.30pm to Wales, where Sunday closing remained in force, and the contested county of Monmouthshire, to which Sunday closing was extended. The scrapping of certain exemptions as well as the expansion of Sunday closing indicate a tougher stance, although the provision for 'theatre suppers' did enable some discretionary extension of drinking time to be exercised.

The Licensing Act 1921 therefore abandoned some wartime measures while simultaneously retaining or modifying and retaining others. It created a system of regulations that were looser than during the war, yet tighter than before the war. Interestingly, it also enhanced the discretionary power of licensing justices. How was this nuanced piece of legislation received at the time?

A 'return to freedom'?

The provisions of the new Act appeared in *The Times* under the headline 'Return to Freedom'.[119] The legislation would cease the 'tyranny' of early closing times and, to Englishmen, represent 'a restoration of some, at least, of their ancient liberties'.[120] The 'theatre supper' clause was particularly celebrated; the *Daily Mirror* excitedly reported that 'London's Dull Evenings Come to an End'.[121] For many, the relaxation of wartime controls was welcomed and the retention of some restrictions prudent. But this moderate extension of the liberty to drink was not universally well regarded; the *Daily Express*, for example, consistently argued that restrictions had been justified during the war, but continuing them afterwards amounted to an unwarranted level of state 'interference in the private lives of the people'.[122] The Licensing Act 1921 thus provoked some heated arguments.

As the quote from the *Daily Express* intimates, much of this contestation rested on the accusation that the Act was not liberalising enough. The *Daily Express* attacked the reforms for creating opening hours that were the equivalent of 'Seven Sundays a Week By Law'.[123] MPs Mr O'Grady and Mr Clynes both voiced concerns about the facilities available for working men, particularly those finishing late shifts, to obtain sufficient refreshments.[124] As in 1872, there was a suspicion that it would be the working class who suffered by the new rules. Private clubs were now subject to the same permitted hours as public houses but, while labourers went without a drink later into the night, wealthy people could exploit the 'theatre suppers' provision and continue to drink until late at hotels and restaurants (where they could afford a meal). For Mr Raffan MP, these provisions amounted to 'one law for the rich and another for the poor'.[125] But geography was also a sore point for many people; while *The Times* rejoiced in the possibility that Londoners' liberty to drink would no longer be 'squeezed into D.O.R.A.'s tight-laced corsets',[126] the *Daily Express* complained that there was an 'anomalous situation' between London and the provinces.[127] The *Daily Express* continued: 'People in the provinces are treated like irresponsible children. They are, in effect, ordered to be in bed by ten o'clock'.[128] For some, the liberties (re)granted by the Licensing Act 1921 were insufficient.

These sentiments, regarding licensing restrictions as class based, geographically unjust and supported by an overactive state, are all familiar themes identified in Chapter Three. Unlike the 1872 Act, however, this statute also raised issues related to the separate regulation of Welsh drinking. Mr Forestier-Walker MP tabled an unsuccessful amendment that would have prevented the enforcement of Sunday closing in Monmouthshire, believing such a thing to be 'unthinkable in the 20th century'.[129] It may have been controversial in an officially English county, but MP for Cardiff J.C. Gould took things further by arguing that people in Wales' large industrial towns were also bitterly opposed to the Sunday closing stipulation, which they had lived with since 1881. Welsh town and city folk apparently resented being 'dragged at the heels of the agricultural districts'.[130] The *Manchester Guardian* explored this issue further, revealing that Welsh MPs were 'receiving shoals of telegrams, petitions and letters' from temperance groups, the drinks trade and club owners that all demanded differing alcohol policies.[131] The situation in Wales and Monmouthshire was therefore a further reason for critique of the Act.

The final major source of controversy was again absent from debates surrounding the 1872 reforms. The creation of permitted hours, regional differences and 'theatre suppers' all contributed towards an enhanced regulatory role for magistrates. The difficulties lurking in this reform were not identified until after the implementation of the Act when some London magistrates seemed reluctant to grant 'theatre supper' extensions. In a piece entitled 'A Storm in a Wineglass', the *Manchester Guardian* rather smugly reported that 'the wicked possibility that the cup that seemed to be promised to some Londoners under the new Licensing Act may be snatched from their lips – for a whole half-hour'.[132] These concerns turned out to be more than idle speculation when, in September and October 1921, magistrates in Stoke Newington, Kensington and Tower Hamlets enforced a closing times of 10pm (rather than using their statutory ability to stretch opening until 10.30 or 11pm).[133] Attacking this London lottery, *The Times* complained that: 'Visitors to London in the future will need to be careful when and where they order alcoholic refreshment. What is legitimate in Piccadilly may be a serious offence at Kensington, and what is right in the City may be wrong in Holborn.'[134]

The *Daily Express* was alarmed that the enhanced power of individual magistrates made them targets for undue influence; the newspaper reported the Bishop of London using his influence to lobby magistrates for earlier closing times in Hanover Square in a distinctly displeased tone.[135] For the *Daily Express*, a discretionary magistracy allowed for 'the last dying joke of Dora':[136] the spectre of 'Pussyfoot on the Bench'.[137] These debates about the vulnerability of the magistracy to undue influence resurrected the licensing debates that led to the Beer Act 1830 with the notable exception that, in 1921, magistrates were seen (by some) to be in the pocket of the temperance movement, not the drinks trade. This prominent concern, in addition to the issues of the varied applicability of the Act to different regions, countries and classes, meant that, although hailed as a 'return to freedom', the Licensing Act 1921 was discursively treated as far from satisfactory.

A temperance victory?

Given that it relaxed some restrictions while retaining others and pleased some people while infuriating many, the question that remains is whether the post-war settlement established by the Licensing Act 1921 represents, in any sense, an advancement of the moral regulation project of the temperance movement.

First, it is necessary to point out that this moral regulation project was not a fixed historical entity and frequently adapted in response to the wider context. The high public profile of both the pledge and prohibition campaigns during the war led to repeated accusations that temperance groups were using the 'cloak of war' to further their own ends.[138] Whether they were quite so instrumental is debatable, but the temperance movement certainly revised its central message to better fit the context of war. After the war, the COETS singled out health as being particularly negated by drinking and set about addressing this problem via its 'Merrie England Campaign'. This campaign aimed to improve 'social life, housing, food, hygiene and thrift' and thus conceived the drink problem in environmental terms.[139] In addition to health, the COETS and particularly the UK Alliance highlighted the importance of sobriety to national efficiency. The Alliance's Phillip Snowden claimed that Britons had been 'spending 2½ times more on drink than upon armaments, and the result was 2½ times more destructive'.[140] Snowden thus positioned the temperance movement as 'the greatest anti-waste crusade', which would, ultimately, provide the foundations for 'industrial prosperity and the lasting glory and greatness' of the British people.[141] The temperance movement was not a fixed and wholly utopian phenomenon; it was discursively adaptive and partially ameliorative.

Nevertheless, the Licensing Act 1921 was largely welcomed by temperance sympathisers due to its enhancement of the legal regulation of this moral problem. The *Daily Express* may have regarded the new limitations on opening times as indicative of an interfering, maternal state but, as the Licensing Act 1872 before it, many people considered the new Act as a necessary limitation on the temptation to drink at inappropriate hours. For example, Labour MP Mr Clynes spoke of his approval of the 1921 Act's maintenance of morning closure so that workers were not exposed 'to the temptation of entering public houses in the early hours while on their way to work'.[142] Furthermore, the CCB's brief reign over the alcohol trade provided reasons to re-examine the old idea that the law cannot remake public morals. The widely publicised decline in alcohol consumption during the war years was seized upon by some as evidence that legal intervention can reform the morals of the population. As *The Observer* explained: 'The paid and consistent reduction in public drunkenness which followed the progressive regulations of the Control Board, judged from whatever viewpoint, have proved that oft-repeated adage "You cannot make a nation sober by Act of Parliament" is a fallacy.'[143] While *The Observer*'s view was not universal, *The Times* in 1920 conceded some ground by arguing that the:

> ... episcopal preference of a 'free England' to a 'sober England' has become a faded paradox, a withered flower of speech. We are all agreed that the restriction of licences and of the hours of public drinking, the reform of publichouses, the quality of the liquors offered for sale, are matters in which wise legislation can promote temperance.[144]

Freedom was no longer antithetical to restrictions on drink, as it had been for the Bishop of Peterborough and others. There was an increased tendency to accept the temperance argument that alcohol was a deeply problematic moral temptation, which must, at least, be *restricted* by law.

Although it fell well short of their aspirations, the UK Alliance regarded the Licensing Act 1921 as 'a great advance over pre-war hours'.[145] The more stringent application of restrictions to Wales, Monmouthshire and the English provinces would not necessarily have displeased temperance advocates either. While they aimed for truly national reformation of behaviour, it has been discussed that temperance groups were most popular outside of London. Furthermore, the movement could take heart from the fact that, in certain areas, the magistracy was restricting drinking opportunities to the full extent allowed by statute. By enforcing 10pm closure in large parts of London, these 'pussyfoots on the bench' were responsible for what the *Manchester Guardian* referred to as a 'Temperance Victory'.[146] The newspaper hailed this as an 'indication of the trend of public opinion';[147] 'all the moral forces in the Christian community combined to plead for an earlier hour, and Christian citizenship has won a notable victory'.[148] The 1921 statute represented a 'mild form of local option' implemented, not by direct democratic influence over the drinks traffic through local polls, which Alliance members had long lobbied for, but through the discretionary powers assigned to licensing justices. This was not a resounding, final victory for the temperance movement, but the furthering of (peacetime) restrictions on the temptation of drink was regarded positively. *The Observer* captured this optimistic sentiment by describing the new Act as 'a definite stage in the struggle for a measure of constructive temperance reform as one of the main planks of national reconstruction'.[149]

But it must be remembered that the governance of alcohol did not end at the limits of the law; the British faith in the power of voluntary self-reform, abundantly evident in the Victorian period, continued to be apparent throughout the period from 1914 to 1921. In 1915, *The Times* argued that 'the English race ... very specially abhors extreme measures enacted by law' but is 'willing to follow a voluntary movement free from the flavour of compulsion'.[150] Brewers responded, perhaps unsurprisingly, that the coercive measures of prohibition or local veto were 'alien to the principles of a liberty-loving people'[151] and Mr MacQuisten MP stated that 'there was no temperance in compulsion'.[152] It is worth reiterating *The Times'* 1920 claim[153] that, although people cannot be coerced into temperance, 'wise legislation can *promote* temperance'. As in the Licensing Act 1872, the role of the law is conceived as promoting not enforcing sobriety. While the greater acceptance of legal intervention hints at the growing influence of prohibitionist ideas, this alliance of legal encouragement and moral compulsion more closely conforms to the tactical preferences of suasionist temperance. This adapted form of collectivised, national and increasingly medical temperance continued to strongly resonate with the governance of drinking in Britain during this era.

The apogee of the temperance movement

During the period from 1914 to 1921, the temperance project took two steps forward followed by only one step back. War led to a tightening of restrictions on the retail and consumption of alcohol and, while peacetime saw some restrictions relaxed, others remained. The pledge campaign did not outlast the First World War, but the model of governance of which it formed a crucial part, embodying legal restriction as well as moral compulsion, was consolidated and strengthened by the whole episode of war. Public discourse clearly shows that teetotalism, as a form of self-denial, was widely constructed as a positive moral action, which should be encouraged through restrictive legal interventions and not enforced by prohibitive laws. The discursive feature is reflective of a broadening belief, apparent even among those who did not practise teetotalism or support prohibition, that alcohol was essentially problematic. This problematisation of all forms of alcohol, in addition to a faith in restrictive legal regulation, a valuation of behavioural self-reform and the salience of the notion of 'the struggle', reveal the discursive fingerprints of moral suasionist temperance. Debates about drink from 1914 to 1921 continued therefore to be shaped by the ideas, beliefs and values of the Victorian temperance movement.

These findings contradict the idea that this period saw a complete redefinition of the drink problem. Of course, public discourse was not constant and the turn of the 20th century saw the increasingly environmental definition of social problems and the growing acceptance of higher levels of state intervention. Moreover, there is ample evidence that war did inflate the importance of the issue of national efficiency. But public discourse on alcohol was still overwhelmingly conceived within attitudinal frameworks that owed a formative debt to the moral regulation project initiated by the temperance movement. To return to the question of whether this period witnessed a moral panic about alcohol, it is necessary to give a nuanced answer. If a moral panic is defined, following Cohen, as a largely unitary, isolated historical episode then the period 1914–21 would not fit this description. If, however, a moral panic is viewed as a high point within a longer-term current of moralisation then, clearly, this period matches the definition. War gave new urgency to the struggle for sobriety, but the demands of this geopolitical context were mediated through the older discursive frameworks of the temperance movement. The remaining chapters explore what happened to efforts to morally regulate drinking after the heyday of the temperance movement.

Notes

1   Shiman, *Crusade Against Drink*; Harrison, *Drink and the Victorians*.

2   See, for example: Barr, *Drink*, pp 301-303; Nicholls, *Politics of Alcohol*.

3   Greenaway, *Drink and British Politics since 1830*, p 91.

4   Ibid, p 97.

5   Cohen, 'Folk Devils and Moral Panics', p 9.

6   Critcher, 'Widening the Focus'.

7   Hier, 'Thinking Beyond Moral Panic'.

8   Wiener, *Reconstructing the Criminal*, p 12.

9   Ibid, pp 337-338.

10   Ibid, p 12.

11   Nicholls, *Politics of Alcohol*, pp 153-155.

12   'The Government and Licensing Reform', *Manchester Guardian*, 19 January 1914.

13   'The Curse of Drink', *Daily Express*, 27 February 1914.

14   'Women's Total Abstinence Union', *Manchester Guardian*, 8 May 1914.

15   Valverde, *Diseases of the Will*.

16   'The Free Churches. National Sobriety: Pledge to Support the Government', *Manchester Guardian*, 11 March 1915.

17   Croydon, H.H., 'To the Editor of *The Times*: Temperance Policy', *The Times*, 3 May 1915.

18   Ibid.

19   Nicholls, *Politics of Alcohol*, p 154.

20   Ibid, p 155.

21   Schrad, *The Political Power of Bad Ideas*.

22   See, for example: Smith, Robinson, 'To the Editor of *The Times*', *The Times*, 16 July 1919.

23   Surgeon Sir A. Pecree-Gould, 'Food versus Beer: Demand for Prohibition During the War', *Daily Express*, 23 March 1917.

24   'The Free Churches. National Sobriety: Pledge to Support the Government', *Manchester Guardian*, 11 March 1915.

25   'The Aims of Government', *Manchester Guardian*, 5 September 1918.

26 See: Brown, 'Joseph Chamberlain'.

27 Anderton, W. Stanley, 'The Drink Problem: To the Editor of the *Manchester Guardian*', *Manchester Guardian*, 5 May 1915.

28 'The Reform of the Drink Traffic', *Manchester Guardian*, 17 January 1917.

29 'German Beer for Britons!', *Daily Express*, 13 April 1915.

30 'Partnership with the Devil!', *Daily Express*, 14 April 1915.

31 'Matters of Moment: The Barley-water Mow', *Daily Express*, 9 April 1915.

32 'Class Distinctions: Mr Tillet on Liquor Control', *Manchester Guardian*, 13 December 1915.

33 'Partnership with the Devil!', *Daily Express*, 14 April 1915.

34 'The King's Example', *The Times*, 7 April 1915.

35 Ibid.

36 Gutzke, David W., *Protecting the Pub: Brewers and Publicans against Temperance*, Suffolk: Boydell and Brewer, 1989, p 1.

37 Blocker et al, *Alcohol and Temperance in Modern History*.

38 Nicholls, *The Politics of Alcohol*, p 155.

39 Green, S.J.D., *The Passing of Protestant England*, Cambridge: Cambridge University Press, 2011, p 143.

40 Nicholls, *The Politics of Alcohol*, pp 36-45, 153-155.

41 The Central Control Board was created by the Defence of the Realm (Amendment) Act 1915 and governed the sale and supply of alcohol during wartime.

42 Ibid, pp 155-156. Also: Greenaway, *Drink and British Politics*, p 98.

43 Nicholls, *The Politics of Alcohol*, pp 36-45.

44 Ibid, pp 155-156.

45 'Treating' refers to the practice of buying a drink for another person.

46 Croydon, H.H., 'To the Editor of *The Times*: "A teetotal war"', *The Times*, 26 September 1914.

47 'Duration of War Pledge', *Daily Mirror*, 28 October 1914.

48 Chapman, E.F., 'To the Editor of *The Times*: Social Welfare in War Time', *The Times*, 14 October 1914.

49 Unusual in the sense that regulating who a person may buy a drink *for* had never been attempted before.

50 Nicholls, *The Politics of Alcohol*, pp 155-158.

51 Baynes, A. Hamilton, 'Reform by State Purchase: To the Editor of *The Times*', *The Times*, 17 November 1919.

52 Batty, Robert B., 'To the Editor of the *Manchester Guardian*: Drink and the War', *Manchester Guardian*, 12 October 1914.

53 Mitra, S.M., 'To the Editor of the *Manchester Guardian*: Prohibition in Military Clubs', *Manchester Guardian*, 6 April 1915.

54 Batty, 'Drink and the War'.

55 Wilson, George B., 'Drink and the War: To the Editor of the *Manchester Guardian*', *Manchester Guardian*, 21 November 1914.

56 Willesden, W.W., 'A Great Opportunity: To the Editor of *The Times*', *The Times*, 24 March 1915.

57 'Earlier Closing: A Demand for Drastic Steps', *Manchester Guardian*, 11 March 1915.

58 Croydon, '"A teetotal war"'.

59 'Partnership with the Devil!', *Daily Express*, 14 April 1915.

60 The cartoon can be viewed at: www.cartoons.ac.uk/browse/cartoon_item/anytext=lusitania?page=1 .

61 'Conference on the Reform of Temperance in Corn Exchange', *Preston Guardian*, 16 November 1872.

62 'Scotland and the Drink Question', *Manchester Guardian*, 20 April 1915.

63 Ibid.

64 Dransfield, F., 'Drink and the War: To the Editor of the *Manchester Guardian*', *Manchester Guardian*, 21 November 1914.

65 'Shorter Hours for Public Houses', *Manchester Guardian*, 4 November 1914.

66 Gow, Gertrude S., 'To the Editor of *The Times*', *The Times*, 7 October 1914.

67 Ibid.

68 Ibid.

69 Ibid.

70 Chapman, 'Social Welfare in War Time'.

71 Harford, Charles F., 'To the Editor of *The Times*: The Liquor Problem', *The Times*, 31 March 1915.

72 Bishop of Durham, 'A Great Opportunity: The Clergy and the Pledge', *The Times*, 19 March 1915.

73 London, A.F., 'To the Editor of *The Times*: Drink or War Loan?', *The Times*, 24 December 1915.

74 'Lord Kitchener's Pledge', *Daily Express*, 2 April 1915.

75 'German Beer for Britons', *Daily Express*, 13 April 1915.

76 'Barley Water or Beer for Britons', *Daily Express*, 9 April 1915.

77 'Restrictions for MPs', *Daily Express*, 1 March 1917.

78 Hilton, *Age of Atonement*.

79 'The King's Lead', *Manchester Guardian*, 15 April 1915.

80 See: 'Lord Kitchener's Pledge', *Daily Express*, 2 April 1914; 'The King's Example', *The Times*, 7 April 1915.

81 Milne, F., 'To the Editor of the *Manchester Guardian*: Drink and the War', *Manchester Guardian*, 21 November 1914.

82 Aggregate national alcohol consumption, as recorded by Excise figures, did fall sharply during the First World War. However, with so many young men abroad at the time, this trend does not necessarily reveal greater sobriety on the part of those who remained behind.

83 Batty, 'Drink and the War'.

84 London, 'Drink or War Loan?'.

85 'The Strength of Britain', *Daily Express*, 25 January 1917.

86 De L.G., W.H., 'To the Editor of *The Times*: France and her Wines', *The Times*, 20 November 1915.

87 'Duration of War Pledge', *Daily Mirror*, 28 October 1914.

88 Curtail, 'To the Editor of the *Manchester Guardian*: Temperance and the War', *Manchester Guardian*, 4 March 1915.

89 London, 'Drink or War Loan?'.

90 Ibid.

91 Bishop of Durham, 'A Great Opportunity'.

92 Hunt, *Governing Morals*.

93 See: Weber, *The Protestant Ethic*.

94 Archibald, W.F.A., and Ross, R.E., 'To the Editor of *The Times*: Work and Alcohol', *The Times*, 1 April 1915.

95 'Parliament and the King's Pledge', *Manchester Guardian*, 21 April 1915.

96 'Barley Water or Beer for Britons', *Daily Express*, 9 April 1915.

97 This finding is reminiscent of Durkheim's separation of morality into the obligatory and the desirable (mentioned in Chapter One). Abstinence from alcohol was not made universally obligatory through law, but it was widely held to be a morally desirable form of behaviour.

98 Wartime restrictions and the pledge campaign are also explored in: Yeomans, Henry, 'Providentalism, the Pledge and Victorian Hangovers: Investigating Moderate Alcohol Policy in Britain, 1914-1918', *Law, Crime and History*, 2011, vol 1, pp 95-108.

99 It is beyond the methodological scope of this book to examine whether or not this dual approach of legal moderation coupled with moral compulsion was a deliberate government policy. But it seems reasonable to suppose that without it, it is likely that harsh alcohol policies would have been seen as more necessary.

100 'Post-War Liquor Control', *The Times*, 4 December 1918.

101 Collier, M.D.W., 'A Medical Memorial: To the Editor of *The Times*', *The Times*, 1 August 1919.

102 Pooles, Edmund G., 'Drink in 1915: To the Editor of *The Times*', *The Times*, 13 March 1916.

103 'Manchester Licences', *Manchester Guardian*, 25 January 1918; 'Less Intemperance among Women', *The Times*, 26 December 1917.

104 Picton-Turbervill, Beatrice, 'Prohibition Propaganda: To the Editor of *The Times*, *The Times*, 23 July 1919.

105 Ibid.

106 Rouse, W.H.D., 'Beer: To the Editor of *The Times*', *The Times*, 27 May 1919.

107 Ibid.

108 'Our King's Speech', *Daily Express*, 15 February 1921.

109 These polls were created by the Temperance (Scotland) Act 1913 but their implementation was postponed due to war.

110 'State Control of Liquor', *The Times*, 8 May 1917.

111 Ibid.

112 'The Public House of the Future', *The Observer*, 5 October 1919.

113 Ibid.

114 Cantaur, Randall, Cardinal Bourne, Francois, Selbie, W.B., and Booth, W. Bramwell, 'Advantages of Present Restriction: To the Editor of *The Times*', *The Times*, 3 December 1918.

115 'Post-War Liquor Control', *The Times*, 4 December 1918.

116 'Public House as Social Centre', *The Times*, 18 November 1919.

117 'The New Phase of the Liquor Question', *Manchester Guardian*, 15 May 1921.

118 'The Licensing Bill: House of Commons', *The Times*, 23 July 1921.

119 'The Return of Freedom', *The Times*, 21 July 1921.

120 Ibid.

121 'London's Dull Evenings to Come to An End', *Daily Mirror*, 21 July 1921.

122 'Give Us Back Our Liberty', *Daily Express*, 21 July 1921.

123 'Seven Sundays a Week By Law', *Daily Express*, 23 July 1921.

124 Ibid. And: 'Parliament: The Licensing Bill', *The Times*, 23 July 1921.

125 'Parliament: The Licensing Bill', *The Times*, 23 July 1921.

126 'New Drink Hours', *The Times*, 21 July 1921.

127 'Give Us Back Our Liberty', *Daily Express*, 21 July 1921.

128 Ibid.

129 'Parliament: The Licensing Bill', *The Times*, 23 July 1921.

130 'Doom of the Bona Fide Traveller in Drink Bill', *Daily Mirror*, 23 July 1921.

131 'Wales and the Licensing Bill', *Manchester Guardian*, 27 July 1921. The position of club owners was generally that, given that their premises were excluded from the Welsh Sunday Closing Act, they did not want any relaxation of restrictions on their public-house competitors.

132 'A Storm in a Wineglass', *Manchester Guardian*, 30 September 1921.

133 '10 pm. Closing of Publichouses', *The Times*, 20 October 1921; 'Hours for Drinks in London', *The Times*, 3 November 1921.

134 'Hours for Drinks in London', *The Times*, 3 November 1921.

[135] 'Drink Hours Muddle', *Daily Express*, 22 October 1921.

[136] 'Joke in an Act', *Daily Express*, 30 August 1921.

[137] 'Pussyfoot on the Bench', *Daily Express*, 29 September 1921.

[138] 'The Truth about Alcohol and the War', *Daily Express*, 14 December 1916.

[139] Harford, Charles, 'Towards Permanent Reform: To the Editor of *The Times*', *The Times*, 24 May 1919. See also: Harford, Charles, 'An Argument to the Sober: To the Editor of *The Times*', *The Times*, 16 July 1919.

[140] 'A Year's Drink Bill', *Manchester Guardian*, 19 October 1921.

[141] Ibid.

[142] 'Parliament: The Licensing Bill', *The Times*, 23 July 1921.

[143] 'Licensing Bill (No. 2): A Very Substantial Advance', *The Observer*, 21 August 1921.

[144] 'The Liquor Poll in Scotland', *The Times*, 28 September 1920.

[145] 'Prohibition Work in Britain', *Manchester Guardian*, 17 October 1921.

[146] 'London Licensing Sessions: A Temperance Victory', *Manchester Guardian*, 18 December 1921.

[147] Ibid.

[148] Ibid.

[149] 'Licensing Bill (No. 2): A Very Substantial Advance', *The Observer*, 21 August 1921.

[150] 'The King's Example', *The Times*, 7 April 1915.

[151] 'Mitchell and Butler's Ltd: The Licensing Problem', *Daily Mirror*, 14 August 1920.

[152] 'Parliament: The Licensing Bill', *The Times*, 23 July 1921.

[153] 'The Liquor Poll in Scotland', *The Times*, 28 September 1920.

FIVE

An age of permissiveness?

Introduction

The previous chapters have explored the emergence of temperance attitudes to alcohol in England and Wales and analysed their influence over the development of a model of governing alcohol consumption based around legal restriction and moral compulsion. It has been argued that the law, particularly the Licensing Acts 1872 and 1921, as well as public attitudes, as evidenced through public discourse, were profoundly affected by the temperance movement's project to morally regulate alcohol. The First World War provoked this social movement into a furious assault on the consumption and trade in alcohol, but these events proved to be something of a 'last hurrah' for mass, organised temperance campaigning. The public profile and political clout of temperance groups declined significantly in the first half of the 20th century.[1] Concomitantly, the prominence of alcohol as a public issue waned after the First World War and, as Greenaway comments, 'drink had a low political salience in mid-20th century Britain'.[2] A brief trawl through news coverage relating to drinking from the 1920s to the 1950s corroborates this conclusion by yielding a quantity of results that is significantly smaller than for preceding or succeeding years.[3] Moreover, there were few significant reforms made to laws affecting alcohol between 1921 and 1960. Legislation, demonstrations, exhortations, lobbying and pledging were not as frequent or as forceful as they had been a generation earlier.

It is feasible that the decline in public anxiety about alcohol during this period is indicative of the rise of popular permissiveness. The inter-war and post-war years are often viewed as periods of secularisation. S.J.D. Green documents how, in the inter-war years, church attendance lessened, Sunday School enrolment dropped markedly and the divorce rate increased.[4] Valverde describes how the belief that morality consists of purification through the suppression of desire fell out of fashion as Freudian ideas recast pleasure-seeking as normal behaviour.[5] By the 1960s, proscriptive religious-based attitudes towards sex (outside of wedlock) were publicly questioned, recreational drug use expanded in popularity and drink laws began to be relaxed. The 1960s have thus been described as an 'age of permissiveness'[6] and, given these earlier related trends, the period stretching back to the 1920s might be interpreted as revealing a similar demise of active, regulatory interest in the behaviour of others. This chapter examines whether it is accurate to describe the inter-war and post-war years as an age of permissiveness. Had the wave of moral regulation unleashed by the Victorian temperance movement finally broken? Or was this merely a low point in the historical tide of moralising about drink? In order to answer these questions, public attitudes and the regulation of alcohol from the aftermath of the Licensing Act 1921 until the next period of significant legal reform in the 1960s are examined.

New frontiers, 1921–45

It is widely noted that the Second World War did not produce the frenzy of drink restrictions and orgy of alcoholic self-denial that the First World War had instigated. Levels of public opprobrium and regulatory interventions aimed at drinking did not come close to matching the intensity seen during the First World War.[7] But why? Was there something different about the Second World War? Or had something changed in the intervening years? Exponents of the 'rational model' of understanding drink regulation would see no need to spend time investigating the apparent easing of anxieties about drink in this period. Alcohol consumption fell to historically low levels during much of the early 20th century. Consumption began a gradual decline in the 1890s and, following some more drastic fluctuations around the First World War, resumed its downward trend.[8] Thom notes that, between 1900 and 1904, average annual consumption of pure alcohol per capita was 10.9 litres whereas between 1930 and 1934 it was only 4.2 litres.[9] This average consumption placed Britain fairly low in a ranking of quantity of drink consumed in European countries and, similarly, the number of alcoholics in England was believed to be comparatively low.[10] Convictions for drunkenness in the 1920s and 1930s were far below their pre-First World War levels[11] and there was some evidence that hospital admissions for common alcohol-related illnesses also declined.[12] As Glover puts it, 'The drunk ... staggered off the streets' during the inter-war years.[13]

Existing academic literature provides some supplement to this 'rational' explanation by highlighting other relevant developments in the 1920s, 1930s and 1940s. The rise of the disease model of addiction in the inter-war years[14] and projects of 'pub improvement' have been investigated. The latter phenomenon may shed some light on the rather muted response to drink in the Second World War. Encouraged by the practices of the ongoing state-run Carlisle Scheme, some breweries and other associations initiated their own projects of 'pub improvement'. By redecorating, improving sanitation, serving food and other changes, efforts were directed towards making public houses more orderly and respectable places.[15] This newfound concern for improving drinking facilities may demonstrate a growing belief that, while not necessarily a positive, public houses could be made into morally neutral environments. Between 1937 and 1938, Mass Observation's[16] research focused on public houses. Interestingly, this study was not preoccupied by drunkenness or immorality and, instead, stressed the importance of pubs as hubs of social life.[17] It also noted that pubs were not an exclusively male domain and were often used by women. So, existing literature shows that, while consumption was generally low, the role of pubs and drinking within non-problematic forms of behaviour was increasingly acknowledged in the inter-war years.

The introduction to this chapter described how drinking attracted less public discussion in the inter-war and post-war years. But, despite declining consumption and increasing acceptability, newspaper archives reveal that drink remained a topic capable of commanding a fair degree of public attention. During the Second World War, for example, the average number of articles per year on alcohol, drinking or drunkenness in *The Times* was 622; lower than during the First World War yet still around two per day.[18] Falls in consumption and harm do not explain why alcohol continued to attract such frequent commentary. The usefulness of 'rational' explanations is also complicated by the occurrence of other compelling social changes during this period. Notably, the late 19th century and first half of the 20th century was a period during which forms of governance shifted away from classical liberalism. In a sense, the pledge campaigns of the First World War exemplified this heuristic shift by showing that individuals, although generally regarded as free-thinking, were not seen as fully socially autonomous as their fate was national, collective and determined, at least in part, by the morality of other individuals of the same nationality. The pledge campaign aligned with the broader situation in which the pressures of total war had highlighted the salience of social interdependencies. The expansion of the electoral franchise in 1918 and 1927 is often depicted in this light as recognition of the great and necessary service that ordinary men and women were prepared to perform for their country.[19] The individualism and libertarianism of classical liberalism was increasingly subordinated to a governing ideology based around the vision of a more inclusive, integrated society. As well as recognising that drinking was still a public issue in this period, it is also important to situate the divergent responses to drink in the two world wars within this shifting governmental context.

This changing context was relevant to the period studied in the last chapter – 1914–21 – but 'welfare liberalism' or 'new liberalism' became more prominent in the 1920s, 1930s and 1940s.[20] The expansion of the probation service, especially in the wake of the Criminal Justice Act 1925, and the criminalisation of many psychoactive substances in the Dangerous Drugs Acts 1920 and 1923, show the state's increased willingness to intervene in behavioural issues in attempts to normalise desirable behaviour and/or proscribe the undesirable.[21] These examples reinforce Sulkunen's description of welfarism in this period as an inclusive but individualised form of government. Sulkunen presents the state as pastoral as it sought to protect and strengthen the whole flock (or population) while maintaining an interest in each individual sheep (or citizen).[22] The greater mutuality of individual and nation state meant that more extensive regulation of problematic individual behaviour as well as expanded political rights were necessary. This enhanced governmental preoccupation with the behaviour of others, however, only makes the apparent rise of permissiveness in regards to alcohol during the period more puzzling. This section pursues an explanation by exploring public attitudes to alcohol and legal developments from 1921 to 1945.

A 'new movement of thought'

In the inter-war period, downward statistical trends in alcohol consumption and alcohol-related harm were sometimes cited by contemporaries in a loosely congratulatory sense. Praise for the apparent spread of alcoholic moderation was not uncommon; an MP commented in 1923 that the British population was 'getting more temperate every day through the common sense of the people'.[23] This position is a historical novelty that contrasts sharply with the public attitude, usual for the rest of the period studied in this book, that drinking is a worsening social problem. The weakening of this default pessimistic attitude deprived the temperance movement of a key discursive weapon that they had employed in previous campaigns. Membership of temperance groups declined during this period[24] and remaining societies became divided between those supporting the local option, national prohibition or other ameliorative solutions. The Temperance (Wales) Bill would have established the local option for Wales and Monmouthshire but was rejected by Parliament in 1924.

A form of the local option was already being operated in Scotland but, partly inspired by US events, full national prohibition was gaining support. In 1922, Edwin Scrymgeour of the Scottish Prohibition Party was elected MP for Dundee. Supported by groups including the Rechabites, Scrymgeour criticised attempts to reduce or restrict drinking and, in 1923, unsuccessfully proposed a Private Member's Bill that would have enacted full prohibition.[25] The Temperance Council of the Christian Church, by contrast, supported more Sunday closure, reduced trading hours and other ameliorative restrictions on the drinks trade.[26] Lacking a common agenda and fractured by internal divisions, the moralistic voice of the temperance movement was diminished in volume.

While drink was not the incendiary issue it once had been, it was still connected to significant behavioural concerns in the inter-war period. Briggs et al report that, in the early 1930s, approximately six and a half thousand people were dying and two hundred thousand were being injured on Britain's roads every year.[27] Much of this harm was attributed to drink-driving. *The Times* featured letters discussing the difficulty of proving drunkenness in court[28] and the *Manchester Guardian* regularly covered convictions for drink-driving in the 1920s and 1930s.[29] Reflecting these issues, a revised 1935 version of the Highway Code contained an enjoinder to all road users (not merely motorists) to ensure that 'alertness or sense or caution is not affected by alcohol or fatigue'.[30] Drink-driving was actually criminalised under Section 12 of the Licensing Act 1872, which stated that the offence of being drunk and disorderly applied to anyone 'who is drunk while in charge on any highway or other public place of any carriage, horse, cattle, or steam engine'. But legal regulation of drink-driving was adapted by the Criminal Justice Act 1925, which stipulated that those convicted of being 'drunk while in charge on any highway or public place of any mechanically-propelled vehicle' shall receive a driving disqualification of at least 12 months, and the Road Traffic Act 1930, which created the new offence of driving or attempting to drive when 'under the influence of drink or a drug to such an extent as to be incapable of having proper control of the vehicle'. Alcohol-related criminality still retained a high public profile.

Other familiar historical problems were remoulded in this period too. Female drinking had long been viewed as more morally suspect than male drinking and, as in the 18th century, was sometimes seen to be having a disastrous social effect. In the 1920s and 1930s, female drinking was strongly linked to maternal neglect of children. Moss describes how, in an effort to prevent children acquiring habits of swearing, drunkenness or sexual impropriety, the Children Act 1908 had banned young people under the age of 14 from entering the bar-room of a licensed premises unaccompanied by an adult. This was, Moss asserts, intended as a protective measure but a string of prosecutions for child neglect in the 1920s and 1930s suggest that the effect of this law was to encourage parents to leave their children outside pubs while they went inside to drink.[31] Pub improvement, to some extent, offered remedies to this problem and some premises opened family rooms or children's play areas.[32] The wider significance of this episode is to illustrate the repositioning of female drinking within a modified moral discourse on drinking. In an era where a loosely eugenic concern for the future strength of the nation pervaded public life, female drinking was deemed problematic in respect to its potentially contaminating effects on the next generation.

Importantly, it was precisely this new generation who became the target for the most prominent concerns about alcohol in the inter-war period. Previously, drinking by young people had not been regarded as a separate or particularly pressing issue. But, by 1923, many people agreed with J. Scott Lidgett, whose letter to the *Manchester Guardian* asserted that 'one of the deplorable tendencies arising out of war conditions … is the increasing use of public-house bars by young people of both sexes'.[33] Lidgett went on to argue that 'the use of alcohol is unnecessary and particularly full of peril in the adolescent period' and his words were echoed in many other references to the 'dangerous age of adolescence'[34] or claims that 'the age from fourteen to eighteen was the most difficult in a boy's life or girl's life'.[35] It was essential, therefore, that adolescents were kept 'morally straight'[36] and away from the problems that alcohol could cause. Lidgett linked juvenile drinking to arrests, *The Times* connected it to disease and illegitimate births,[37] while *The Observer* described how young people were lured into pubs by wirelesses playing loud music and there learned habits of heavy drinking and gambling.[38] The assertion that drinking *will* lead to drunkenness and other immoral behaviour resonates, in some respects, with older teetotal temperance beliefs. An obvious difference, however, is the limitation of drink's corrosive effects to young people. Scrymgeour agreed that 'the public-house was a contaminating centre, and therefore objectionable to people up to eighteen years of age' but sarcastically commented that 'after that, presumably, any man or woman could enter safely'.[39] While Scrymgeour's views on adult drinking were not widely held in the 1920s, public discourse was typified by the idea that drinking during adolescence, at least, was very much a 'slippery slope'.

Whether connected to the behavioural effects of war conditions or not, public discourse in the 1920s exhibited ample evidence that youth or adolescence, as a period of the human lifespan, had been identified and problematised. Furthermore, the emergence of youth drinking as a public issue, as with female drinking in this period, can be connected to a temporal anxiety about national future. At a conference of the National Union of Teachers, the need to diminish the 'considerable evil' of adolescent alcohol consumption was discussed in reference to the 'future of the country'.[40] The National Union of Teachers was among the first bodies to endorse a ban on the sale of alcohol to young people under the age of 18 and it gathered 116,000 signatures on a petition to this effect.[41] *The Observer* saluted such developments as welcome evidence of a 'new movement of thought', which focused on anything that may serve to 'imperil or to retard a full development of national efficiency'.[42] While teachers, the Temperance Council of Christian Churches and the national press seemed very much behind such a measure, there were a number of critics. As well as the prohibitionists already mentioned, trade representatives queried how publicans were supposed to differentiate between 17- and 18-year-olds and some MPs argued that their own adolescent drinking had done them no harm.[43] The 'new movement of thought' and the demand for a ban on 18s purchasing alcohol, however, proved resilient to these detractions. *The Times* put it thus:

> In the practically unanimous opinion of those in a position to judge of the evil effects on boys and girls of the existing facilities, the change is urgently called for. During the trying years of adolescence it is unquestionable that the habit of drinking, particularly in the environment of a public-house, has a poisonous effect on the young of both sexes. It exercises an exciting and unhealthy stimulus on the animal side of their nature, and, by weakening their powers of self-control, is the direct cause of much misery.[44]

In 1923, a Private Member's Bill aiming to reform age restrictions relating to alcohol was introduced to Parliament. Chapter Three described how the first national age-related qualification on the sale of alcohol was created by the Licensing Act 1872. The Intoxicating Liquors (Sales to Children) Act 1886 then prohibited sales for on-premises consumption of any other alcoholic drink to persons below the age of 13. This age limit was raised to 14 by the Intoxicating Liquors (Sales to Children) Act 1901.[45] The 1923 Bill, which was introduced to Parliament by temperance-advocating Nancy Astor, proposed to raise the age limit so that young people under the age of 18 were forbidden from purchasing alcoholic drinks for consumption on licensed premises. In the House of Commons, Astor spoke of being the mother to five sons and the difficulties in keeping them 'morally straight' during the 'the very difficult time' between the ages of 14 and 20. Invoking temporal anxieties about national future, she claimed that '[t]here could be nothing worse for a country than to have drunkenness amongst the adolescents' and further argued that her Bill would benefit the 'health and morality of the community'.[46] Legal restrictions, Astor insisted, would help young people develop self-control in the long run.[47] Astor's Bill passed successfully through Parliament, with strong cross-party support, and it became an offence for licensed premises to 'knowingly' sell any form of alcoholic drink to someone under the age of 18 for consumption on the premises.[48]

While not seeking to restrict off-licence sales, the Intoxicating Liquors (Sales to Persons Under Eighteen) Act 1923 marked something of a new departure in regulatory terms. It was observed at the time that the fact that this legislation was proposed by Britain's first female MP, and followed swiftly on the heels of the enfranchisement of women over the age of 30, may not have been a coincidence.[49] It may, perhaps, have embodied a maternalistic concern for child protection. But it also signified the state's willingness to use legal interventions in an effort to safeguard the future efficiency, health and morality of the nation. *The Observer* explained that 'in a healthy state which preserves through all vicissitudes and external changes a will to advance, the orbit of governmental action and responsibility is not a fixed orbit'.[50] In these historical circumstances, where the influence of drink was believed to be corrupting and contaminating future generations during the vulnerable period of adolescence, it was seen as widely acceptable for the state to provide a legal substitute for the self-control that young people under the age of 18 may not yet have learnt to exercise.[51] Briggs et al explain how high numbers of fatalities on the roads led to the police focusing on drink-driving and other offences in a more preventative way.[52] Similarly, the child-oriented and protective dimensions of the Intoxicating Liquors (Sales to Persons Under Eighteen) Act 1923 demonstrate that it was also an attempt to govern the future, in this case, through the regulation of alcohol consumption by young people.

It is important that there was evidence, at the time, that young people needed little assistance in remaining 'morally straight'. In Parliament, Home Secretary William Bridgeman explained that 64,000 people were convicted of drunkenness in 1921 and only 2,174 were under the age of 21. He provided similar figures for 1919 and 1920 showing that young people under the age of 21 constituted a small proportion of drunkenness convictions, before adding that the number of young people under the age of 18 who were convicted was even lower.[53] However, as has been consistently asserted in this book, 'rational' trends in consumption and measurable incidences of harm are never sufficient explanation for variations in public attitudes and the regulation of alcohol. The most important legal reform to alcohol regulation in the inter-war years – the Intoxicating Liquors Act 1923 – cannot be explained fully without reference to changing public attitudes. Specifically, the old teetotal temperance idea of a 'slippery slope' was repositioned within a less overtly moralistic context in which temporal anxieties about the national future were rife. The result was preventative, child-focused regulation. This discussion of female drinking, drink-driving and particularly youth drinking in the inter-war years shows that, despite the decline of organised temperance, the use of alcohol by certain social groups continued to be moralised and subjected to new forms of legal censure.

Official responses to the Second World War

In early 1939, the COETS considered expanding its mission to incorporate the amelioration of gambling problems[54] and the Salvation Army claimed that this problem had surpassed drink and was now 'the greatest social evil'.[55] Undoubtedly, anxiety about alcohol was somewhat blunted during the inter-war years, although the last section has shown that certain forms of alcohol consumption were subject to new or adapted forms of censure. So, did war conditions prompt regulatory change, as they had from 1914 to 1918?

The legal regulation of alcohol was not dramatically intensified during the Second World War. Glover records that imports of wine were restricted and the production of spirits was limited.[56] Treating, however, was not banned, beer was not subjected to rationing[57] and opening times were not uniformly reduced. There was some local implementation of earlier closing times; the Manchester licensing justices, for example, created a new closing time of 9.30pm.[58] But, Home Secretary Herbert Morrison discouraged this practice and suggested that, wherever possible, local authorities should allow pubs to trade until 11pm.[59] In a number of areas, concerted efforts were also made to provide social alternatives to the pub. There were calls for milk bars to be set up in Carlisle (which was still under state management)[60] and a night cafe was established in Manchester.[61] But, elsewhere the responses were markedly different. Troubled by the apparent spread of illicit 'bottle parties' and 'near-beer parlours', the Metropolitan Police permitted a bar in London's West End to sell alcoholic drinks until 2am.[62] Later in the war, similar experiments with late opening were reported in Wales.[63] This demonstrates that, unlike in the First World War, there was little national consensus that reduced opening hours were necessary or desirable.

The government's primary reform of alcohol regulation during the Second World War involved significant tax hikes. Several war Budgets introduced successive increases in the excise duties imposed on the trade in beer, wine and spirits. Glover calculates that, by the end of the war, beer was taxed at a rate six times higher than it had been before the war and around 22 times higher than it had been in 1914.[64] As a result of a voluntary agreement between brewers and the government, the strength of many types of beer also fell in 1941 and 1942. The scarcity of certain resources did contribute to temporary beer shortages during some periods of the war but, overall, both pub-going and beer production seem to have increased during the war.[65] As well as profiting from the tax revenues that these trends yielded, the government also used pubs as bases from which fundraising campaigns, such as 'War Weapons Week', could operate.[66] While attributing a certain importance to pubs as part of the war effort, the government did attempt to tighten the enforcement of age restrictions. In 1943, the Home Office insisted that all on-licensed premises displayed a sign reading reminding patrons that young people under the age of 18 were forbidden from buying or consuming alcohol in their establishments.[67] Such a measure, which involved no reform other than a compulsory reminder of what the Licensing Act 1923 allowed and disallowed, was decidedly lenient.

Some of the differences in how alcohol was dealt with in the two world wars could be linked to the attitudes of some key players. Britain in the Second World War, for example, was presided over by the 'prodigious imbiber'[68] Winston Churchill rather than temperance-sympathising David Lloyd George. But this attitudinal shift was too profound to be reduced to individual personalities. Herbert Morrison resisted a series of calls for tighter drink restrictions and stated that 'the Government attach importance to giving the public reasonable opportunity for recreation consistent with the war effort'.[69] On other occasions, Morrison reminded his opponents that 'social conditions were better than in the last war'[70] and insisted that new restrictions would only be created when the obtainable information supports such a move.[71] Lord Woolton, Minister of Food, voiced similar sentiments. He argued, in May 1940, that 'if we are to keep up anything approaching the normal life of the country beer should continue to be in supply'.[72] Furthermore, when pressured to provide the public with greater information on existing licensing laws and the 'evil results of excess', Ministry of Information spokesperson, Ernest Thurtle, argued that it was not the government's duty to 'lecture the public on the good or evil effects of alcohol'.[73] The dominant governmental attitude during this period was that drinking was not necessarily a problematic behaviour and so, in the absence of compelling contrary information, general restrictions need not be altered.

More startlingly, as well as maintaining that drinking was not inherently wrong, Churchill's government also tried to use alcohol to aid the war effort. It is widely acknowledged that ensuring a good supply of beer to the troops became a serious governmental concern during the Second World War.[74] Glover reports that, in 1944, Churchill personally ordered that British troops under fire in Italy were supplied with at least four pints of beer each per week.[75] It was even suggested, in 1942, that drinkers may be capable of serving their country better than abstainers. Minister for Air, Archibold Sinclair, controversially proposed that not being able to mix with drinkers made abstainers less suitable for service in the Women's Auxiliary Air Force.[76] Drinking among civilians was seen to be important also and many people saw it as the government's responsibility to ensure that available beer was equitably distributed to troops and civilians alike. In January 1944, the *Daily Mirror* attacked the government's record on drink:

> If the Government really thinks that drinking beer is morally wrong and physically harmful, let it say so and forbid its consumption altogether.... If, on the other hand, the Government regards beer as the national beverage, and as a necessity to thousands of workers in wartime, let it see that sufficient is brewed to meet the needs of the population.[77]

The newspaper demanded that the government increase production, rectify distribution problems and fix prices to ensure the availability of alcoholic drinks. More than simply being regarded in a morally neutral way, beer, perhaps alcohol in general, was viewed by some as a necessary or beneficial substance.

The *Daily Mirror*, however, was angered by the government's failure to resolve problems with the supply of drink. Suspecting that this failure may have been driven by more than simple incapability, the newspaper stated that 'those in authority regard the men and women who consume alcoholic beverages as belonging to the more sinful section of mankind'.[78] This position presents a challenge to the idea that, in dominant governmental attitudes, drinking was becoming more acceptable during this period. But, if the *Daily Mirror*'s assertion held any validity, it held less than the same statement would have commanded during the First World War. Indeed, in August 1944, the Parliamentary Secretary to the Ministry of Food, W. Mabane, was forced to defend the government's actions and insist that 'everything possible was being done to distribute beer equitably among consumers'.[79] While the extent of change may not have been enough for the *Daily Mirror*, the mere fact that Mabane was forced to make such a statement is indicative of a significant historical shift. The prospect of a government spokesperson claiming that every effort was being made to increase the availability of beer would have been almost unthinkable during the fevered atmosphere of the First World War. Building on the growing acceptability of drinking during the inter-war years, permissiveness had developed to the point where beer-drinking and pub-going were seen by the government as, in some circumstances, worth protecting.

Public attitudes and 'moral failures'

How did this new governmental posture relate to wider public attitudes? In some respects, the outbreak of war in 1939 instigated the same attitudinal reaction to alcohol that had occurred in 1914. Again, temperance groups quickly drew attention to the amount of resources that were used to manufacture alcoholic drinks. Representatives of the UK Alliance, the Band of Hope and the Friends Temperance Union all argued that valuable cereal crops were being wasted in the manufacture of beer and, in the interests of the war effort, should be used as food instead.[80] Many commentators also echoed debates from the previous war by decrying the alleged increase in drunkenness. For example, the Dean of Manchester, Garfield Williams, wrote to the *Manchester Guardian* in November 1939 to report an apparent increase in drunkenness during daytime.[81] The Dean's version of events was disputed by some, not least because arrests for drunkenness fell in Manchester during this period.[82] Nevertheless, a belief that valuable foodstuffs were being wasted in the production of the beer that was intoxicating a large number of people was marked. This situation led Isaac Foot MP to assert that 'in every sphere of national service strong drink was fighting on the side of the enemy'[83] and to designate it as a 'fifth column' in Britain.[84] This description of drink as an enemy within, using a term coined during the Spanish Civil War, shows that some people still regarded drinking as a potentially suicidal national habit. While the vocabulary no longer concerned U-boats and 'greatest foes', some commentaries on the Second World War exhibited the same concern for self-destruction that Lloyd George had expressed during the First World War.

But the particular circumstances of the Second World War raised some new drink-related issues. Drink-driving became acutely problematic during the blackouts, which began in September 1939. *The Times* reported on a number of prosecutions for driving under the influence of alcohol during the blackouts. One case involved a one-eyed drink-driver who, missing full headlights as well as his left eye, had trusted his passenger's word when told to turn left only to mount the curb as there was actually no turning there.[85] Drinking during the blitz raised further problems too. The *Manchester Guardian* described a publican's fear of an early morning air raid, which would cause drinkers to empty from pubs into the street. 'Every lad,' he explained, 'would try to show off before his girl by being awkward with the police, and every girl would feel compelled to draw attention to herself by fainting or going into hysterics.'[86] Whether or not the publican's fears materialised is not recorded, but the arrival of drunk people in crowded air raid shelters was a persistent cause for complaint.[87] While drink-driving and public drunkenness were not new concerns, the Blitz and the blackouts gave them new urgency.

In other respects, discourse on alcohol during the Second World War diverged more drastically from discourse on alcohol during the First World War. While the First World War prompted concerted efforts to maximise the military, industrial and moral capabilities of the nation, anxieties from 1939 to 1945 were instigated more by a perception that war was lessening moral restraints on behaviour. In 1943, the Archbishop of Canterbury stated that 'it is inevitable that the circumstances of the war should multiply temptations and diminish the safeguards'.[88] The Bishop of London identified the effects of this corrosive process as a decline in honesty, a 'landslide in sexual morality' and an increase in drunkenness.[89] Interestingly, this 'moral failure'[90] was associated almost exclusively with young people. There was a palpable sense, at the time, that the alleviation of traditional social controls, coupled with an abundance of well-paid jobs, led to immorality among young people specifically. Magistrate Edgar Gates cited the causes of the youth problem as a 'general increase of freedom enjoyed by young people, the weakening of parental control by the conditions of this war, the money which young people easily earn'.[91] It seems odd in retrospect to speak of young people enjoying 'greater freedom' at a time when the threat to their lives and wellbeing was so prominent.

However, at the time, the enhanced opportunities for leisure that more money and less parental supervision bought were, in the wake of the emergence of youth drinking as a major public issue in the 1920s, a substantial source of wartime public anxiety.

Within this general anxiety about youth drinking, young women were once again singled out for specific attention. Female pub-going appeared to increase during the war and, in some areas, the number of women prosecuted for drunkenness also rose.[92] The Bishop of Sodor argued that increased drinking 'exposed the victims to peril' and the Archbishop of Canterbury stated that even a 'comparatively small amount of drinking' led to the 'removal of self-control and habitual inhibitions'.[93] Speaking to a temperance society, Magistrate Freda Corbet explained that even a little drink means that:

> ... a certain exhilaration comes over you and a 'don't careness'.... Then all the sweet modesty and coyness of womanhood is overcome by any if you are not very careful.... It is not when a girl is drunk that the danger time comes ... but when she had just a few drinks and can't control her emotions.... Then men are very difficult to resist.[94]

The men in question were often identified as American servicemen who would 'treat' girls to drinks. The end result of increased female drinking was believed by many to be 'sexual immorality'[95] on a large scale. Unwanted pregnancies and an increase in venereal disease were often cited as evidence of this.[96] Young women were, in other cases, accused of failing in their maternal responsibilities. The *Manchester Guardian* ran a story on 'Birmingham Beer Babies' who were, until the age of five, apparently given alcoholic drinks by their mothers to help them sleep.[97] Drinking was not so much attacked as immoral in itself, but targeted more for its apparent causation of other social problems such as sexual promiscuity and bad parenting.

The regulatory agendas that arose from these anxieties about the effects of drinking on young men and women are another contrast between the two wars. Of course, there were some similarities: temperance activist Henry Carter called for a ban on the 'wasteful and perilous custom of treating' and a re-formation of the Liquor Control Board.[98] Other commentators called for 'restraint and self-discipline'[99] or even, in the words of the Baptist Union Assembly, 'a more militant faith in Christ' and 'a reaffirmation of the Puritan note in our witness and life'.[100] But such calls were no longer typified by a utopian faith in the ability of temperance crusades to purify the nation and were usually characterised by a more ameliorative desire for greater education of the population. Despite the evangelical zeal of its rhetoric, the Baptist Union Assembly's only concrete demands were for a ban on treating and for more education and training about drink, sex and Christian ideals. Some news reports criticised the adequacy of education about alcohol currently on offer in schools[101] and others attacked BBC coverage for not correctly depicting the dangers of drink.[102] Similarly, in its report on 'Birmingham Beer Babies', the *Manchester Guardian* posited that the solution lay in little more than better education of young people about alcohol.[103] The near-utopian faith in prohibition or nationalisation had receded as calls for more or better education became ubiquitous.

The decline of utopian aspirations can be situated in relation to the broader waning of the spirit of evangelicalism. While documenting more general currents of secularisation, Green refers specifically to the 'strange death of puritan England' during this period.[104] The doctrine of atonement, in which refuge from the depravity of humankind could only be found by people individually striving to make themselves and those around them more virtuous, had, it is contended, faded.[105] Green cites contemporary comments from A.L. Rowse and George Orwell who both celebrated the feeling that, with the apparent lessening of puritanical strictures, they were no longer compelled to constantly think about how to do good.[106] This situation correlates with the demise of utopian temperance campaigns, which, in earlier periods, had sought to totally remake the nation's relationship with alcohol. Additionally, diagnoses of current social problems may well have been affected by these changes. During the First World War, there was a widespread perception, consistent with evangelical sentiments, that the nation was mired in depravity and, weighed down with the immorality of drink, was sinking fast. By the time of the Second World War, however, the problem was not what we were but, rather, what we might become. As the Archbishop of Canterbury and others articulated, the perceived danger came from disruptions to the equilibrium instigated by 'moral failures'. The greater freedoms and relaxed social controls that war was seen to engender were positioned as a threat. The decline of evangelicalism was connected to the advent of an attitudinal situation in which depravity was envisaged as a potential more than an actuality.

Isaac Foot still feared that the inherent, embodied depravity of a 'fifth column', an enemy within, would be our national undoing.[107] But more typical public attitudes were coloured by a fear of external threats, including the military threat from Germany and the sexual threat from American servicemen, as well as temporal threats related to what might happen if present social and moral conditions were changed by war. This altered moral landscape was partly shaped by the weakening of the evangelical spirit that had been a significant factor in instigating the campaigns against drink in the 19th century and in constructing the fear of a drunken 'enemy within' during the First World War.

Reflections, 1921–45

Alcohol and drinking declined as major public issues during the period from 1921 to 1945.[108] Consumption was decreasing for much of this period but this section has demonstrated that deeper attitudinal shifts also affected the way in which alcohol was understood and regulated. In the First World War it was believed to be necessary to morally fortify the nation with teetotalism in order to lift it from depravity and save it from defeat. Valverde identifies that this ethos of purification declined shortly after[109] and this section has shown that, by the Second World War, drinking was increasingly acceptable as a more ethically confident nation aspired mainly to avoid damaging disruptions to the existing order. These subtle changes were connected to secularisation but, more particularly, to the demise of evangelicalism. The belief that radical, purifying surgery was needed to address Britain's internal, inherent national depravities had faded. This factor helps explain why, despite the rise of more welfarist forms of government, new interventions in drinking behaviour were scarce in the 1920s and 1930s and resisted by the government during the Second World War. Where new regulations were implemented or demanded, they tended to be preventative and targeted in nature. Drinking by young people, particularly girls, and drink-driving became new frontiers that had to be strengthened with preventative regulation during this period. Particularly in regards to restrictions on young people drinking, the logic was temporal and characterised by a desire to prevent individual 'moral failures' that might produce a collective national slide down a slippery moral slope. The ethos of purification had thus been replaced by an ethos of protection. Changes in attitudes and legislative reticence do not, therefore, indicate that drinking was wholly acceptable. Rather, they show that the primary fear of external and temporal threats supported the use of future-oriented regulations that targeted those whose drinking was deemed to be the most potentially problematic.

The growth of targeted regulation

After a downward trend that originated in the 1890s, alcohol consumption began to increase after the Second World War. There was also evidence that the commonality of drunkenness and alcohol-related mortality were rising.[110] The immediate post-war years, however, saw little departure from the model of regulating drink that had arisen in the inter-war years and been consolidated from 1939 to 1945. The 'drink problem' failed to attract the level of public attention to which it had been subjected in the 19th century. The Licensing Act 1953 gave local authorities greater control over the structural conditions of licensed premises, but this was hardly a sweeping reform. More radical proposals were unsuccessful or limited in scope. Clement Attlee's Labour government legislated for the extension of state management to all licensed premises operating in the 'new towns', but the incoming Conservative government scrapped these provisions in 1951 before they came into effect.[111] The Licensing Act 1949 enabled premises providing music and dancing to apply for licences to trade alcohol until 3am, but this only applied within London.[112] Apparent increases in consumption and harm did not, therefore, immediately result in either public alarm or the development of more restrictive alcohol policies.

It was not until the 1960s that significant changes, via a series of Acts of Parliament, would be made to the way in which alcohol was regulated. By this point, it was clear that the governmental context was shifting. A reconceptualisation of the role of government in personal behaviour might have been occurring during the Second World War. Ernest Thurtle's rejection of the idea that the government should lecture people about right and wrong implied the salience of a more libertarian governmental position towards personal behaviour.[113] This position became more prominent in 1957 when the Wolfenden Report famously recommended the decriminalisation of (male) homosexuality.[114] Judge and conservative moralist Lord Devlin was critical of these proposals, arguing that society is based on shared values and so the criminalisation of behaviour that contravenes these shared values is justified by the need to prevent social disintegration.[115] The liberal jurist H.L.A. Hart defended the Wolfenden Report from Devlin's critique. For Hart, the state could only legitimately intervene in an individual's behaviour if their actions harmed others; hence, the law should not seek to regulate consensual sexual relationships. Hart drew extensively on J.S. Mill's 'harm principle' and Devlin's anti-thesis closely paralleled the thoughts of Fitzjames Stephens, with whom Mill famously argued in the 19th century.[116] Interestingly, Devlin's position also corresponded to the portrait of society painted by sociologist Emile Durkheim, in which shared norms and values were functionally necessary in order to prevent the slide into the normless, pathological condition of anomie.[117] It was this societal vision that gave rise to the concept of 'moral regulation' as a set of beliefs or attitudes that provide social cohesion.

The Hart–Devlin debate thus resonated with earlier debates about the role of the state in issues of personal morality. Devlin effectively aligned himself with Victorian temperance activists, particularly prohibitionists, who believed that a system of moral regulation could not sustainably exist without legal enforcement. For Devlin and the prohibitionists, maintaining social cohesion was thus an adequate justification for the enforcement of morality. For Hart and Mill, as with Lord Stanley (discussed in Chapter Three), individual liberties were sacrosanct and could only be negated when 'the harm principle' allowed. In respect of homosexuality, Hart won the argument and gay sex was decriminalised in the Sexual Offences Act 1967. The state thus appeared to be retreating from issues of personal behaviour, abandoning the fortifications of moral regulation and falling back to less aggressive, more utilitarian lines. So, how did this governmental context affect drinking? Was there a similar retraction of alcohol regulation from the 1960s onwards?

This section explores the attitudinal and legal dimensions of the 'drink problem' that existed in the 1960s. It particularly focuses on the major reforms of drink laws in this period enacted by the Licensing Act 1961, the Licensing Act 1964 and the Road Safety Act 1967. It is worth noting that, although a fairly prominent issue within public discourse on drinking in the 1960s, alcoholism is only dealt with briefly here. This is because it cannot be analysed fully without being situated in regard to medicine and public health more broadly. Hence, alcoholism will be explored more fully in Chapter Seven.

Baby boomers as 'baby boozers'

The 1960s are commonly seen as having witnessed something of a national rebirth. Gone was the austerity of the post-war years; in popular parlance, the decade has become synonymous with social change. From The Beatles to the Campaign for Nuclear Disarmament, popular culture and political protest were transformed as the post-war 'baby boomers' came of age. Questioning established values became commonplace and sexual behaviour in addition to the use of recreational drugs became the subject of particularly inflammatory debates. These social upheavals provided the backdrop for further developments within public debates about alcohol. This was partly manifested in the growth of anxiety about alcoholism. In 1961, alarming estimates placed the number of British alcoholics at 200,000 to 350,000.[118] Worse, in 1965, the World Health Organization approximated that there were 300,000 to 500,000 alcoholics in the country, of whom 100,000 were said to be 'socially crippled'.[119] This new concern was tied to the increasing recognition that alcoholism, as a pattern of behaviour that is habitual or compulsive, is distinct from drunkenness. This shift, which related to the rise of the 'disease model' of addiction, will be explored further in Chapter Seven. At this stage it is pertinent to note that greater prosperity and the challenging of traditional moral boundaries coincided with acute public fears about excessive, unrestrained forms of alcohol consumption.

More than alcoholism, however, public fears about unfettered conduct were attached to the behaviour of young people. Youth culture, as something recognisably separate from dominant culture in terms of attitudes and social practices, began to emerge in Britain after the Second World War. It was in the context of this emerging category of youth that Stan Cohen examined the construction of young Mods and Rockers as 'folk devils'[120] and this moralistic atmosphere, unsurprisingly, had implications for drinking. In the early 1960s, an increase in drunkenness convictions among the general population was widely reported by the press[121] and soon it became common to refer specifically to 'the disturbing increase in drunkenness among young people'.[122] In 1964, the *Daily Express* described Mods and Rockers clashing in Clacton under the headline '97 Leather Jacket Arrests'. The arrests were for fighting and vandalism as well as drunkenness, but a local café owner quoted by the newspaper was clear that '[i]t was a case of too much beer and boredom in most cases'.[123] When, in 1964, the House of Commons debated the issues of juvenile delinquency and hooliganism, Labour MP George Thomas linked the worrying trend to drinking.[124] Similarly, the Attorney-General Sir John Hobson claimed that 'most juvenile crime was committed under the influence of alcohol' and 'the more opportunity youths had of indulging in drink the more likely they were to get into trouble'.[125] *The Guardian* featured a column by former teacher Arthur Bart, who argued that disorder and vandalism committed by young people often 'goes with drink' as well as motorbikes and scooters.[126] The moral panic Cohen identified was closely connected to young people's consumption of alcohol and its apparently detrimental effect on public order.[127]

But anxieties about youth were not limited by reference to drink. The use of other intoxicants became increasingly controversial as the decade wore on; in 1964, the House of Commons discussed the problem of 'purple hearts', a type of amphetamine that was leading many young people into a 'thoroughly murky world of black-marketeering and intimidation'.[128] Sexual behaviour also received attention and there were serious political debates about how strip clubs were, according to Cyril Black MP, 'defaming national life'.[129] Eric Fletcher MP supported Black's proposal that such premises be outlawed by arguing that they were 'conducive, not only to depravity, but to crime'.[130] Extra-marital relations, gambling[131] and beat music were all implicated as part of a broader social decline responsible for corrupting a generation of young people.[132] *The Times* reported on a new craze of 'coffee clubs', which did not serve alcohol but allowed young people to socialise late into the night, thus providing a new 'opportunity for young people to get into trouble'. Customers were described as 'teenage tramps' of the sort usually seen 'thumbing lifts at the entrances to motorways, equipped with sleeping bag, long hair, and a guitar'.[133] A vivid picture of problematic youth emerged from public discourse but, importantly, it was youth rendered problematic by more than just drink.

As had been the case during the Second World War, this generational moral decline was commonly explained as the result of rising affluence. In 1957, Prime Minister Harold Macmillan boldly told the country that they had 'never had it so good'[134] yet, for many, this new prosperity was not cause for celebration. Conservative MP J.H. Cordle claimed that 'the wind of change of our affluent society has brought in its wake a gust of lust which this country has never seen before'.[135] Cordle was concerned primarily with indecent imagery and, writing in the *Daily Mirror*, Dr H. Mackenzie-Wintle made the related point that high wages for under-educated teenagers contributed to an increase in illegitimate births.[136] John Hobson linked economic prosperity to increased alcohol consumption and youth crime, describing how 'there is far greater temptation in an affluent society';[137] in the House of Commons, James Griffiths highlighted the amount of money young people have;[138] and, in the House of Lords, the Bishop of Carlisle claimed there has 'never been a generation of young people who had so much money and time to spend on pleasurable pursuits'.[139] There is an element of class snobbery to this debate, which the teacher writing in *The Guardian*, quoted earlier, elucidated aptly. Affluence among the young was not a problem two or three decades previously when its behavioural effects were limited to 'the confident, light-hearted destructiveness' of the 'young gentlemen of Oxford and Cambridge'.[140] Wider prosperity, however, was the root of many social problems.

Increasing affluence was accompanied by a burgeoning consumer culture. The increased prominence of advertising within public discourse is marked if newspapers from from the 1910s and 1920s are compared with those from the early 1960s. From a contemporary standpoint, alcohol adverts contained some eye-opening messages. A 1965 advert for Cossack vodka claimed that the product will improve your life: 'Don't you feel marvellous? People who drink Cossack Vodka do.' Perhaps attempting to appeal to those who wished to conceal their drinking from others, the advert then claimed that the product contained 'No sweetening. No flavouring. No smell. So? You feel fine! Good morning!'[141] The connection of alcohol to self-betterment was not unusual at the time and other adverts featured in newspapers asserted that 'a WHITBREAD makes the most of you'[142] or that 'the world is a happier place' when one mixes Rose's Lime Juice with gin or vodka.[143] But did the majority of people possess the moral fortitude to resist these powerful messages? A 1963 advert for Gordon's gin asserted that the product was 'cooler, fresher – tempting!'[144] and the level of concern about young people's drinking indicated the belief that most people did not possess sufficient self-control to resist such advertisements. Prosperity increased the leisure opportunities of ordinary people in the 1960s but also exposed them to temptations that, it was widely believed, they struggled to resist.

The drinking habits of young people as well as, to some degree, the issue of alcoholism, were prominent in the 1960s. To many, the 'baby boomers' were becoming a generation of violent, disorderly 'baby boozers'. Existing concerns about young people's drinking, which have been documented from the 1920s onwards, were intensified as discernible youth cultures began to emerge. Moreover, in this period of economic growth, the ascetic suspicion of personal prosperity visible during the Second World War was massively heightened. Affluence was commonly constructed as antithetical to a good moral order, inferring that, as in ascetic alcohol discourse from the Victorian period (discussed in Chapter Two), thrift and self-control were the dominant behavioural ideals. But, unlike the Victorian period when drink was viewed as a singular, gigantic social threat, drugs, sex and gambling took their place alongside alcohol as targets of overlapping forms of moral regulation. The 1960s, in this sense, intensified rather than altered attitudes towards alcohol that had been prevalent since the 1920s. Drinking, particularly by young people, was problematic in the 1960s but it was only one ingredient in a more general porridge of social anxieties about personal behaviour.

'Don't ask a man to drink and drive'

Within this mesh of interconnected moral concerns, it is possible to discern another distinctly drink-related issue. As with youth, concerns about drink-driving that emerged in the inter-war years proliferated after the Second World War. Car ownership more than doubled between 1950 and 1960 and continued to increase steeply throughout the 1960s.[145] The potential for drink-driving was thus magnified. In 1961, public debate of drink-driving concentrated largely on the provisions of the new Licensing Bill. Contained within provisions allowing restaurants to apply for liquor licences was the genesis of some acute concerns. The problem was where these restaurants were geographically situated and, as Cyril Black explained, the Bill suggested 'it would not be possible for a Bench to refuse licences on the M1 and similar motorways'.[146] These worries were taken seriously and, in Parliament, an amendment was tabled that would have prevented licences being granted to premises located on motorways. Conservatives also tabled an amendment to prohibit the sale of alcoholic drinks on coaches due to the fear that this practice may result in the coach driver drinking. Although these proposals were withdrawn or defeated, the salience of the issue of drink-driving within public debates about licensing reform is notable.

In addition to these issues of safe licensing, there was the supplementary problem of how to enforce the statutory criminalisation of driving while drunk. The prohibition of drink-driving was reinforced by the Road Traffic Acts 1960 and 1962 but the problem for enforcement agencies was that the law did not specify exactly what constituted drunkenness. Usually, it was necessary for the arresting officer to contact a police doctor who would then be tasked with ascertaining whether or not the person was fit to drive. As many arrests for this offence were late at night, it was often difficult for the police to contact a doctor. Moreover, even if a doctor was contacted, the time lapse was sometimes such that the driver was able to sober up. Often, therefore, cases were either dropped or the prosecution hinged on the word of the driver against the word of the arresting officer. In these circumstances, the defence would usually opt for a Crown Court trial as juries were notoriously reluctant to convict drink-drivers. Writing in *The Guardian*, the chief constable of Manchester Police, John McKay, reported that in drink-driving cases 'only 3.4% of those tried in the magistrates' courts were acquitted; but 61.6% of those committed to the Crown Court received no conviction'.[147] The problem, he complained, was that there were 'shades of drunkenness' and, in the absence of concrete evidence, drivers would usually receive the benefit of the doubt.

This 'benefit of the doubt' was symptomatic of a broadly permissive attitude towards drink-driving. A light-hearted tone was apparent in much public discourse on the subject. In 1964, the *Daily Mirror* reported on the case of 'giggling Wong', an unusually ticklish Chinese man who could not be examined by the police doctor following his arrest for drink-driving due to him breaking down in fits of laughter upon being touched.[148] Likewise the concern of Cyril Black and others for the effects of alcohol on drivers was far from universal. A letter in *The Times*, for example, claimed that impatience among drivers was the cause of more accidents than drink[149] and Lord Arran, quoted in the *Daily Express*, argued that the poor condition of roads was a more significant factor.[150] Research findings discussed in *The Guardian* compounded the problem; it was reported that most road offenders were unremorseful and their actions were tolerated by others.[151] Minister of Transport, Ernest Marples, complained about such attitudes, lambasting people who failed to regard driving while unfit as a 'social crime'.[152] Marples did, however, believe that attitudes were changing and the appearance in November 1964 of an early Christmas anti-drink-driving campaign supports this. The advert pictured a person trapped beneath a wrecked car under the headline 'Don't ask a man to drink and drive'.[153] As well as revealing a gendered view of drink-driving, this campaign evidences the increasing public or official condemnation of this behaviour. Generally permissive attitudes towards drink-driving were increasingly being challenged in the early 1960s.

Legal reforms in the 1960s

In many ways, the Licensing Acts 1961 and 1964 were liberalising measures. The Licensing Act 1961 permitted restaurants and hotels to apply for licences. This was contentious at the time; it was feared that cafes may become dens of drunken iniquity and hives of the 'barbaric' practice of 'vertical drinking'.[154] In order to quell related fears that proprietors may apply for restaurant licences in order to run a drink-led business, Minister of State for Home Affairs Dennis Vosper had to affirm that only the serving of 'substantial refreshment' would warrant a liquor licence.[155] As well as creating restaurant licences, the Licensing Act 1961 also extended permitted hours during which pubs could trade from eight to nine per day, meaning that premises across the country could open until 11pm if the licensing justices acquiesced (otherwise closing time would likely be 10.30pm). Moreover, the special certificates that London clubs providing music and dancing could apply for under the Licensing Act 1949, were implemented nationwide. This meant that such premises could open until as late as 2am in most of the country and 3am in the West End of London. Off-licences were governed by different rules and, although also subject to modification by magistrates, the Licensing Act 1964 allowed such premises to sell alcohol from 8.30am until 11pm. These liberalising measures could be equated with the retraction of state influence and enhancement of individuals' moral autonomy in respect to drinking.

The state's retreat from the domain of moral absolutes was perhaps most apparent in the reform of Welsh Sunday closing laws. Implemented in Wales in 1881 and Monmouthshire in 1921, the Licensing Act 1961 replaced Sunday closing with a system of local polls. For many people, this was a system of moral absolutes; the Act was 'pernicious' and 'insidious'[156] and it was calculated to 'undermine the Lord's Day in Wales which is one of the bulwarks of our moral and spiritual heritage'.[157] But, as Labour MP John Parker made clear, some people regarded the issue as a matter of 'religious principle ... an attempt by sabbatarians to force their religious observances on other people'.[158] Labour's Rhys Thomas was more colourful in his argument, arguing that the provision was a necessary part of 'liberalizing and emancipating the people of Wales from the cold and chilly grasp of the modern fringe of puritanism'.[159] Given the context of the Wolfenden Report, this secularised rejection of morally driven state interferences was fashionable. Although it is worth highlighting that, for many contemporaries, this issue was a matter of Church against Chapel, a permissive Anglicanism comfortable with secular government facing a puritanical Non-conformism.[160] The more individualist, harm-driven liberalism of Hart and Wolfenden was conflicting with the evangelically inspired mission of moral improvement that had occupied paternalistic liberals, such as Joseph Chamberlain, in earlier decades. It was in light of this ideological face-off that *The Guardian* described the new Sunday closing polls as confronting 'the Liberal ideal with the Non-conformist conscience'.[161] The issue was not so much the state's retreat from moral issues but its adoption of one form of liberal morality above another.

That said, this new governance was not always permissive and interventions were pursued in some spheres. The increased prominence of alcoholism as a public issue accompanied the establishment of advice centres run by the National Council on Alcoholism in various cities and the Department of Health's efforts to create specialist treatment units.[162] More notably, licensing reforms tightened controls on youth drinking. The Intoxicating Liquors Act 1923 had fixed the age for purchasing alcohol to be consumed on licensed premises at 18. The Licensing Bill 1961 initially proposed no changes to these age limits, meaning that anyone above the age of five would be legally able to purchase alcohol for consumption off licensed premises. However, Cyril Black MP proposed banning young people under the age of 18 from any purchase of alcohol and, despite highlighting that in only nine of 1,120 cases of young persons convicted of drunkenness was there any evidence of off-licence involvement, government minister Dennis Vosper was forced to re-examine the issue.[163] The result was that Section 21 of the Licensing Act 1961 brought off-licence sales into line with on-licence sales, setting the legal age for purchasing alcohol at 18.[164] This measure was then consolidated in the Licensing Act 1964 and 18 has ever since remained the age at which alcohol can be legally purchased in England and Wales.

Both the 1961 and 1964 Acts were formulated in the midst of heightened unease about youth behaviour. As already established, earlier age prohibitions on alcohol purchase and consumption were advanced mainly within a welfarist ethos of protection. The Intoxicating Liquors Act 1923, as discussed earlier, was justified largely in preventative terms. But by the 1960s these preventative or protectionist rationales were becoming mixed with a more punitive preoccupation. Many people agreed with Labour MP Charles Royle's diagnosis when he stated that 'a great deal of crime we are experiencing today among young people is due to drink'.[165] Just as the moral panic that Cohen identified began to construct youths as 'folk devils', references to 'young thugs' and 'hooligans' became more frequent in public discourse.[166] The tightening of age restrictions must be viewed within a context in which young people were no longer vulnerable minors requiring protection or tested adolescents who needed assistance in remaining 'morally straight'. Increasingly, young people were viewed as a violent, disorderly menace from which the general population must be shielded.

The tightening of restrictions was also apparent in regards to drink-driving. From 1964 onwards there was considerable debate about replacing the system whereby a police doctor was needed to verify a person's drunkenness with a fixed scientific measure. Dr A.J. Howard called for a statutory limit to be created 'above which a *prima facie* case is established of critical impairment'.[167] Howard suggested that the limit should be 100 milligrammes (mg) of alcohol per 100 millilitres (ml) of blood although, as he acknowledged, this would mean that the legal limit would be different in every person (depending on their tolerance of alcohol). Support for a statutory limit was soon provided by the Lord Chancellor and John McKay, who welcomed the prospect of a tougher stance as '[o]ne should not expect a sinner to become a saint just because he was driving a car'.[168] In 1965, the British Medical Association recommended a blood–alcohol concentration of no more than 80mg per 100ml of blood. Although seen as too tolerant by *The Observer*, which claimed that the average person would be able to legally consume five pints of beer or 12 whiskies prior to driving,[169] the British Medical Association's recommendation was enacted in the Road Safety Act 1967. This Act also made it an offence for any person to refuse to give a blood or urine specimen without 'reasonable excuse' and, in the same year, the government approved police use of breathalysers to indicate the level of intoxication. The ability of the police to enforce drink-drive laws was increased by the replacement of discretionary powers with evidential limits and testing equipment.

The increasing problematisation of youth drinking and drink-driving within public discourse was soon reflected in the prohibition of alcohol sales to young people under the age of 18 and the replacement of the vague, discretionary system of policing with tougher frameworks for dealing with drink-driving (as a strict liability offence). The growth of interventions targeting alcoholics in this period demonstrates a similar trend. Despite its chronological proximity to the Wolfenden Report, the state's retraction from the issue of personal alcohol consumption was only partial. Restaurant licences, longer drinking hours and Sunday polls in Wales indicate a degree of relaxation. But the intensification of legal regulation, especially around young people and driving, suggests that alcohol law was becoming more targeted rather than simply more relaxed.

Paint it Black

What was the role of temperance groups within this reformulated drink question? When the Licensing Bill 1961 was presented to the House of Commons it contained a clause that would enable liqueur chocolates to be sold by unlicensed persons. For Cyril Black this was a dangerous proposal and, to prove his point, he revealed to the House a 15-inch chocolate egg, which, he claimed, 'could contain enough liquor to intoxicate a considerable number of members'![170] This intervention was both amusing and unsuccessful, given that the relaxation of rules on selling liqueur chocolates was upheld. But Black was not a maverick eccentric and held a number of important positions, including chairman of the Moral Law Defence Association, member of the all-party Parliamentary Temperance Group and president of the Band of Hope temperance society. Black sided with Lord Devlin in the debate about homosexuality, arguing that these 'unnatural practices, if persisted in, spell death to the souls of those who indulge in them' as well as destruction for the great nations who weaken their 'moral responsibility' by legalising them.[171] It has already been mentioned how Black raised objections to licensing reforms relating to the licensing of strip clubs, the licensing of roadside premises and off-licence sales to young people under the age of 18. All of these points provoked considerable debate, and controversy surrounding the latter point resulted in the amendment of the Bill. Does this mean that Black's moralising agenda was prominent in the 1960s?

Organised temperance underwent a mild revival during the 1950s and 1960s. The Parliamentary Temperance Group was formed in 1955 and, by 1960, had almost one hundred members.[172] Press coverage of alcohol issues during this period also reveals a surprising amount of references to temperance organisations of varying sorts. A meeting of the National Temperance Federation to discuss the Licensing Act 1961 was reported in *The Guardian* in January of that year[173] and, the following month, the same newspaper printed a personal advert from the Federation which read: 'The Licensing Bill provides for: MORE drinking and LESS control, MORE road accidents and LESS safety, MORE crime and LESS sobriety, FIGHT IT! By writing to your MP.'[174]

Both the Sons of Temperance Friendly Society, originally formed in New York in 1842, and the UK Alliance, formed in Manchester in 1853, were vocal in their criticism of the 1961 Act. The Sons of Temperance argued that relaxing drinking laws was tantamount to encouraging greater consumption and, by 1963, secretary of the UK Alliance H. Cecil Heath was claiming that the Licensing Act 1961 had been a disaster that had brought the nation 'almost to the point of "free trade in drink"'.[175] In this instance, Heath was commenting on research that found that arrests for drunkenness were twice the pre-war average. The research, which was discussed in *The Times* and *The Guardian*,[176] had been commissioned by the UK Alliance, Heath's own organisation. By a variety of means, temperance groups managed to occupy a discursive position where their views would be continued to be heard and afforded a fair degree of credence.

Importantly, it was not only within the rhetoric of temperance groups that drinking habits were located within a narrative of moral crisis. In April 1964, the House of Commons discussed recent incidents of youth disorder in Clacton. The Home Secretary, Henry Brooke, noted that youth crime appeared to be rising in other countries too and that part of the blame must lie with the parents. But Brooke was also keen to point out that the 'moral outlook' of society was negatively affecting young people. He claimed that 'we all are playing our part in creating that moral atmosphere of society' and so increasing youth crime must be recognised 'as a condemnation of us all'.[177] H. Cecil Heath echoed these comments when, addressing the topic of drink-driving, he stated that the nation's problems 'were predominantly moral and spiritual rather than economic in character'.[178] Both of these diagnoses indicated a deficiency in moral values that had allowed dysfunctional social conditions to develop and both encompassed a desire for a new moralisation of drinking (or at least a moralisation of drivers and young people). This moralisation could be realised through an educational drive that brought voluntary behavioural change or, as Heath specified, it could be necessary to make certain behaviours crimes 'subject to severe penalties'.[179] These comments show that the confidence in the moral solidity of the nation that had been apparent in the Second World War had given way to a potent sense of moral crisis. While their proposals differed somewhat, Heath, Brooke and others were all effectively promoting new forms of moral regulation to quell these problematic behaviours.

These new attempts at moral regulation were not teetotal in nature, but were, to a fair extent, temperance-inspired. At a meeting of the National Temperance Federation, Reverend Dr Vine claimed that 'the campaign was not to promote the witness for total abstinence, magnificent as that was. It was to resist social evils'.[180] In this reformed discourse, the social evils targeted were the behaviour of youth and driving while under the influence. For temperance adherents, alcohol was still an evil substance; but in the 1960s they narrowed their focus to certain groups or activities. In doing so, they helped prepare the ground, attitudinally speaking, for greater government interventions; cries from the *Daily Mirror* and the Royal Automobile Club – that new drink-driving laws were 'an unjustifiable interference' with the rights of sober drivers – seemed to fall on deaf governmental ears.[181] Similarly, although rejected in 1961, Section 167 of the Licensing Act 1964 implemented Cyril Black's demand that young people under the age of 16 be banned from purchasing chocolate liqueurs. The tightening of laws relating to young people drinking and drink-driving also support the idea that temperance groups exerted a degree of influence over legal reforms as well as public attitudes. This enhanced problematisation of drink-driving and youth drinking corroborates the idea that by the end of the 1960s a form of moral regulation project had emerged that was framed within a new sense of moral crisis but entwined with the older Victorian temperance movement. In the 1960s, therefore, public attitudes towards alcohol were painted a distinct shade of Cyril Black.

Reflections on the 1960s

So, in the 1960s there was no retreat from the regulation of drinking comparable to the decriminalisation of gay sex. The libertarian Wolfenden Report coincided with a period in which more liberty was granted to some drinkers at the same time as being removed from others. These changes positioned some forms of drinking as generally acceptable while more extensively problematising other forms. Sulkunen calls this regulatory formation 'consequentalism' and defines it as 'the idea that policy should be justified not by judgments of the intrinsic value of different lifestyles, but on the basis of what follows from them'.[182] Sulkunen's narrative is therefore consistent with Lord Wolfenden's preferences: regulation is concentrated on behaviours that engender harmful outcomes rather than, in this analysis, alcohol consumption per se. But, while Sulkunen's argument may apply to drink-driving, it is less suitable as a characterisation of the regulation of drinking by young people in this period. While youth drinking might be perceived to be connected to more harmful outcomes than adult drinking, the production of evidence contradicting this belief was insufficient to prevent the imposition of new restrictions in both 1923 and 1961. The evidence was not entirely conclusive but, even if it had been, it would have stood at odds with a prevailing discursive climate in which continued temperance activities and a general perception of a moral crisis conspired to produce an increasingly moralistic and punitive attitude towards the behaviour of young people. The problem of youth drinking was, therefore, defined by the age of its participants more than its potentially harmful consequences.

This new, mid-20th-century version of the British drink problem was influenced by older discursive and regulatory forms. Continuing temperance attitudes, campaigns and the salience of an ascetic suspicion of wealth both indicate that changes in the 1960s were, to some degree, rooted in the Victorian period. The project to morally regulate alcohol had also altered significantly since the 19th century as a result of historical processes begun in the inter-war years. Specifically, efforts to reform all drinking or all drinkers had been replaced by targeted forms of legal and moral censure.

Conclusion

Much of the period discussed in this chapter is peculiar. Alcohol consumption was not a major public issue for much of the mid–20th century as the demise of evangelicalism, and the emergence of more inclusive forms of welfarist government provided a context in which some explicitly moral concerns could be regarded as not urgent or pressing. Notably, drinking as a social practice was viewed as widely legitimate to the extent that, during the Second World War, government spokespersons defended and promoted the role of beer in morale-boosting recreation. But this peculiar period represents only a point of low tide within efforts to morally regulate alcohol consumption. The organised temperance movement and the evangelical culture that had supported it declined in the first half of the 20th century but new forms of moralisation were slowly being fashioned from the pieces of the old. Youth drinking and drink-driving emerged in the inter-war period and became, amid wider perceptions of moral crisis, significant public issues in the 1960s. This was, therefore, more a period of gestation than it was of demise. While drinking was subject to diminished moral denunciation and limited legal innovation for much of the 1920s, 1930s and 1940s, it was clear by the 1960s that a reshaped project to morally regulate drinking had been born.

This governmental strategy was a revision rather than a rewrite. Temperance groups were still active in their condemnations of forms of drinking. They were sometimes (and sometimes not) joined in this task by government ministers, but increasingly also by those concerned about road safety, young people and the moral health of the nation generally. Many older legal restrictions remained in place, although important adaptations were made. The Road Safety Act 1967 increased restrictions on drinking and driving and the Licensing Act 1961, in particular, increased many people's liberty to drink while simultaneously increasing restrictions on drinking by young people. So, the model of governing drinking through legal restrictions and moral compulsion, established in 1872, remained in place, albeit in a form that had been moderately altered. The advent of a dominant permissiveness might be seen to challenge this governmental model. But, while liberalising measures may indicate a permissive attitude towards drinking in the mid–20th century, enhanced restrictions on particular groups and specific activities show that this was limited to certain people in certain situations. If this was an age of permissiveness, the permissiveness apparent was only partial or exclusive. The next two chapters also show that any sense of permissiveness would be historically short-lived. In

1961, the Bishop of Carlisle said that 'the battle of temperance was always only won temporarily and the dangers inherent in intoxicating drinks remained'.[183] Tensions may have calmed during much of the mid-20th century, but the 1960s had already seen the first engagements in what was to become a much bigger conflict about the role of alcohol in British society.

Notes

[1] See: Thom, *Dealing with Drink*; Greenaway, *Drink and British Politics*, pp 130-132.

[2] See: Greenaway, *Drink and British Politics*, p 150.

[3] A search for the keywords 'alcohol AND crime' between 1922 and 1960 on *The Times* archive yielded 107 hits. The same keyword search for the previous 38 years, 1884 to 1921, produced 417 hits. For the succeeding period from 1961 to 1985 (when the archive ends), 272 hits were recorded. A similar pattern was revealed by other keyword searches; 'drink AND disorder' produced 585 hits for 1884–1921 but only 148 hits for 1922–60.

[4] Green, *Passing of Protestant England*, pp 135-179. Although there is some contention regarding the continuing importance of religion (especially in certain geographical areas), it is hard to refute the suggestion that religious organisations were exerting *less* influence over people's lives than in the preceding century. See Green's *Passing of Protestant England* for further discussion.

[5] Valverde, *Diseases of the Will*, pp 96-97.

[6] 'Conversation with Derek Rutherford', *Addiction*, 2012, vol 107 (5), p 893.

[7] Brown, Pete, *Man Walks Into Pub*, London: Pan Macmillan, 2004; Jennings, *The Local*, pp 209-210.

[8] Plant and Plant, *Binge Britain*, p 29; Jennings, *The Local*.

[9] Thom, *Dealing with Drink*, pp 20-21.

[10] Ibid.

[11] Jennings, *The Local*, p 194; Briggs, John, Harrison, Christopher, McInnes, Angus, and Vincent, David, *Crime and Punishment in England*, London: UCL Press, 1996, pp 195-196.

[12] 'Parliament', *The Times*, 20 July 1923.

[13] Glover, Brian, *Brewing for Victory: Brewers, Beers and Pubs in the Second World War*, Cambridge: Lutterworth Press, 1995, p 4.

[14] Thom, *Dealing with Drink*; Valverde, *Diseases of the Will*; Baggott, *Alcohol, Politics and Social Policy*.

[15] See: Nicholls, *Politics of Drink*; Jennings, *The Local*; Greenaway, *Drink and British Politics*.

[16] The Mass Observation was a social research project, begun in the 1930s, which examined everyday life. It included a number of observations of pubs and drinking behaviour.

[17] Nicholls, *Politics of Drink*; Barr, *Drink*.

[18] A search for 'alcohol OR drink OR drunk' in *The Times* yielded 4,195 hits for 1914–18 and a slightly higher 4,355 for 1939–45. The mean number of articles per year thus equalled 839 hits per year for 1914–18 and 622 per year for 1939–45. The same search in *The Guardian/Observer* archive yielded 5,235 hits for 1914–18 and a slightly lower 4,790 hits for 1939–45. The mean number of articles per year for *The Guardian/Observer* was 1,047 for 1914–18 and 684 for 1939–45.

[19] For example, Millicent Garret Fawcett said that 'Women, and especially, I believe, young women, have been eager aspirants to enrol themselves for every kind of national service. Show them what wants doing from a national point of view, and they are ready to do it in this country' ('Votes for Women at 21', *The Times*, 4 October 1927).

[20] See: Hobhouse, Leonard, *Liberalism and Other Writings*, Cambridge: Cambridge University Press, 1994.

[21] See: Seddon, Toby, *A History of Drugs: Drugs and Freedom in the Liberal Age*, Abingdon: Routledge: 2010; Garland, David, *Punishment and Welfare*, Aldershot: Gower, 1985.

[22] Sulkunen, *The Saturated Society*, pp 141-158.

[23] 'Parliament: Lady Astor's Bill', *The Times*, 14 July 1923; 'Sexual Morality and Drinking', *The Times*, 22 October 1943.

[24] Greenaway, *Drink and British Politics*, p 130.

[25] 'Prohibition at the Next Election?', *Manchester Guardian*, 12 March 1923; 'Private Members' Bills', *Manchester Guardian*, 17 February 1923.

[26] Green, *Protestant England*, p 172.

[27] Briggs et al, *Crime and Punishment*, p 207.

[28] For example: Wilson, Gordon, 'Definition of Drunkenness: To the Editor of *The Times*', *The Times*, 18 October 1927; Eccles, W. McAdam, 'Alcohol Before Driving: To the Editor of *The Times*', *The Times*, 16 January 1934.

[29] For example: 'Driving after Taking Drinks', *Manchester Guardian*, 18 July 1928; 'Motorists Fined', *Manchester Guardian*, 13 September 1932.

[30] 'Important Changes in the Highway Code', *The Times*, 11 May 1935.

[31] Moss, Stella, '"A Grave Question": The Children Act and Public House Regulation, c.1908-1939', *Crimes and Misdemeanours*, 2009, vol 3 (2), pp 98-117.

[32] Ibid.

[33] Lidgett, J. Scott, 'Education and Licensing Reform: To the Editor of the *Manchester Guardian*', *Manchester Guardian*, 27 February 1923.

[34] 'House of Commons: Big Majority for Lady Astor', *Manchester Guardian*, 10 March 1923.

[35] 'Parliament: A Liquor Bill', *The Times*, 10 March 1923.

[36] Ibid.

[37] 'A Sensible Reform', *The Times*, 7 March 1923.

[38] 'The Drinking Age', *The Observer*, 25 February 1923.

[39] 'Prohibition at the Next Election?', *Manchester Guardian*, 12 March 1923.

[40] 'The Dual System in Education', *Manchester Guardian*, 5 April 1923.

[41] Percy, Eustace, Fisher, Herbert A.L., Snowden, Philip, and Wintringham, M., 'Lady Astor's Bill: To the Editor of the *Manchester Guardian*', *Manchester Guardian*, 6 March 1923.

[42] 'The Protection of Youth', *The Observer*, 24 June 1923.

[43] 'Parliament: A Liquor Bill', *The Times*, 10 March 1923.

[44] 'A Sensible Reform', *The Times*, 7 March 1923.

[45] Under this statute, young people under the age of 14 could still buy alcoholic beverages but only in quantities less than one pint, which were contained in a sealed bottle and not consumed on the premises.

[46] 'House of Commons: Big Majority for Lady Astor', *Manchester Guardian*, 10 March 1923.

[47] 'Drink Ban for Youth', *The Times*, 10 March 1923.

[48] An exception was made that enabled over-16-year-olds to purchase and consume non-spirits alcoholic drinks if they were to be drunk with a meal to be eaten away from the bar room.

[49] 'For Women and Children', *Manchester Guardian*, 21 August 1923.

[50] 'The Protection of Youth', *The Observer*, 24 June 1923.

[51] 'As a stand-by for the young in the difficult period of adolescence it will prove a valuable addition to the law of the land' ('A Serious Measure', *The Times*, 14 July 1923).

[52] Briggs et al, *Crime and Punishment*, p 208.

[53] 'House of Commons: Big Majority for Lady Astor's Bill', *Manchester Guardian*, 10 March 1923.

[54] 'Drink and Gambling', *Manchester Guardian*, 7 February 1939.

[55] 'Drink Now a Lesser Evil', *Manchester Guardian*, 12 January 1939.

[56] Glover, *Brewing for Victory*.

[57] Green, *Protestant England*, pp 143-143.

[58] 'Drink Hours Curfew', *Manchester Guardian*, 21 September 1940.

[59] 'Questions to Ministers', *Manchester Guardian*, 17 October 1941.

[60] Chance, Robert, 'Youth and Drink: To the Editor of *The Times*', *The Times*, 8 December 1943.

[61] 'Drinking Among Young People', *Manchester Guardian*, 27 November 1943.

[62] '2 A.M. Drinks Test in Piccadilly', *Daily Express*, 22 April 1940.

[63] 'More Drinking by the Young', *Manchester Guardian*, 22 November 1944.

[64] Glover, *Brewing for Victory*, pp 33-39.

[65] Ibid, pp 85–110.

[66] Ibid, p 30.

[67] 'Drinking Among Young People', *Manchester Guardian*, 31 March 1944.

[68] Green, *Protestant England*, p 143.

[69] 'Questions to Ministers', *Manchester Guardian*, 17 October 1941.

[70] 'Drink in War-Time', *Manchester Guardian*, 9 January 1942.

[71] 'Drinking by the Young', *Manchester Guardian*, 17 November 1943.

[72] Glover, *Brewing for Victory*, p 14.

[73] 'Information and Alcohol', *Manchester Guardian*, 9 November 1943.

[74] Glover, *Brewing for Victory*; Jennings, *The Local*; Green, *Protestant England*.

[75] Glover, *Brewing for Victory*, p 123.

[76] 'W.A.A.F. Police Appointments', *Manchester Guardian*, 26 March 1942.

[77] 'Drink Racket', *Daily Mirror*, 25 January 1944.

[78] Ibid.

[79] 'Shortage of Beer Explained', *The Times*, 16 August 1944.

[80] 'Churches and the Drinks Trade', *Manchester Guardian*, 8 April 1940; 'Drink Problem in Wartime', *Manchester Guardian*, 15 October 1941; 'Foodstuffs and Drink Trade', *Manchester Guardian*, 2 March 1942.

[81] 'Drunkenness in Manchester: To the Editor of the *Manchester Guardian*', *Manchester Guardian*, 6 November 1939.

[82] Heap, A. Leathey, 'War-Time Drinking: To the Editor of the *Manchester Guardian*', *Manchester Guardian*, 23 November 1939.

[83] 'Drinking by the Young', *Manchester Guardian*, 13 June 1944.

[84] Ibid; 'Drinking by Young People', *Manchester Guardian*, 11 November 1940.

[85] 'A Motorist with One Eye Fined £10', *The Times*, 25 September 1939.

[86] Artifex, 'The Drink Nuisance', *Manchester Guardian*, 10 September 1940.

[87] Ibid; Carter, Henry, 'Drink in War-Time', *Manchester Guardian*, 17 September 1941.

[88] 'Dangers of Increased Drinking', *Manchester Guardian*, 14 October 1943.

[89] 'Sexual Morality and Drinking', *The Times*, 22 October 1943.

[90] Reed, C., 'Juvenile Drinking: To the Editor of the *Manchester Guardian*', *Manchester Guardian*, 28 October 1943.

[91] 'Drinking Among Young People', *Manchester Guardian*, 9 October 1943.

[92] 'Drinking by Women in Salford', *Manchester Guardian*, 3 January 1944.

[93] 'Dangers of Increased Drinking', *Manchester Guardian*, 14 October 1943.

[94] 'Women J.P on "That Exhilaration"', *Daily Mirror*, 18 March 1944.

[95] 'Dangers of Increased Drinking', *Manchester Guardian*, 14 October 1943.

[96] See: 'Sexual Morality and Drinking', *The Times*, 22 October 1943.

[97] 'Juvenile Drinking Evil in Birmingham', *Manchester Guardian*, 22 December 1943.

[98] Carter, Henry, 'Drink and Youth: To the Editor of *The Times*', *The Times*, 23 December 1943.

[99] Chance, Robert, 'Youth and Drink: To the Editor of the *Manchester Guardian*', *Manchester Guardian*, 15 January 1944.

[100] 'Youth and Drink Habit', *Manchester Guardian*, 6 May 1944.

[101] Austin, D., 'Education and Drink: To the Editor of the *Manchester Guardian*', *Manchester Guardian*, 14 May 1943; Brown, Joseph, 'Education and Drink: To the Editor of the *Manchester Guardian*', *Manchester Guardian*, 17 May 1943.

[102] Listener, 'The B.B.C. and Alcohol: To the Editor of the *Manchester Guardian*', *Manchester Guardian*, 4 February 1944.

[103] 'Juvenile Drinking Evil in Birmingham', *Manchester Guardian*, 22 December 1943.

[104] Green, *Protestant England*, pp 135.

[105] Hilton actually sees the demise of evangelicalism as beginning in the 1870s. See: Hilton, *Age of Atonement*, pp 5-6.

[106] Green, *Protestant England*, p 140.

[107] 'Drinking by the Young', *Manchester Guardian*, 13 June 1944.

[108] Indeed, much of the source material in this section comes from the traditionally temperance-sympathising *Manchester Guardian* as the other newspapers studied (especially the more populist *Daily Express* and *Daily Mirror*) devoted distinctly less column inches to the topic of alcohol.

[109] Valverde, *Diseases of the Will*, p 97.

[110] Baggott, *Alcohol, Politics and Social Policy*, p 32.

[111] Nicholls, *The Politics of Alcohol*, pp 191-192.

[112] Barr, *Drink*, pp 158-159.

[113] 'Information and Alcohol', *Manchester Guardian*, 9 November 1943.

[114] Committee on Homosexual Offences and Prostitution, *Report of the Committee on Homosexual Offences and Prostitution* (Wolfenden Report), London: Her Majesty's Stationery Office, 1957.

[115] Harcourt, 'The Collapse of the Harm Principle'.

[116] Ibid.

[117] Durkheim, *Suicide*.

[118] Ibid; Petschek, Willa, 'Alateens', *The Observer*, 17 September 1961.

[119] McGlashan, Colin, 'Helping the Man in the Shabby Suit', *The Observer*, 17 October 1965.

[120] Cohen, *Folk Devils and Moral Panics*.

[121] 'Drunkenness Convictions Twice Pre-War Average', *The Guardian*, 9 May 1963; 'Drink Convictions up by 10,000', *The Times*, 9 May 1963.

[122] 'Buying from Off-Licences', *The Guardian*, 19 April 1961.

[123] '97 Leather Jacket Arrests', *Daily Express*, 30 March 1964.

[124] 'Parliament – Monday April 27', *The Times*, 28 April 1964.

[125] 'Affluence a Cause of Crime Wave', *The Times*, 5 February 1964.

[126] Bart, Arthur, 'A Handful of Headlines', *The Guardian*, 8 August 1964.

[127] It is worth noting that, in some sense, this moral panic was self-justifying. Speaking in Parliament, Mr Gurden MP claimed the fact that newspapers 'seemed almost daily to contain reports of incidents of hooliganism' as justification for governmental consideration of the issue. See: 'Parliament – Monday April 27', *The Times*, 28 April 1964.

[128] 'Harder for the Unauthorised to get "Pep Pills"', *The Guardian*, 1 May 1964.

[129] 'Ban on Striptease Rejected', *The Guardian*, 21 April 1961.

[130] Ibid.

[131] 'Churches Told: Hit Harder at Betting', *Daily Express*, 4 December 1961.

[132] 'Music Blamed for Rowdyism', *The Guardian*, 10 February 1965.

[133] 'Teenage Trouble in "Coffee Clubs"', *The Times*, 12 May 1965.

[134] 'More Production the Only Answer', *The Times*, 22 July 1957.

[135] 'No Ban on Club Drinks for Under 18s', *The Guardian*, 20 June 1961.

[136] 'Tempting for Teenagers', *Daily Mirror*, 3 October 1961.

[137] '"Affluence a Cause of Crime Wave"', *The Times*, 5 February 1964.

[138] 'Motorways Likely to be Dry', *The Guardian*, 6 June 1961.

[139] 'Parliament: Peers' Ideas on Licensing Reform', *The Times*, 5 July 1961.

[140] Bart, Arthur, 'A Handful of Headlines', *The Guardian*, 8 August 1964.

[141] 'Cossack's Vodka', *Daily Mirror*, 19 March 1965.

[142] 'Whitbread', *Daily Mirror*, 26 August 1961.

[143] 'Rose's Lime Juice', *Daily Express*, 27 March 1961.

[144] 'Gordon's Gin', *Daily Express*, 11 June 1963.

[145] The number of licensed vehicles on British roads more than doubled between 1950 and 1960 and continued a steep upward trajectory throughout the 1960s and 1970s. See: Department for Transport, 'Licensed Vehicles by Tax Class, Great Britain, Annually, 1909 to 2011', 2012, http://webarchive.nationalarchives.gov.uk/20120913084528/http://www.dft.gov. uk/statistics/tables/veh0103/

[146] 'Five MPs Attack Licensing Bill', *The Guardian*, 25 January 1961.

[147] 'Alcohol Limit as the Test', *The Guardian*, 22 December 1964.

[148] 'The Testing of Giggling Wong', *Daily Mirror*, 24 March 1964.

[149] Sparrow, Gerald, 'Four out of Five', *The Times*, 28 December 1965.

[150] 'Peers Blame Roads', *Daily Express*, 6 February 1964.

[151] 'Drivers Against the Law', *The Guardian*, 12 May 1963.

[152] 'Last Chance for Drunken Drivers', *The Guardian*, 5 June 1964.

[153] 'Don't Ask a Man to Drink and Drive', *Daily Express*, 26 November 1964.

[154] 'Standing to Drink: Bar Barbarism?', *The Guardian*, 15 February 1961.

[155] 'Licensing Bill Amendments', *The Guardian*, 9 February 1961.

[156] 'Sunday Opening Opposed', *The Guardian*, 23 January 1961.

[157] 'Archbishop Resigns Vice-Presidency', *The Times*, 13 February 1961.

[158] 'Sunday Option in Wales', *The Guardian*, 17 March 1961.

[159] 'Right to Drink in Welsh Clubs', *The Times*, 22 March 1961.

[160] 'Dangers of Disunity', *The Guardian*, 24 February 1961.

[161] 'War of Attrition over Sunday "Pint"', *The Guardian*, 5 October 1961.

[162] New Centre for Advice to Alcoholics', *The Guardian*, 23 July 1963; Perfect, P., 'Letters to the Editor: Help for Alcoholics', *The Guardian*, 20 April 1965; 'Special Units for Treating Alcoholics', *The Guardian*, 10 December 1963.

[163] 'Motorways Likely to be "Dry"', *The Guardian*, 6 June 1961.

[164] It should be noted that, under the provisions of Section 169 of the Licensing Act 1964, it is permissible for a person aged 16 or 17 to be served 'beer, porter, cider or perry for consumption at a meal in a part of the premises usually set apart for the service of meals which is not a bar'.

[165] 'No Ban on Club Drinks for Under 18s', *The Guardian*, 20 June 1961.

[166] '16 Sent to Prison for Part in Riot', *The Guardian*, 22 August 1961.

[167] '"Intimidation" Reports Upset Conference', *The Times*, 15 June 1964.

[168] 'Alcohol Limit as the Test', *The Guardian*, 22 December 1964.

[169] 'Comments', *The Observer*, 21 February 1965.

[170] 'Liquor Not to be Sold on Coaches', *The Times*, 26 April 1961.

[171] *Hansard*, House of Commons Debate, 26 November 1958, vol 596, cols 365–508.

[172] Baggott, *Alcohol, Politics and Social Policy*, p 9; Blocker, Jack S., Fahey, David M., and Tyrell, Ian R., *Alcohol and Temperance in Modern History: An International Encyclopaedia*, Santa Barbara, CA: ABC-CLIO, 2003, p 303.

[173] 'Five MPs Attack Licensing Bill', *The Guardian*, 25 January 1961.

[174] 'Personal', *The Guardian*, 6 February 1961.

[175] 'Drink Convictions up by 10,000', *The Times*, 9 May 1963.

[176] Ibid; 'Drunkenness Conviction Twice Pre-War Average', *The Guardian*, 9 May 1963.

[177] 'Neither Riot nor Warfare', *The Guardian*, 28 April 1964.

[178] 'Drink Slogan Ideal – For Others', *The Guardian*, 29 March 1963.

[179] Ibid.

[180] 'Five MPs Attack Licensing Bill', *The Guardian*, 25 January 1961.

[181] 'Snap Breath Tests of Drivers Attacked', *The Times*, 22 December 1965; 'Snap Drink Test Shock for Drivers', *Daily Mirror*, 22 December 1965.

[182] Sulkunen, *The Saturated Society*, p 143.

[183] 'Parliament: Peers' Ideas on Licensing Reform', *The Times*, 5 July 1961.

SIX

Alcohol, crime and disorder

Introduction

Chapter Five traced the lessening in efforts to morally regulate the use of alcohol in the inter-war period before identifying the beginnings of a recovery in the 1960s. What was the fate of this renewed moral regulation project? Simple keyword searches reveal that the number of references to 'alcohol or 'drink/drinking/drinker(s)' in *The Times* and *The Guardian* rose more or less exponentially between 1965 and 2000.[1] There was also a flurry of legislative activity affecting alcohol around the turn of the millennium. Both of these points imply that public anxiety about drinking was returning to almost Victorian heights. So, how can historical developments in the ways in which we understand and regulate alcohol consumption help make sense of increased public unease about drinking in the late 20th and early 21st centuries? Interestingly, this period of intensifying concerns coincided with further declines in organised temperance. Although revived somewhat in the 1960s, temperance groups had ceased to have any visible presence within public discourse on alcohol by the turn of the 21st century. So, had any remnants of temperance sentiments survived within public attitudes to alcohol? And what of the regulatory processes identified within the 1960s? Did liberalisation, targeted restrictions and resurgent moralising discourse continue to shape the way alcohol was governed?

This chapter examines public attitudes and alcohol regulation in the late 20th and early 21st centuries with a specific focus on the topics of crime and disorder. Particular attention is paid to the late 1980s and 2003–10 as these were periods in which major reforms to alcohol laws were made. Events since 2010 will be considered in Chapter Seven, which, with a concentration on the issues of addiction and public health, covers a roughly parallel timeframe.

The narrative of deregulation

Crime and disorder became major public issues in the late 20th and early 21st centuries. In the 1970s, Hall et al politicised the concept of a 'moral panic' by arguing that the public reaction to 'mugging' had been manipulated by dominant social groups in response to, and in order to divert attention away from, structural social and economic problems.[2] More recently, Bauman has proposed that public fears and anxieties, understood to be an inextricable feature of globalised consumer society, are frequently connected to the politicisation of crime and the escalation of exclusionary, incarcerative penal policies.[3] It is widely acknowledged that law and order have become major electoral issues in Britain, especially since the election of Margaret Thatcher's first administration in 1979.[4] The public salience of issues of personal safety and security, as well as their perceived centrality to the practice of government, are both illustrated by recent criminological discussions of 'governing through crime'.[5] This burgeoning political concern for crime and disorder provides a fertile breeding ground for moralising discourse. Indeed, it is within this era of ongoing, intense scrutiny of personal behaviour that some commentators have argued that moral outrage or moral panics have become routine or endemic.[6]

While wider social changes led to an enhanced late-20th-century preoccupation with some aspects of personal behaviour, the connection of alcohol to crime and disorder is a much older issue. In 1758, the *London Chronicle* wrote that:

> Besides impairing the understanding, destroying the health, and shortening of life by intemperance in general; what broils, quarrels, and duels does Excessive Drinking, in particular, frequently occasion? How like idiots or madmen does it make many appear and act? What number of scandalous and fatal amours hath it betrayed multitudes into? What friendships hath it dissolved; and how many murders, even of the dearest friends, hath it occasioned?[7]

These concerns were amplified in the 19th century; for the author of a letter published in *The Times* in 1830, drink was implicated in the 'the worst cases of murder, street robbery, housebreaking, seduction, and suicide'.[8] Prohibitionist F.W. Farrar's approving quotation of Mr Justice Denman's remark that 'drunkenness is the parent of all crime' shows that for temperance advocates the scope of unruliness attributed to alcohol was even broader.[9] Drink was at the root of almost all violence, aggression or damage to property; it was, as H.H. Croydon argued in 1915, 'the most prolific source of poverty, disease and crime'.[10] In order to tackle this troublesome relationship, the Church of England Temperance Society established police court missions in the 1870s, which aimed to wean offenders off drink and thus prevent reoffending.

Such voluntary evangelical efforts contributed to the eventual creation of state-employed probation officers in the Probation of Offenders Act 1907.[11] The temperance movement increased the seriousness with which alcohol's criminogenic properties were regarded and helped to establish new forms of intervention. But the association of alcohol with crime and disorder long predates the British temperance movement.

It is important to stress that, although the association has long been recognised, the precise relationship between alcohol and crime remains unclear. Of course, some categories of offence are alcohol related in their definition: drink-driving offences, public drunkenness and various licence infringements are, by nature, drink-related crimes. But a swathe of other criminal acts, covering offences against the person and property, can also, in some instances, be connected to drinking. In these instances, causality is never entirely concrete. For example, if a person assaults another after a bout of drinking, is alcohol the cause? If so, why does drinking cause violence in some people some of the time but not in other people or on other occasions? This pattern might be explained by the idea that the frequent coincidence of drinking and violence is a product of circumstance rather than causation. It might also be explained by the common belief that alcohol is a disinhibitor; meaning that consumption releases aggressive, violent or sexual impulses that are usually restrained. Following this logic, it could be the case that, depending on what impulses are lurking in different individuals' psyches, drinking affects everyone differently.[12] It has also been argued that drunkenness is a largely subjective experience during which people act out their own expectations of what drunkenness will entail. If, therefore, people associate drinking with violence, these two behaviours will coincide in their actions.[13] Of course, in legal terms, the individual is responsible for their actions regardless of the level or form of intoxication that they experience or the cultural expectations that they attach to this experience. But, in explanatory terms, the link between alcohol and crime remains uncertain.

Lack of certainty allows the relationship between drinking and crime to be contested. This deficiency in clear knowledge about what precise causal mechanisms connect alcohol to crime facilitates discursive conflict and historical fluctuation in regards to how the relationship is understood.[14] After calming somewhat in the inter-war years, the connection of drink to crime and disorder began attracting more attention in post-war society. The last chapter examined how alcohol consumption was identified as a contributing factor within wider discourses on road safety and youth (mis)behaviour. The tightening of certain restrictions in the 1960s did not eradicate public or political concerns about the dangers of drink. Thom investigates an interesting, although fairly short, period of political interest in homeless, habitual drinkers as recidivists during the late 1960s and early 1970s.[15] More generally, concerns about the effects of drink on crime were compounded by a sustained increase in average consumption. There were notable fluctuations in consumption over the course of the 1970s, 1980s and 1990s and there is some divergence in consumption levels reported in different sources. Nonetheless, the general trend was upward during the late 20th century.[16] In the absence of clear causal knowledge about alcohol-related crime, increasing consumption could be identified as a worrying trend in its own right.

Amid tightening targeted restrictions, the Licensing Act 1961 had extended the hours and the type of premises at which most people could consume alcohol. The efficacy of relaxing some restrictions, especially while consumption was increasing, was questioned as it jarred with a populist conservative faith in the necessity of moral regulation, as expressed by Cyril Black and others. Policy makers did not, however, abandon this regulatory strategy. In 1972, the Erroll Committee made the case for further reform of licensing. Arguing that demand should be the most important determinant of drink regulation, the committee proposed a number of liberalising measures, including the reduction of magisterial discretion, the extension of the hours in which alcohol could be sold and the lowering of the legal age for purchasing alcohol to 17. In 1973, the Clayson Report into Scottish licensing laws made similarly liberalising recommendations, many of which were implemented in the Licensing (Scotland) Act 1976. This Act abolished the local polls that the temperance movement had finally wrested from the legislature in 1913 as well as transferring licensing powers from the licensing courts to local councils and allowing for some extension of opening hours. In England and Wales, the recommendations of the Erroll Committee were rejected. In 1976, Kenneth Clarke MP's Private Member's Bill unsuccessfully proposed an extension to opening hours.[17] Statutes that relaxed certain licensing restrictions were, however, passed by Parliament in the 1980s, 1990s and 2000s.

Many commentators seek to explain these licensing reforms and their apparent effects by employing a narrative of deregulation. Various academics have highlighted how the relaxation of certain licensing restrictions has been harnessed by national and local government in order to foster a vibrant night-time economy. This night-time economy provided an engine for the regeneration of some urban areas and helped to create jobs, growth and, through various forms of taxation, valuable revenue for governments. However, the night-time economy is also accused of encouraging forms of heavy drinking or 'binge drinking', which are associated with violence, vandalism and public disorder. Hayward and Hobbs argue that the economic value of the night-time economy blinded policy makers to the social cost incurred.[18] By allowing free market logic to dictate alcohol policy, governments are frequently accused of contributing to the manufacture of what Measham and Brain have called 'a new culture of intoxication'.[19] Liberalisation, according to Moriarty and Gilmore, is partly responsible for an 'epidemic in binge drinking'.[20] For Martin Kettle, writing in *The Guardian*, the consequences of these policies have been a 'national menace' and further liberalising measures can only 'mean more drinking. And more noise. And more fighting. And more accidents'.[21] It is widely contended that the result of deregulation is increased drinking, rising levels of public disorder and more alcohol-related crime.

So, the relationship of drink to crime is well established historically. But, despite the rather hazy causal connection of the two phenomena, liberalising legal measures and a general politicisation of law and order have conspired to make this relationship more controversial in recent decades. The popular narrative of deregulation contends that relaxing legal rules worsens the crime and disorder problems that result from drinking. But is it right to characterise the reform of alcohol regulation in the late 20th and early 21st centuries as deregulation? And does regulatory change help to explain the rising tide of public anxiety about drinking? The next section examines these questions in regard to the 1980s before subsequent sections consider their implications for the 2000s. As probably the most significant reform to drink laws since at least 1921, particular attention is paid to the fallout from the Licensing Act 2003.

Acceptable in the 1980s?

Subsequent to the reforms of the 1960s, the next major reforms to the legal rules governing alcohol in England and Wales were enacted in the Licensing Act 1988. This Act scrapped the statutory requirement that public houses close from 3pm until 5.30pm on weekdays. Margaret Thatcher's government, which passed the 1988 reform, articulated its desire to remove 'unnecessary and outdated' restrictions.[22] As Chapter Four discussed, afternoon closure was created during the First World War and made permanent by the Licensing Act 1921. It was recognised in the late 1980s that this restriction originated during a bygone national emergency and so its removal garnered a fair amount of support.[23] The new Act also stipulated that off-licences could begin selling alcoholic drinks at 8am, 30 minutes earlier than previously permitted. Afternoon closure remained on Sundays but, reportedly following some parliamentary errors, it was reduced in length by one hour.[24] Furthermore, the Licensing Act 1988 amended closing times so that all pubs could open until 11pm, rather than just those in London or those outside of London that had been granted permission to do so by the licensing justices. This legislation, therefore, continued the liberalisation of opening times that had begun in 1961. Excluding Sundays, it was now possible for all public houses to open from 11am to 11pm.

A leader column in *The Guardian* was sanguine about the likely effects of this change, commenting that Scotland had apparently not suffered adversely following the implementation of similar reforms in 1976.[25] Others, however, were more disturbed by these regulatory changes. Football hooliganism had become a significant public issue in the 1980s and British newspapers reported on trouble at the European Championships held in West Germany in the summer of 1988. Violent disorder caused by 'tribes of football hooligans' occurred after England matches in Stuttgart and Dusseldorf.[26] Hooliganism also affected domestic football and, as a broader social problem, was commonly associated with an emergent issue of rural violence and disorder. Disorder was not restricted to inner cities; gangs of hooligans were reported to roam around 'the watering holes of Surrey' as well as outside football grounds.[27] These problems were widely understood as related to drinking. 'Yobbo man'[28] and 'lager louts'[29] emerged as (mis) behavioural motifs during this period and were situated as threats to the moral order. Home or abroad, rural or urban, it seems that young men plus alcohol was regarded as the principal recipe for violence and disorder.

For many people, the logical response to this situation was a desire for stricter legal controls on drinking. The government, however, rejected several restrictive proposals, such as the ban on alcohol advertising recommended by 1987's Masham Report[30] or the city centre detoxification units requested by police.[31] Reforms that were implemented, such as the extension of pub opening hours, were viewed as likely to 'increase the temptation for alcohol excess'.[32] The Royal College of Physicians pointed out that countries with more relaxed drink laws tend to consume more alcohol. They argued that 'all the evidence points to the fact that increasing the accessibility to alcohol by whatever means increases its consumption'.[33] Diane Hayter of Alcohol

Concern argued that, as a result of licensing reforms, 'people will stay in pubs all afternoon and there will be more broken homes, more accidents on the roads and more days taken off work'.[34] Hayter and others were intuitively evoking the 'availability theory'[35] of alcohol consumption. The availability theory states that greater availability of alcohol equals greater consumption and inflated social harm. Following this logic, the Licensing Act 1988 could only worsen existing problems with young male behaviour as manifested in rural disorder and football hooliganism.

While the availability of drink was being increased generally, it was, in some situations, also being actively decreased. Drinking at football matches was seriously curtailed by the Sporting Events Act 1985. This legislation followed the death of 39 Juventus fans at their European Cup Final match against Liverpool. The fans were killed when crowd trouble led to a stampede and the collapse of a wall in Heysel Stadium, Brussels. In the aftermath, immediate attention was concentrated on crowd violence perpetrated by drunk Liverpool fans as the apparently principal cause of the disaster.[36] As a writer for *The Times* put it, 'alcohol, boredom and desire to increase territory all played their part'.[37] Thatcher had already labelled football hooligans an 'enemy within'[38] and, after Heysel, she again likened them to the perpetrators of picket-line violence and Northern Irish terrorism. Her government was certainly swift in its response: new legal rules were proposed less than a week after Heysel and passed through Parliament with cross-party support. The Sporting Events Act 1985 made being drunk at a 'designated sporting event' an offence, criminalised possession of alcohol at or on the way to a 'sporting event' and prohibited sales of alcohol at stadia in areas that were in sight of the pitch.[39] Alcohol and misbehaviour at football matches were, in dominant understandings, intertwined.

Further drink restrictions were created by the Licensing Act 1988. Section 10 prevented the granting of further licences to garages. This provision was the result of an amendment tabled in the House of Lords following concerns about drink-driving. Approximately one hundred and fifty garages possessed licences in 1988 and the government, contrary to House of Lords' pressure, insisted that there was no evidence connecting these garages to drink-driving.[40] While the government did manage to ensure that garages with an existing licence would not lose it, this legislation was amended to prevent new licences being granted to garages. Age controls, additionally, were amended so that the word 'knowingly' was removed from the description of the offence of selling alcohol to a young person under the age of 18. 'Knowingly' had been on the statute books in this regard since 1923 and its deletion removed the opportunity for licensees or their employees to avoid prosecution by pleading ignorance. Some MPs argued that this new rule went too far and meant that licensees would be regarded as guilty until they could prove their innocence.[41] Under Section 16 of the Act, the accused could still mount a defence on the grounds that they had exercised 'due diligence to avoid the commission of such an offence' or 'had no reason to suspect that the person was under eighteen'. Nevertheless, this subtle change of wording did make it incumbent on those working in licensed premises to ascertain the age of their customers. Keen not appear 'soft' on 'yobbos' and 'lager louts', Home Secretary Douglas Hurd used these developments to proclaim that the Licensing Act 1988 was 'not merely a liberalizing measure ... but that it also strengthens the law on young drinkers'.[42]

These restrictive actions were not, however, considered sufficient to protect the government's credibility from the criticism, articulated from the standpoint of the availability theory, that extending opening times would worsen existing problems. So, the Home Office also urged the police and courts to fully utilise the powers at their disposal. In July 1988, the Home Office announced a six-point plan 'to stop brawling by drunken youths'.[43] Hurd spoke of 'a new generation of young criminals who mug, rob and rape without the slightest trace of remorse for their victims'.[44] Asserting that violent crime was increasing, he further added that contemporary violent crime was distinct because 'offenders, particularly young offenders, often had no feelings at all towards their victims'.[45] 'There are teenagers in this country,' Hurd continued, 'a minority but still too many who display a moral brutishness which seems to make them incapable of any kind of imaginative sympathy with their victims.'[46] This unfeeling, criminal generation was to be tackled through:

- the full employment of police and court powers to revoke licences from disorderly premises;
- more extensive use of existing powers to temporarily close licensed premises in areas where disorder is anticipated;
- greater application of court powers, granted by the Licensed Premises (Exclusion of Certain Persons) Act 1980, to ban violent offenders from specified premises if their offences had been committed in a licensed establishment.

In summer 1988, a Home Office circular containing these and other similar exhortations was sent to all police forces and the Chancellor, Lord MacKay, told an audience of magistrates that failing to do their 'duty' in punishing offenders and troublesome premises would 'risk serious damage to your country'.[47] More rigorous application of existing sanctions, rather than fresh legislation, was the government's legal response to remorseless, brutish, drunken criminals.

But the way in which Mackay, Hurd and others understood and sought to respond to this problem went beyond the purely legal. Churches had attributed the Heysel disaster to the 'moral and religious decline of the nation, of which lack of discipline is the chief factor'[48] and, similarly, the Home Secretary conceptualised the issue of alcohol-related crime and disorder in 1988 as Britain's 'moral underachievement'.[49] Hurd sought to enlist the help of parents and schools to help 'teach children self-discipline and respect for others'[50] and ministers considered widening the (newly created) national curriculum to cover 'social education' and 'duty to the community'.[51] The roots of this 'moral decline' were identified by Hurd as boredom and expectations of excitement, which he linked to television.[52] Others conformed to the ascetic moralising tradition by rooting behavioural problems in affluence: football hooliganism was described by Thatcher as a 'disease of a prosperous society';[53] a letter in *The Observer* described hooligans as 'newly affluent gangsters, relieving the tensions built up by their newly fashionable white collar jobs';[54] a Labour MP linked rural violence to "'loadsamoney' lager louts".[55]

Some favoured poverty as an explanation: Labour leader Neil Kinnock identified unemployment and hopelessness as contributing to hooliganism.[56] But all sides of the public debate understood the problem in Durkheimian terms as a lack of concrete behavioural norms. Arguments around lax moral boundaries, a deficit in empathy among the affluent and an absence of attainable goals for the poor living in poverty all indicate that problems with young male, alcohol-related behaviour were constructed in public debates as a deficiency in moral regulation.

So, in the 1980s, licensing reforms gave greater liberty to drink to most people in most social situations. However, drinking was far from universally acceptable. Anxieties about youth behaviour apparent in the 1960s had been remoulded into specific unease about alcohol-related violence and disorder perpetrated by drunk young men. Hence, the legal regulation of youth drinking and drinking at football matches was tightened during this period and, importantly, there was a clear sense that stricter discipline needed to be instilled in all social spheres to help combat a generational moral decline. A relaxation of controls on opening times was, therefore, accompanied by the proliferation of targeted alcohol restrictions and a wider intensification of the project to morally regulate certain forms of alcohol use.

The 'new culture of intoxication'

In some respects, the period following the 1980s saw a continuation of the same discursive and regulatory patterns. The Licensing (Sunday Hours) Act 1995 removed the statutory compulsion for pubs to close in the afternoon on Sundays. Licensing liberalisation was once again accompanied by ongoing public concerns about 'lager louts'. However, Measham and Brain have argued that anxieties about youth drinking are not completely misplaced and that what, why and how young people drink changed markedly around the turn of the millennium.[57] Documenting a rise in sessional consumption, or 'binge drinking', they posit that this trend was partly attributable to the rave scene of the late 1980s and early 1990s, which normalised the recreational pursuit of different psychoactive states. Measham and Brain also regard the heightened commodification of alcohol, in 'alcopops' or 'shots', and the development of dance bars and theme pubs in a competitive night-time economy as significant. In a consumer culture where, it is explained, individuals define themselves through acts of consumption, a behavioural trend towards 'determined drunkenness'[58] has thus purportedly arisen. It is this 'new culture of intoxication',[59] this apparent trend of binge drinking, that has dominated public discourse on alcohol in recent years. Moreover, it provided the discursive backdrop to arguably the most significant reform of alcohol laws since 1872: the Licensing Act 2003.

This section explores how binge drinking has been problematised in reference to crime and disorder. The point is not to question Measham and Brain's assertions about the rise of a 'new culture of intoxication'; rather it is to scrutinise their partial vindication of the public anxieties about current drinking practices. While, of course, behavioural change does occur, this cannot and does not provide sufficient explanation for public attitudes towards alcohol. So, how can the manner in which drinking has been understood and regulated since 2003 be explained?

Civilising the alcoholic nation

In April 2000, the government's White Paper *Time for Reform* was published. Its aims were to reduce alcohol-related crime and disorder, reduce alcohol misuse, encourage tourism and promote self-sufficient rural communities. Echoing the views of the Erroll Committee, the

White Paper set out plans to achieve these aims by 'modernising' the licensing system and reducing unnecessary regulation.[60] This was the basis of what became the Licensing Act 2003 and perhaps the most important measure through which this legislation sought to achieve modernisation was through the abolition of licensing justices. Section 3 of the Act transferred the responsibility of dealing with applications for the grant or renewal of licences from magistrates to local councils, who were required to create licensing committees of 10 to 15 members. By shifting the function of licensing from the appointed judiciary to political authorities, this reform represents an effective end to the system of granting licences that the Wine and Beerhouse Act 1869 had established and a crucial revision of the separation of governmental powers. Although it is probably too early to appreciate the historical significance of this change, the 2003 reform may in time prove to be as important as the Victorian rejection of free-trade-inspired alcohol governance in favour of a system of magisterial control.

In other respects, the Licensing Act 2003 was more clearly liberalising. Under Section 18, it is apparent that when dealing with applications for licences the presumption is in favour of their grant, assuming that the application has been properly completed and no 'relevant representations' are made. If 'relevant representations' are made, which largely constitute the expression of concerns about the suitability of the applicant or the likely effects of granting a licence made by 'interested parties' or 'responsible authorities',[61] further conditions can be attached to the licence, such as the stipulation that door supervision must be provided. Barring such complications, however, the murky process of magisterial discretion was replaced with a basic presumption that, if applied for, a licence should be granted. But the most eye-catching part of the legislation was its failure to specify any permitted hours of trading or mandatory closing times. Under Section 17, applications for licences must specify during which hours it is intended that alcohol will be sold and licensing commissions can accept, amend or reject these applications (subject to aforementioned considerations). It is, however, quite possible for applicants to apply for a licence for up to 24 hours per day. When these new rules were implemented in November 2005, the Licensing Act 2003 meant that, for the first time since the 1830s (when the hours of the newly created beerhouses were restricted), there were no statutory restrictions on the times during which alcohol could be sold.[62]

Removing statutory limits on opening hours was a controversial move. In January 2003, *The Guardian*'s Martin Kettle wrote that 'we are Britain, and we are an alcoholic nation....We drink too much, too fast and too young'.[63] He went on to attack the government's response to this problem: 'The worst thing the government can do is what it is trying to do – an honest subtitle to the licensing bill would read "the licensing bill is designed to extend the culture of public drunkenness and all the miserable consequences that flow from it".'[64] Kettle was equally critical in May of that year when he claimed that 'only the most sozzled end of the drinks industry now denies that Britain has a drink problem. Or that the heart of the problem is binge drinking by young people, including by under-age drinkers, in the centre of towns'.[65] But Kettle aside, debate about the new drinking regulations was distinctly muted when the legislation passed through Parliament in 2003. The newspaper coverage from this period suggests that the most contentious part of the Act at the time was not the prospect of '24-hour drinking' but the changes made to the rules regarding the provision of live music.[66]

Concern about drinking rose exponentially during 2004. The *Daily Mail* reported that alcohol consumption had risen by 50% since 1970 and this increase was responsible for 'a massive rise in crime, violence and disease'.[67] The newspaper went on to claim that 'many city centres turned into virtual no-go areas late at night by drunken yobs'[68] and the cost of drinking to the criminal justice system was placed at anywhere between £1 billion and £7 billion.[69] During this period, press stories about alcohol abounded with references to 'thuggery and intimidation', 'lager loutettes' and 'feral children'.[70] Friday and Saturday were reportedly times of 'mayhem', when 'the girls in high heels will be puking up' and 'the police vans will be full'.[71] The government responded by announcing a crackdown on irresponsible licensees who encourage binge drinking. Despite Home Office Minister Hazel Blears' confident declaration that this would 'put an end to no-go city centres – reclaiming them for decent, law-abiding citizens',[72] public anxiety about drinking showed no sign of abating.

It was into this simmering cauldron of social unease that the implementation of longer opening hours was added in 2005. Although muted in 2003, politicians, magistrates, police chiefs and journalists were now vocal in their dismay at the legal reforms. The *Daily Telegraph* reported that the British Transport Police had serious concerns over a likely increase in violence[73] and *The Observer* highlighted how many magistrates as well as senior police officers believed the new laws would increase rape and sexual assault.[74] Shadow Secretary for Culture, Media and Sport, Theresa May, said that 'longer drinking hours will mean more crime and disorder';[75] Liberal Democrat MP Mark Oaten described the plans as 'madness';[76] and Charles Harris QC said that the Licensing Act 2003 was 'close to lunacy'.[77] Glen Smyth of the Metropolitan Police Federation commented that: 'Most nights of the week our officers are overwhelmed by a sea of drunken, violent, vomiting yobs who when they're not fighting each other are falling through shop windows. That's now. What's it going to be like when we have a licensing free-for-all?'[78] Crime and disorder were already popularly seen as 'out of control' and this situation could only be worsened by enabling people to drink later into the night.

In the face of mounting uproar about an apparently dangerous policy, Tony Blair's government was accused of 'staggering complacency' and practising 'the politics of neglect' by Conservative MP and barrister Edward Garnier.[79] In response to this fierce criticism, the government argued that the Licensing Act 2003 would civilise British drinking culture. Allowing later opening would have the effect of staggering closing times, thus reducing the build-up of people on the streets at 11pm and thereby diminishing disorder. It was also claimed that new rules would reduce drunkenness by ending the rush to drink as much as possible before last orders. Culture Secretary Tessa Jowell therefore stated that licensing reform 'will make towns and cities safe for all, not a free for all'[80] and Home Secretary Charles Clarke spoke of creating a 'civilised kind of life as exists in continental Europe'.[81] But the idea of Europeanising British drinking was seen by many as preposterous. Frank Dobson MP claimed that the English 'have been binge drinkers since time immemorial',[82] the actor Tony Booth publicly declared that the British drink in 'a more primitive, frightening, Anglo-Saxon way' than our European neighbours[83] and Charles Harris QC stated that after drinking British people become 'pugnacious and bellicose' and 'fight at the slightest provocation'.[84] The government's logic was rejected in derisory terms and the tone of most public discourse surrounding the licensing reforms remained severe and near-hysterical.

So, the transferral of licensing powers from magistrates to local councils attracted little attention and, by 2005 at least, the overwhelming majority of discussion of the Licensing Act 2003 focused on opening times. The discourse is also notable for the palpable sense of dread that came to typify anticipation of longer opening hours. In 2003, Martin Kettle's outraged commentary on the reforms was unusual. But by the end of 2005, this brand of alarming fatalism had become a sort of discursive white noise; no longer exceptional, it was an omnipresent shrill sound discernible in any public arena in which alcohol was discussed.

'Whoops, no apocalypse'

The provisions of the new Act were implemented in November 2005 and, despite widespread anxiety about pending disaster, the practical changes were quite limited. Of the 184,000 licensed premises in England and Wales at this time, only 700, mainly supermarkets, were granted 24-hour licences.[85] The vast majority of licensed premises opted for rather modest extensions to their trading hours. Hadfield and Measham draw on government data to report that Saturday night drinking time was extended by an average of just 21 minutes. They also show that only 1% of premises that did not previously open later than midnight chose to do so under the new rules.[86] The Department of Culture, Media and Sport's evaluation of the Licensing Act 2003 found no uniform detrimental effects[87] and Home Office aggregate statistics show that national crime levels continued their downward trend from 2005 onwards.[88] Round-the-clock drinking and the attendant mayhem predicted clearly did not materialise; drinking habits actually changed very little, prompting the British Beer and Pub Association to (rather smugly) comment 'whoops, no apocalypse'.[89] Given its limited practical effects, the reaction to the new Licensing Act 2003 fits the classic definition of a 'moral panic'; a disproportionate reaction prompted by an exaggerated sense of threat.

It must also be recognised that the reaction to the liberalising 'politics of neglect' represents broader government actions in an inaccurate or, at best, partial way. To expand, while certain provisions of the Licensing Act 2003 were liberalising, many others were not. Section 155 increased the police's power to confiscate alcohol from young people and Section 160 gave the police anticipatory as well as reactive powers to close premises. Under this provision and with a magistrate's approval, the police can close licensed premises in any area 'where there is or is expected to be disorder' for up to 24 hours.[90] These enhanced police powers were entirely typical of New Labour's approach to criminal justice. The Criminal Justice and Police Act 2001, for example, had given the police the power to hand out 'on-the-spot' fines to persons caught committing a range of relatively low-level offences. Several drink-related offences, including the offence of simple drunkenness created by the Licensing Act 1872, were listed as targets for immediate fines (usually £80) under Section 1 of the Act. Handing the police sentencing powers has been controversial and serious questions have been raised about the delivery of justice and implications for the rule of law.[91] More pertinent for this book is that such reforms demonstrate that, while certain restrictions have been relaxed, new powers have enabled the stricter policing of other drinking regulations.

As the police's anticipatory power to close licensed premises in certain areas shows, many of New Labour's new drink restrictions were also future oriented and spatially defined. In addition to 'on-the-spot' fines, the Criminal Justice and Police Act 2001 created Designated Public Place Orders (DPPOs). DPPOs enable local authorities to delimit certain areas, typically town and city centres, within which restrictions can be placed on public drinking. It is not illegal to drink alcohol within such areas but the police can ask people to cease consuming alcohol in these areas. Failure to comply with such a request constitutes a criminal offence under Section 12 of the Act. As a result of Section 30 of the Anti-Social Behaviour Act 2003, local authorities can also create Dispersal Orders, which allow police officers, within designated areas, to require groups of two or more people to leave the designated area immediately if the behaviour of the group 'has resulted, or is likely to result, in any members of the public being intimidated, harassed, alarmed or distressed'.[92] Further to these anticipatory powers, the Violent Crime Reduction Act 2006 allows courts to impose Drink Banning Orders on individuals who have been convicted of an offence while the under the influence of alcohol. These civil orders can prohibit an individual from consuming alcohol or entering licensed premises and so hypothetically prevent future offending. The Act also enables local authorities to reclaim some of the costs of additional law enforcement from areas in which alcohol-related disorder is common (although reports suggest that these powers have rarely been utilised).[93] Especially in regards to public drinking, the discretionary powers of police, the sentencing options of the judiciary and local authorities' ability to spatially restrict drinking all proliferated under New Labour.[94]

These new powers have largely been used on the 'feral children' who occupy 'no-go areas'. While dispersal notices can be given to people of any age, a report by Crawford and Lister found that they are most commonly used on young people.[95] Other new regulations have more explicitly targeted the behaviour of young people. The Licensing (Young Persons) Act 2000 outlawed so-called 'proxy-buying' of alcohol, where an adult buys drinks for a young person under the age of 18 from an off-licence (Section 169C). The Licensing Act 2003 raised the age at which a person can enter licensed premises unaccompanied by an adult from 14 to 16 and the Criminal Justice and Police Act 2001 also amended the Licensing Act 1964 so that the police are authorised to carry out 'test purchasing'.[96] Test purchasing is a means of checking that licensees are trading legally, which entails police sending a person under the age of 18 into a licensed premises to attempt to buy alcohol. Under the mandatory code created by Gordon Brown's government, drinks retailers are also obliged to ask anyone who looks as if they may be aged under 18 for identification. Many large retailers, including Tesco, Asda and Morrison's, currently operate a more rigorous 'Challenge Twenty-Five' policy whereby people suspected of being under that age, even if they are not suspected of being under 18, must provide identification before they can purchase alcohol. The New Labour years, from 1997 to 2010, thus witnessed an intensification of attempts to restrict young people's access to alcohol.

The New Labour Government also increased the responsibility placed on licensees and their staff (paid or unpaid). The Licensing Act 2003, for example, highlighted the duties of licensees and bar staff by creating new offences of:

- allowing disorderly conduct on licensed premises (Section 140);
- selling or allowing the sale of alcohol to someone who is already drunk (Section 141);
- allowing unaccompanied children (under the age of 16) to be on the licensed premises without taking 'reasonable steps' to ascertain their age (Section 45).[97]

The mandatory code of Brown's government was implemented between April and October 2010 and contained several further restrictions on the drinks industry. 'Irresponsible promotions', such as 'all you can drink for £10' or 'women drink for free', were banned. Licensed premises were also required to provide free tap water and offer smaller measures of beer, wine and spirits (alongside larger measures).[98] The Licensing Act 2003 may have increased the hours during which alcohol can be sold, but accompanying and subsequent regulations have stressed the legal responsibilities of licensees and bar staff as well as reducing, to some extent, their commercial freedoms.

As well as failing to appreciate the negligible practical impacts of changes to opening times (which, admittedly, are easier to recognise in retrospect), the moral panic surrounding the Licensing Act 2003 was also based on a misconceptualisation of New Labour's drink policies. From 1997 to 2010, changes to England and Wales' alcohol laws were clearly not all about liberalisation and, in a number of significant ways, the regulation of drinkers and drink-sellers was significantly increased while the powers of the police and local authorities also grew. There has certainly not been a total deregulation of the drinks industry; partial liberalisation has been accompanied by greater legal restrictions.

Recent changes to how alcohol is legally regulated are, therefore, best described as a bifurcated process.

A moral panic about drinking and licensing

Despite Measham and Brain's argument, it is difficult to find much that is worthy of vindication in the public reaction to the Licensing Act 2003. Styles of drinking may or may not have changed, but it is clear that public attitudes towards the licensing reforms bore little relation to the nature or extent of the threat to social order that the legislation posed. Average alcohol consumption had actually begun to decline by 2005[99] and, due to their limited practical effect, extended opening times were unlikely to have much impact on this trend. The direction of change in regard to the legal rules governing drinking was, moreover, bifurcated rather than simply deregulatory. Rational, behavioural accounts are, therefore, limited in their capacity to explain public anxieties about alcohol from 2003 to 2005. This episode could legitimately be described as a 'moral panic'. But, importantly, if it is a moral panic, where did it come from? How does it relate to the long history of public attitudes towards that which have been explored in this book?

The attitudinal heritage of Victorian temperance

If the practical effects of licensing changes were limited and the narrative of deregulation is overstated, how can this outburst of anxiety in 2005 be explained? This section considers how the bifurcated process of changing the way alcohol was governed related to moral regulation and also considers the relevance of the Victorian temperance movement as a historical influence over public attitudes to alcohol.

The drunk man of Europe

While opening hours were being extended in November 2005, a parallel news story revealed traces of an underlying morality that affects attitudes to alcohol. The story revolved around the attempted prosecution of Ruairi Dougal for rape at Swansea Crown Court. The case against Dougal fell apart when the complainant admitted in court that she had been too drunk to remember whether she had consented to sex or not.[100] As later affirmed by the Court of Appeal in *R v Bree* [2007],[101] drunken consent is still consent and, in the absence of clear evidence that consent was not given, the defendant could not be convicted. For some this was simply an issue of reliable evidence (or lack of it), but for others such cases demonstrated the salience of the view that women who are intoxicated bear at least some responsibility for any harm they suffer while intoxicated. Lawyer Marion Smullen complained that juries are reluctant to convict in rape cases where the victim is (voluntarily) intoxicated.[102] Furthermore, in 2008, *The Guardian* reported that the Criminal Injuries Compensation Authority had been cutting payments to rape victims who were drunk at the time the crime was committed. This situation echoes the Victorian period; in a rape case that came before Judge Willes in Northampton in 1856 there were said to be 'some doubts' over whether 'the offence of rape could be committed upon the person of a woman who had rendered herself perfectly insensible by drink'.[103] A woman's decision to drink continues to represent the wilful lowering of her moral profile; the consequences deriving from this decision are thus regarded as at least partially her fault.[104] Within this web of culpability and respectability, alcohol use becomes a definer of the victim's moral worth.

Echoes of Victorian ideas were also apparent in debates about licensing reforms. Focusing solely on the liberalising aspects of the legal changes, public discourse tended to paint the Licensing Act 2003 as set to open the floodgates of crime and disorder. On the eve of extended opening hours coming into effect, *The Sun* reported in battle-ready terms the creation of a 'field hospital' in Newcastle-upon-Tyne to handle the imminent 'casualties of 24-hour drinking'.[105] Employing vocabulary that usually denotes unavoidable physical catastrophes, *The Sun* spoke of casualty units being 'swamped' by victims of alcohol-related violence and accidents[106] as well as 'the inevitable swarm of drunken youngsters' who bring disorder to the streets.[107] Of course the press may be prone to sensationalism, but it was not just the *Daily Mail* that believed that 'the binge is about to become an uncontrolled riot of drunkenness'.[108] David Blunkett MP described the Licensing Act 2003 as 'a leap in the dark' that risked worsening crime problems[109] and Mark Oaten MP claimed that 'when the problem is running out of control in our town centres, extending drinking hours to twenty four hours a day is madness'.[110] In all of these comments, a preoccupation with rationality and control, as well as the threat that drink poses to an apparently fragile social order, is palpable. Evoking the memory of the 'slippery slope' that temperance activists described, many people felt that the line between order and chaos was as thin as a few extra hours of drinking time.

References to 'swarms' and being 'swamped' also serve to depict this liberalising legislative disaster in entirely deterministic terms.

In the 'rising tide' of alcoholic excess,[111] Tessa Jowell was cast as 'the Ministerial equivalent of "King Canute"' trying vainly to prevent the inevitable.[112] The implication that longer drinking hours unavoidably mean more crime and disorder embodies the availability theory. Plant and Plant provide some support for the availability theory, including by citing the increase in alcohol consumption and certain alcohol-related harms that followed the proliferation of drink-selling premises enabled by the Beer Act 1830.[113] Sumner and Parker argue that the availability theory rests on the assumption that alcohol is a disinhibiting drug that, when consumed, unlocks a Freudian dungeon of aggressive, violent and sexual impulses.[114] Although their research was funded by the drinks industry, Sumner and Parker's point resonates with reactions to the prospect of longer opening hours; David Davis MP warned of 'anarchy on the streets'[115] and John Yates of the Association of Chief Police Officers talked of a likely increase in rape and sexual assault.[116] Allowed unrestricted access to alcohol therefore, humans will swiftly descend a slippery slope, act on their innate urges and commit bestial acts. Without legal fetters, people will quite literally become the 'urban savages'[117] of Charles Harris QC's rhetoric.

The contemporary availability theory therefore parallels the temperance idea of a slippery slope and, in either case, the first sip of alcohol or the unrestricted availability of alcohol is made problematic by a critical lack of self-control. Chapter Three found that public perceptions of a deficit in self-control were prominent in the Victorian period and, although lessening in the inter-war years and becoming associated mainly with young people (as Chapter Five explored), are again widely evident in contemporary discourse. In 2010, *Daily Express* columnist Theodore Dalrymple argued that Britain is rapidly becoming 'a nation without sufficient self-respect to control itself'.[118] For Victorian temperance activists, this situation could be rectified by the adoption of the teetotal pledge or, for those sceptical of individuals' fortitude, the implementation of prohibition. Contemporary solutions also attempt to inculcate self-control. In 2008, the government launched a major anti-binge drinking campaign, which, in the words of then Home Secretary, Jacqui Smith, aimed to 'challenge people to think twice about the serious consequences of losing control'.[119] The campaign featured television adverts depicting young people vomiting, damaging their property and injuring themselves before text asks:'you wouldn't start a night like this, so why end it that way?'[120] Once again, the development of self-control is the preferred means of halting the slide towards drunkenness, savagery and victimisation.

It should be stressed that this deficiency in self-control is associated almost exclusively with British people. It was described earlier how the government's ambition of creating a 'civilised' European drinking culture was criticised by Tony Booth and Charles Harris. Given the parallels with temperance discourse being drawn, Booth and Harris' comments can be reinterpreted as demonstrating an almost puritanical disgust with the recreational habits of the British. Equally, references to 'booze Britain'[121] and 'binge Britain'[122] have become almost ubiquitous features of discourse on alcohol, serving to emphasise that Britain is the depraved exception to the general European rule of sobriety. Comparisons with other, apparently more civilised, countries further reinforce this idea; Geethika Jayatilaka of Alcohol Concern said that 'extending licensing hours are more likely to turn our town centres into Faliraki than Florence'[123] and academic Victor Robinson asserted that 'we are not a Mediterranean people and have not been socialised into the respect for alcohol those cultures have'.[124] Europe, and particularly Southern Europe, is constructed as a beacon of civilisation standing in stark contrast to Britain's alcoholic depravity. This discursive framework resonates strongly with the nationally self-deprecatory temperance commentaries of the Victorian period, which Chapter Two rooted in the self-repulsion of evangelical Protestant beliefs.

The idea that Britain alone is mired in a swamp of drink and debauchery corresponds to temperance activist Sir Wilfrid Lawson's belief that he lived in 'a world full of sin, of wrong, and of injustice'.[125] The overriding tone of 2005's surfeit of apocalyptic commentaries was not, however, generally despondent and many rallied for concerted action against alcohol consumption. Writing in *The Observer*, liver specialist Professor Roger Williams depicted the situation as extremely serious and spoke of the numerous 'adverse consequences of our drinking culture'.[126] But reflecting the pervasive belief of the temperance movement that it is imperative to struggle against these overwhelming evils (described in Chapters Two and Three), Williams' belief in the grave seriousness of the current situation becomes an impetus towards action. Williams thus calls for higher drinks prices, warning labels on bottles and cans, and more money for preventative educational programmes and treatment facilities. An article in *The Sun* reflects this position, stating simply that 'doing nothing isn't an option'.[127] The language used to discuss the contemporary 'drink problem' may be secular, but the attitudes resonate with the evangelical notion of the struggle.

Of course, this idea of Britain as peculiarly debauched, as the drunk man of Europe, ignores the alcohol problems faced by many other

European countries. In actuality, research has found that levels of alcohol-related mortality, liver disease and overall consumption are not especially high in Britain when compared with more 'civilised' European countries.[128] *The Independent* was probably the only newspaper to pick up on this point in 2005, arguing that the government's plan to reproduce the drinking culture of other European countries may make things worse; 'if we do end up with a wet drinking culture, the toll in terms of health problems will be grave' as consumption and harm will likely rise.[129] Despite this evidence to the contrary, the Victorian idea that Britain alone is typified by a dysfunctional relationship with alcohol remains. This belief receded somewhat during the patriotic bombast of the First World War and remained subdued during the mid-20th century. It was apparent, to some degree, in descriptions of drunk English football fans rioting in Europe during the 1980s, and public discourse studied from 2003 to 2010 shows abundant signs of a resurgent faith in Britain's exceptional alcoholic depravities.

The reaction to the extension of opening times in 2005 therefore shows considerable qualitative affinities with Victorian, temperance-influenced discourse on alcohol. The similarities are also more pronounced and more specifically attached to alcohol than in the vividly moral and noticeably ascetic discourse of the 1960s. The connection of drink to respectability, the idea of a slippery slope of consumption and the belief in a national deficit of self-control as well as a national surplus of depravity all illustrate the manifold interpretive links of contemporary alcohol discourse with the evangelically inspired rhetoric of the 19th century. Evangelical ideas, Chapter Two argued, were important in the transition from moderationist to teetotal temperance and, although receding in influence somewhat from the 1920s to the 1960s, they remain a discernible component of attitudes to drinking to this day. In this attitudinal and heuristic universe, the arrival of 24-hour licensing, the provision that dominated discussion of the Licensing Act 2003, cannot possibly elevate Britain to the level of consumptive sophistication displayed by its near neighbours. In the absence of sufficient self-control, the reforms could only be understood as sure to worsen existing problems by removing remaining (legal) constraints on our essential national depravity.[130]

'Please drink responsibly'

When the booze-fuelled apocalypse failed to materialise, anxiety about alcohol did not go away. References to the 'new menace'[131] of binge drinking were still common and the *Daily Telegraph*'s statement that 'alcohol-fuelled violence and gratuitously vicious behaviour have become part of our national life' was fairly typical of public discourse on drink in 2006 and 2007.[132] In 2008, the British Medical Association publicly referred to the 'binge drinking epidemic'[133] and the Archbishop of Canterbury claimed that there is 'a whole culture of alcohol abuse which this country has failed to tackle'.[134] The continuation of concerns about drinking is a reminder that 2005 was not an isolated outburst of anxiety in the form of the classic, exceptional moral panic described by Stan Cohen. This was a high point of concern within longer-term processes of moralisation, which, as the qualitative connections presented in the last section show, stretches back to the 19th century. Building on this point, this subsection considers the extent to which the contemporary governance of alcohol can be considered a project of moral regulation.

Chapter Three argued that the crucial discursive innovation of the temperance movement was the problematisation of alcohol and, through tightening of legal controls, the period 1864 to 1872 saw this idea pass into law. It has already been stressed that liberalisation only formed one part of New Labour's approach to drinking, but it is important to highlight the grounds on which this liberalisation was justified. The government did not argue, as Victorians often did, that beer and wine are harmless and so many existing restrictions are unnecessary. Under Section 4 of the Licensing Act 2003, licensing authorities must consider four licensing objectives when dealing with applications:

- the prevention of crime and disorder;
- the improvement of public safety;
- the prevention of public nuisance;
- the protection of children from harm.

Many of the social problems associated with alcohol, including crime and disorder, are therefore at the heart of the reform and the centre of the new licensing system it established. Additionally, while opposition parties attacked the Licensing Act 2003, they opposed the means the New Labour Government chose to deal with alcohol rather than contesting the categorisation of alcohol as a problem. For example, many Conservatives (at the time) favoured alternative policies such as London Mayor Boris Johnson's ban on drinking on London transport introduced in 2008. The 2003 Act may have represented a challenge to the availability theory of drinking but it actively reproduced the conception that alcohol is inherently problematic.[135]

Alcohol's enjoyable, non-harmful effects are rarely acknowledged in public discourse.[136] New restrictions mean that the sort of adverts that in the 1960s proclaimed that 'a WHITBREAD makes the most of you' are not permitted, and my research found no light-hearted equivalents of the 'giggling Wong' story. That said, certain forms of consumption are considered broadly legitimate. While rejecting the idea of minimum unit pricing (which will be discussed in more detail in the next chapter), in 2009 the Work and Pensions Secretary, James Purnell, said that it would penalise the 'responsible majority' of drinkers.[137] David Poley, chief executive of the drinks industry representative, the Portman Group, echoed this political message claiming that pricing controls would 'have a marginal effect on harmful drinkers but force hard-working families to pay more for a drink'.[138] 'Moderate' drinking is, therefore, permissible for most people who can be trusted to control themselves and not contribute to any social problems.[139] This is the new official behavioural ideal: the hard-working family-person who enjoys a drink occasionally but heeds the increasingly widespread warning on the bottle that exhorts him or her to 'drink responsibly'.[140] As with the Victorian model of the respectable, sober working man, such rhetoric is a classic example of what Foucault calls a 'dividing practice' and a key feature of moral regulation projects.[141]

The counterpoint in this dividing practice is the irresponsible, harmful drinker. As Matthew Elliott of the Taxpayers Alliance explained in the *Daily Telegraph*: 'Responsible drinking in local pubs has been a cornerstone of British society for centuries. Binge drinkers who wreak havoc should be targeted.'[142] It is these binge drinkers who are commonly blamed when, to quote the *Daily Mail*, 'gutters are awash in blood and vomit', when 'sodden, brutal excess' turns town centres into 'no-go areas for families'.[143] In line with the emergence of the issue of youth in the mid-20th century, these problematic binge drinkers are portrayed as young. As Martin Kettle explained in 2003, 'the heart of the problem is binge drinking by young people, including by under-age drinkers, in the centre of towns'.[144] By 2007, the government expressed a similar position in its alcohol strategy document *Safe, Sensible, Social*. The government pledged to concentrate attentions on the 'significant minority who don't know when to stop drinking' and defined this minority as constituted by drinkers under the age of 18, 18- to 24-year-old binge drinkers and harmful drinkers.[145] Critcher has argued that the binge drinker 'does not make an impressive folk devil' as their identity is not defined solely in reference to this activity.[146] Nevertheless, it is clear that the press and political discourse tends overwhelmingly to attribute the social problems associated with the 'significant minority' of young binge drinkers.[147] It is certainly feasible that inflamed moralising discourse about youth drinking paved the way, in both the 1960s and the New Labour years, for the tightening of legal restrictions on young people and alcohol described earlier. Certain forms of behaviour committed by particular social groups are problematised discursively and then regulated legally. Ongoing problematisation is then necessary to justify this remodelled social order. This analysis corresponds to Corrigan and Sayer's theory, in which moral regulation provides the attitudinal foundations on which levels and forms of state intervention can be built and defended.[148] But, following Ruonavaara particularly, moral regulation is not just about legitimising state actions but also encompasses attempts to influence the self-formation of others.[149] In 2008, Justice Secretary, Jack Straw, exemplified this point by describing the government's intention to create a 'moral imperative'[150] for young people to avoid alcohol. As with Victorian teetotaller W. Hunt's desire to create a 'moral obligation' of abstinence, the intimation is that the law cannot or should not be the sole arbiter in these affairs and that where the law finishes, at probably the clearest boundary of state influence, moral obligations or imperatives should continue to provide some form of governance. To elaborate, binge drinking or becoming intoxicated is not against the law per se. Nor is it illegal for those over the age of five yet below the age of 18 to consume alcohol. The law, in these respects, remains restrictive and not prohibitive. So in this respect, the government's promotion of the ideal of the 'responsible majority' of hard-working, moderate-drinking family persons is an attempt to govern beyond the law; the process of self-formation is shaped by the implicit condemnation of deviance from the specified norm. For the Victorian temperance movement, respectability without sobriety was ruled out. Likewise, the attribute of responsibility and normalisation through membership of the majority is now constructed as impossible for binge drinkers. Through these mechanisms it is hoped that individuals will become resolved of the need to reform their behaviour.

This form of governance embodies the belief that the individual should be the primary unit of social change. Chapter Three found that the system of regulation established by the Licensing Act 1872 effectively corroborated the assertion by *The Times* that 'no moral work was ever achieved without personal agencies'.[151] In some cases persuasion may be necessary where the individual drinker is not motivated to change; Charles Turner MP was quoted earlier asking workmen 'to discourage intemperance by giving the cold-shoulder'[152] to their heavy drinking colleagues. The government's *Safe, Sensible,*

Social document parallels this strategy by insisting that everyone must take responsibility for creating a 'sensible drinking culture'. Vernon Coaker's ministerial foreword to the document states that:

> Parents and guardians should look at the example they set in their drinking habits, as well as know what their children are up to outside of the home. Friends of anti-social and harmful drinkers must exert influence. Business and industry should reinforce responsible drinking messages at every opportunity.[153]

Persuasion, therefore, remains a crucial means to influence individual action and, perhaps, a substitute for a more interventionist legal regime. Following Ruonavaara's theory, which gives greater recognition to non-legal, non-coercive attempts to influence the behaviour of others, this can be seen as an integral part of moral regulation.

Within the permissible bounds of conduct specified by law, behavioural ideals and persuasive projects are brought to bear on those deemed to be problem drinkers. It must also be noted that official rhetoric continues to separate the choices individuals can make about their own conduct into normatively distinct categories. Just as Henry Bruce, Victorian Home Secretary, structured legally mandated personal choices through his condemnations of drinking, so modern politicians seek to influence such decisions. Tony Blair called heavy drinking a 'new British disease'[154] and Gordon Brown said that 'binge drinking is unacceptable'.[155] Both former premiers thus gave clear moral direction to individual choices about alcohol; the 'right choice' is not legally compulsory but making the 'wrong choice', as Blair and Brown demonstrated, will attract the moral censure of the dominant morality. O'Malley and Valverde state that 'when governments value desired actions as pleasant and undesired as unpleasant, they are attempting to "govern at a distance"'.[156] The concept of 'governing at a distance' or 'governing through choice' is borrowed from Rose and Miller, who see it as a central means through which liberal governments seek to exercise power over spheres of human action that they do not wholly control.[157] The replacement of the older binary oppositions of good and evil with responsible and irresponsible or acceptable or unacceptable therefore shows that discourse about alcohol has become more secularised. But additionally, it is clear that this discursive phenomenon evidences the continued efforts of powerful social actors to govern the behaviour of others.

So, a powerful project to morally regulate the use of alcohol has been identified. It is evidenced in the legitimisation of interventions targeting specific social groups (mainly young people) as well as a wealth of discursive attempts to govern individual choices.

Contemporary projects of moral regulation

The relaxation of opening hours for licensed premises was not just accompanied by the intensification of police powers, responsibilities for licensees and clampdowns on youth drinking and public drinking identified earlier. It also coincided with a broader social context in which moralising discourse has framed a variety of extra-legal attempts to govern the consumption of alcohol, such as the construction of behavioural choices with dividing practices and moral imperatives. These efforts form part of a general project to morally regulate the use of alcohol (through influencing the actions of others in a specific direction). The survival of more historically particular discursive features, such as an evangelical faith in depravity and a problematisation of all forms of alcohol that resulted from the teetotal turn in the 1830s, show that contemporary efforts to morally regulate the use of alcohol also bear some discursive relation to the specific campaigns of the 19th-century temperance movement. This social movement thus left an attitudinal heritage that, to some extent, continues to be visible within public discourse on alcohol.

Conclusion

In some respects, the period covered in this chapter is characterised by an intensification of the regulatory processes that Chapter Five identified in the mid-20th century. Attitudes to alcohol continued to be characterised by a specific concern for the drinking habits of young people. While 'binge drinking' was a new term, its popular and almost exclusive association with the behaviour of young people mean that it was consistent with the discursive tenets that, in earlier periods, identified football hooligans, lager louts or teenage tramps as symptoms of a behavioural malady affecting the young. Chapter Five argued that mid-20th-century permissiveness was never universal and applied only to certain people in certain situations. Equally, the series of reforms to the laws governing the sale and consumption of alcohol during the period studied in this chapter are best described as a bifurcated process. Legislation in 1988, 1995 and 2003 continued the process initiated in 1961 of relaxing restrictions on opening times.

Although some forms of alcohol consumption were thus positioned as broadly legitimate, others were increasingly proscribed. Much legal regulation, particularly that relating to youth drinking, public drinking and drinking at football matches, was tightened during the late 20th and early 21st century.

Of course, historical differences must also be recognised. Drink-driving barely featured in public discourse surrounding the Licensing Act 2003. Thoroughly problematised and subject to increasing legal and moral censure, it has slipped out of view somewhat as an area of discursive contention. Significantly, public discourse on drink has increased in quantity and anxiety. In the 1960s, alcohol was seen to have exercised a seditious influence over rebellious, amoral youths and, in the 1980s, to have disinhibited the aggressive, remorseless young men who attended football matches. But, in these periods, alcohol sat alongside drugs, sex, unemployment, lack of discipline and other factors as a perceived cause of social problems and a symptom of moral decline. The moral panic about binge drinking and licensing reforms in 2005, fuelled by the popular conception that longer opening hours equal greater alcohol consumption and more crime and disorder, show that drinking was understood as a potent and singular social problem in its own right. While anxiety lessened somewhat after 2005, this chapter has shown that alcohol continued to be the subject of alarmed commentaries and new legislative interventions. The position of drink as a singular concern for public-minded moralists distinguishes this period from the mid-20th century and highlights its similarities to the 19th and early-20th centuries. This comparison is further supported by evidence presented, which demonstrates the qualitative affinities between Victorian temperance attitudes and the ideas, beliefs and values that shape more contemporary understandings of alcohol. Moralising discourse surged in volume during this period and its qualitative character indicated a revival of some evangelically inspired Victorian temperance attitudes.

The popular narrative of deregulation largely relies on recent legal reforms as explanation for alarmed attitudes and market forces as explanation for deregulation. This book offers an alternative explanation. First, the relaxation of opening times was not an invention of New Labour but the continuance of a process begun by Harold Macmillan's government in 1961 and continued by Conservative administrations in the 1980s and 1990s. Second, 'deregulation' should be substituted for bifurcation as many other legal restrictions on drinking have been simultaneously created or tightened. Third, condemnations of excessive drinking and the promotion of forms of 'responsible drinking' demonstrate the existence of vigorous projects to morally compel people to make certain behavioural choices. Finally, these points illustrate the endurance of the model of alcohol governance that became prominent in the early 1870s. Legal restrictions and moral compulsion continue to construct individual choices about alcohol. It is worth adding that these conclusions result from historical analysis of the period from the 18th century onwards. The way in which we understand and regulate alcohol cannot be comprehended without knowledge of, for example, the Licensing Act 1872 or the evangelical faith in national depravity that typified Victorian views of drinking. This historically informed analysis allows projects to morally regulate alcohol to be recognised and explained.

Notes

[1]   I searched for 'alcohol OR drink★' at five-yearly intervals from 1965 to 2000. *The Times* recorded a lower number of hits for these keywords in 1975 than in 1970 but every other result across both newspapers showed a consistent upward trajectory. In *The Times* there were 1,159 hits for 1965 and 4,991 for 2000. In *The Guardian*, there were 1,302 hits for 1965 and 5,324 for 2000. Roughly speaking there was a fourfold increase in the total number of references to 'alcohol OR drink★' between 1965 and 2000 across both newspapers.

[2]   Hall, Stuart, Critcher, Chas, Jefferson, Tony, Clarke, John, and Roberts, Brian, *Policing the Crisis: Mugging, the State and Law and Order*, Basingstoke: Macmillan, 1978.

[3]   Bauman, Zygmunt, 'Social Issues of Law and Order', *British Journal of Criminology*, 2000, vol 40 (2), pp 205-221.

[4]   Cavadino, Michael, and Dignan, James, *The Penal System* (4th edition), London: Sage Publications, 2007, pp 26-27; Muncie, John, *Youth and Crime* (3rd edition), London: Sage Publications, 2009, pp 139-140.

[5]   Simon, Jonathan, *Governing Through Crime: How the War on Crime Transformed American Democracy and Created a Culture of Fear*, Oxford: Oxford University Press, 2007, p 4. For a more British perspective, see: Crawford, Adam, 'Governing through Anti-Social Behaviour: Regulatory Challenges to Criminal Justice', *British Journal of Criminology*, 2009, vol 49 (6), pp 810-831.

[6]   Rowbotham and Stevenson, *Behaving Badly*.

[7]   'Postscript: To the Author of the *London Chronicle*', *London Chronicle*, 10 August 1758.

[8]   Homo, 'Abuse of Spirituous Liquor', *The Times*, 4 January 1830.

[9]   Farrar, F.W., 'Drink and Crime', *Fortnightly Review*, 1893, vol 3 (Jan-June), p 790.

[10] Croydon, H.H., '"A Great Opportunity": To the Editor of *The Times*', *The Times*, 8 March 1915.

[11] Nellis, Mike, 'Humanising Justice: The English Probation Service up to 1972', in Gelsthorpe, Loraine, and Morgan, Rod (eds) *Handbook of Probation*, Cullompton: Willan, 2007, pp 25-58.

[12] For a fuller discussion of the link between alcohol and crime, see: Dingwall, Gavin, *Alcohol and Crime*, Cullompton: Willan, 2006.

[13] Fox, Kate, 'Understanding Alcohol', *Four Thought*, BBC Radio 4, 12 October 2011, www.bbc.co.uk/programmes/b015p86z

[14] I have explored the connection of evidence to policy making in regards to alcohol in more detail elsewhere. See: Yeomans, Henry, 'Blurred Visions: Experts, Evidence and Alcohol Policy', in Holmwood, John, and Smith, Alex T. (eds) *Sociologies of Moderation*, Oxford: Wiley Blackwell, 2013.

[15] Thom, *Dealing with Drink*, pp 85-104.

[16] Baggott, *Alcohol, Politics and Social Policy*, p 32; Plant and Plant, *Binge Britain*, p 55; World Health Organization, 'Levels of Consumption, *European Information Systems on Alcohol and Health*, http://apps.who.int/ghodata/?theme=GISAH &region=euro

[17] See: Barr, *Drink*, pp 144-146.

[18] Hayward and Hobbs, 'Beyond the Binge'; see also: Hadfield, *Bar Wars*; Winlow and Hall, *Violent Night*.

[19] Measham, Fiona, and Brain, Kevin, 'Binge Drinking, British Alcohol Policy and the New Culture of Intoxication', *Crime, Media, Culture*, 2005, vol 1 (3), p 262.

[20] Moriarty and Gilmore, 'Licensing Britain's Alcohol Epidemic', p 94.

[21] Kettle, Martin, 'Alcoholic Britain Should Not Be Offered Another Drink', *The Guardian*, 2 January 2003.

[22] 'The Day in Politics: Lords Defeat for Government over Alcohol Sales at Garages', *The Guardian*, 1 April 1988.

[23] 'A Long Drink this Summer', *The Guardian*, 6 August 1988.

[24] 'Lord's Slip Means an Extra Round on Sundays', *The Times*, 23 April 1988; 'Parliament: Drinking Hours Mistake Admitted', *The Times*, 28 April 1988.

[25] 'A Long Drink this Summer', *The Guardian*, 6 August 1988.

[26] Erlichman, James, 'Tipplers on the Retreat Despite Yobbo Man', *The Guardian*, 21 June 1988.

[27] 'Waking up to the Old Demon Drink', *The Guardian*, 21 June 1988.

[28] Erlichman, James, 'Tipplers on the Retreat Despite Yobbo Man', *The Guardian*, 21 June 1988.

[29] 'Demand for More Police Officers', *The Times*, 4 November 1988.

[30] Wintour, Patrick, 'The Day in Politics: Landlords Face Mild and Bitter Changes', *The Guardian*, 19 January 1988.

[31] Fletcher, Martin, 'Under-age Drinking Move', *The Times*, 19 January 1988.

[32] Erlichman, James, 'Tipplers on the Retreat Despite Yobbo Man', *The Guardian*, 21 June 1988.

[33] Wintour, Patrick, 'Government "Fails Drink Abuse Test"', *The Guardian*, 21 June 1988.

[34] Beach, Kathy, 'Views Split in Scottish Fling', *The Guardian*, 20 August 1988.

[35] Plant and Plant, *Binge Britain*, p 124.

[36] For a fuller analysis of the social reaction to the Heysel disaster, see: Young, Kevin, '"The Killing Field": Themes in the Mass Media Responses to the Heysel Stadium Riot', *International Review for the Sociology of Sport*, 1986, vol 21 (2-3), pp 253–266.

[37] Murray, Ian, 'How Alcohol, Boredom and Rivalry Killed Fans and Reputations', *The Times*, 31 May 1985.

[38] 'Yet Another Enemy Within', *The Guardian*, 26 March 1985.

[39] Which occasions were designated as 'sporting events' for the purposes of the Act was left to the discretion of government ministers. Football matches are typically defined as such while spectators of other sports are often still permitted to consume alcohol.

[40] Gunn, Sheila, 'Alcohol Sales Ban at Garages', *The Times*, 1 April 1988; 'The Day in Politics: Lords Defeat for Government over Alcohol Sales at Garages', *The Guardian*, 1 April 1988.

[41] 'Parliament: Licensing Law Change Wins MPs' Approval', *The Times*, 4 February 1988.

[42] Oakley, Robin, and Evans, Peter, 'Hurd Plans Drive Against Lax Landlords and Drink-Crime', *The Times*, 9 July 1988.

[43] Wintour, Patrick, 'New Curbs on Violence', *The Guardian*, 12 July 1988.

[44] Oakley, Robin, 'Schools "Must Tackle Crime"', *The Times*, 12 July 1988.

[45] Ibid.

[46] Ibid.

[47] Evans, Peter, 'Courts Told Not to Shrink from Duty', *The Times*, 16 July 1988.

[48] Longsley, Clifford, 'City with a Sense of Religion', *The Times*, 10 June 1985.

[49] Wintour, Patrick, 'New Curbs on Violence', *The Guardian*, 12 July 1988.

[50] Oakley, Robin, 'Schools "Must Tackle Crime"', *The Times*, 12 July 1988.

[51] Ibid.

[52] Evans, Peter, 'Hurd Urges Action on Drink', *The Times*, 29 June 1988.

[53] Burgess, Charles, 'Sports Writers Brief Thatcher on Riot', *The Guardian*, 1 June 1985.

[54] Davies, David, 'Letters: Affluent Fans Lead Fighting', *The Observer*, 9 June 1985.

[55] 'Demand for More Police Officers', *The Times*, 4 November 1988.

[56] Naughtie, James, 'Year's Exile "Not Enough as PM Seeks New Laws"', *The Guardian*, 1 June 1985.

[57] Measham and Brain, 'New Culture of Intoxication'.

[58] Ibid, p 274.

[59]   Ibid, p 262.

[60]   UK Government, 'Licensing Act 2003 – Explanatory Notes', www.legislation.gov.uk/ukpga/2003/17/contents

[61]   Under Section 13, 'interested parties' are defined as people living or conducting business in the vicinity of the premises or bodies representing such people. 'Responsible authorities' include a variety of persons such as police chiefs, fire authorities and planning authorities.

[62]   The Estcourt Act 1828 stipulated that licensed premises could not open during the hours of morning service on Sunday. But, otherwise, opening times were not restricted until the 1830s. See: Harrison, *Drink and the Victorians*, pp 328-329.

[63]   Kettle, Martin, 'Alcoholic Britain Should Not Be Offered Another Drink', *The Guardian*, 2 January 2003.

[64]   Ibid.

[65]   Kettle, Martin, 'My Name is Britain and I Have a Drink Problem', *The Guardian*, 31 May 2003.

[66]   For example, see: Bridge, Richard, Jones, Cheryl, Rodney, Mike, and Laurie Watt, 'Does Licensing Bill Threaten Freedom?', *Daily Telegraph*, 7 January 2003; Cumming, Tim, 'Stop that Fiddling', *The Guardian*, 28 January 2003.

[67]   Hope, Jenny, 'Raise Drink Prices to Fight Crime and Ill-Health, say Doctors', *Daily Mail*, 5 March 2004.

[68]   Ibid.

[69]   Jayatilaka, Geethika, 'Alcohol Misuse Must Be Tackled If We Are Serious About Cutting Crime', *The Times*, 1 November 2004; Tendler, Stewart, 'Police Fear Car Crime, Drink and Disaffection', *The Times*, 22 November 2004.

[70]   Hinscliff, Gaby, 'Bingeing Women Fuel Crime', *The Observer*, 18 July 2004.

[71]   Elliott, Larry, 'This Crackdown Won't Cut Drink-Fuelled Crime', *The Guardian*, 7 May 2004.

[72]   Bennetto, Jason, 'Alcohol Blamed for Soaring Levels of Violent Crime', *The Independent*, 30 April 2004.

[73]   Alleyne, R., 'New Drinks Law "Delays Disorder for an Hour"', *Daily Telegraph*, 19 November 2005.

[74]   Townsend, Mark, and Hinscliff, Gaby, 'New Drink Laws Spark Rape Fears', *The Observer*, 27 November 2005.

[75]   Travis, Alan, Muir, Hugh, and Crown, Rosie, 'Government Admits New Drinking Hours Could Lead to Increase in Offences', *The Guardian*, 23 November 2005.

[76]   Plant and Plant, *Binge Britain*, p 100.

[77]   Ibid, p 109.

[78]   Hickley, Matthew, 'How Drink Helped Fuel the Rise in Violent Crime', *Daily Mail*, 21 October 2005.

[79]   Ibid.

[80] 'Time Will Tell', *The Sun*, 22 January 2005.

[81] 'Ministers "should rethink 24-hour drinking law"', *Daily Mail*, 13 January 2005.

[82] '24-hour Drinking Reform in Chaos', *Daily Mail*, 17 January 2005.

[83] Plant and Plant, *Binge Britain*, p 108.

[84] 'Violence Fear Over New Drink Laws', *BBC News*, 10 August 2005.

[85] Travis et al, 'Government admits new drinking hours...'.

[86] Hadfield, Phil, and Measham, Fiona, 'After the Act: Alcohol Licensing and the Administrative Governance of Crime', *Criminology and Public Policy*, 2010, vol 9 (1), p 72.

[87] Department for Culture, Media and Sport, 'Evaluation of the Impact of the Licensing Act 2003', 2008, www.culture.gov.uk/images/publications/Licensingevaluation.pdf

[88] Office for National Statistics, 'Crime in England and Wales: Year Ending December 2012', 2013, www.ons.gov.uk/ons/dcp171778_307458.pdf

[89] British Beer and Pub Association, 'Licensing Anniversary YouGov Poll – Whoops No Apocalypse', 2006, www.beerandpub.com/newsList_detail.aspx?newsId=122

[90] The Licensing Act 2003 also created Early Morning Restriction Orders. These have been enhanced by the Coalition Government's Police and Social Responsibility Act 2011 and allow local authorities to restrict opening hours of licensed premises between midnight and 6am.

[91] See: Morgan, Rod, *Summary Justice: Fast – but Fair?*, London: Centre for Criminal Justice Studies, 2008.

[92] It is interesting to note that while the discretionary powers of the magistracy over licensing were being scrapped, the police's discretionary powers to discipline drinkers were being vastly inflated.

[93] Prince, Rosa, 'No Takers for Alcohol Disorder Zones', *Daily Telegraph*, 22 July 2009. The Police and Social Responsibility Act 2011 made similar provisions for local authorities to charge late-night licensed premises for the cost of policing and other arrangements made in connection with drinking between midnight and 6am.

[94] Again, this enhanced discretionary power has been controversial. See: Crawford, Adam, and Lister, Stuart, *The Use and Impact of Dispersal Orders*, Bristol: The Policy Press, 2007.

[95] Ibid.

[96] This change brought statute into line with case law. The Queen's Bench Divisional Court ruled in 1988 that test purchase evidence is admissible in court providing it has been fairly obtained by police (*The Times*, 19 April 1988).

[97] In slightly different forms, these offences are present in Sections 168, 172, and 173 of the Licensing Act 1964.

98 Home Office, 'Tough New Powers to Tackle Alcohol Crime Announced', 2010, http://webarchive.nationalarchives.gov.uk/+/http://www.homeoffice.gov.uk/about-us/news/powers-tackle-alcohol-crime.html

99 Dunstan, Steven, *General Lifestyle Survey Overview: A Report on the 2010 General Lifestyle Survey*, Newport: Office for National Statistics, 2012; 'Alcohol Consumption "Continues to Fall"', *BBC News*, 3 September 2010.

100 Dickson, E. Jane, 'It's Not a Crime for Women to Get Drunk: It's Just Not Very Clever', *The Independent*, 26 November 2005.

101 *R v Bree* [2007] EWCA Crim 256.

102 Dickson, E. Jane, 'It's Not a Crime for Women to Get Drunk. It's Just Not Very Clever', *The Independent*, 26 November 2005.

103 'Midland Circuit', *The Times*, 6 December 1856.

104 This may be the case in instances of male rape also but, in the reports I found, the victims were female.

105 Perrie, Robin, 'Revellers "Field Hospital"', *The Sun*, 23 November 2005.

106 Wooding, David, 'Medics Fear 24-hour Pubs', *The Sun*, 3 January 2005.

107 Kavanagh, Trevor, 'Cops' Late Drink Warning', *The Sun*, 10 August 2005.

108 'A Drink Sodden Law that No One Wants', *Daily Mail*, 12 January 2005.

109 'Blunkett Voiced Concerns over 24-hour Drinking', *Daily Mail*, 16 January 2005.

110 Plant and Plant, *Binge Britain*, p 100.

111 Linklater, Magnus, 'The Terrible Cost of Not Raising Drink Prices', *The Times*, 17 March 2009.

112 Slack, James, and Hinkley, Matthew, 'Drink Crime: It Will Go Up', *Daily Mail*, 16 November 2005.

113 Plant and Plant, *Binge Britain*, p 124.

114 Sumner, Maggie, and Parker, Howard, *Low in Alcohol: A Review of International Research into Alcohol's Role in Crime Causation*, London: Portman Group, 1995.

115 '24-hour Pub Cop Fury', *The Sun*, 8 July 2004.

116 Townsend, Mark, and Hinscliff, Gaby, 'New Drink Laws Spark Rape Fears', *The Observer*, 27 November 2005.

117 Britten, Nick, 'Judge Says 24-hour Drinking Will Create "Urban Savages"', *Daily Telegraph*, 11 January 2005.

118 Dalrymple, Theodore, 'Our Binge Drinking Culture is a Living Hell for Everyone', *Daily Express*, 13 August 2010.

119 'Binge Drinking Adverts Launched', *BBC News*, 4 May 2008.

120 Home Office, 'Alcohol – Know Your Limits', 2008, http://news.bbc.co.uk/1/hi/uk/7457746.stm

121 'Warning Over Booze Britain', *Sunday Express*, 15 April 2007.

122 Taylor, Ben, Hickley, Matthew, and Narain, Jaya, 'A Year On, This is Binge Britain', *Daily Mail*, 16 October 2006.

[123] '24-hour Pub Opening "A Disaster"', *BBC News*, 18 October 2005.

[124] Ibid.

[125] Harrison, *Drink and the Victorians*, p 377.

[126] Williams, Roger, 'Sober Lessons about Drink', *The Observer*, 27 November 2005.

[127] 'Time Will Tell', *The Sun*, 22 January 2005.

[128] World Health Organization, 'Global Status Report on Alcohol', pp 11-12; Burroughs, A., and McNamara, D., 'Liver Disease in Europe', 2003, *Alimentary Pharmacology and Therapeutics*, 2003, vol 18 (3), pp 54-59.

[129] Fickling, David, 'Alcohol Consumption': Raising a Glass to the Health of a Nation', *The Independent*, 28 October 2005.

[130] For further discussion, see: Yeomans, Henry, 'Revisiting a Moral Panic: Attitudes to Alcohol, Ascetic Protestantism and the Implementation of the Licensing Act 2003', *Sociological Research Online*, 2009, vol 14 (2), www.socresonline.org.uk/14/2/6.html

[131] Hickley, Matthew, 'Faliraki UK', *Daily Mail*, 10 February 2006.

[132] 'The Alcohol Culture and a Spiralling Rate of Crime', *Daily Telegraph*, 6 February 2007.

[133] Bates, Daniel, '24-hour Drink Laws Crime Soaring', *Daily Mail*, 23 February 2008.

[134] Beadles, Jeremy, 'Reply Letters and Emails', *The Guardian*, 5 February 2008.

[135] Sulkunen has made a parallel point about liberalising reforms implemented in Nordic countries in the 1960s. These were not driven by respective states embracing intoxication as a positive but efforts to reduce problematic spirits-drinking by improving the quality and availability of beer. See: Sulkunen, *The Saturated Society*, p 104.

[136] This is true in the political and press discourses I examined at least.

[137] Hencke, David, and Sparrow, Andrew, 'Gordon Brown Rejects Call to Set Minimum Prices for Alcohol', *The Guardian*, 16 March 2009.

[138] 'Plans for Minimum Alcohol Price', *BBC News*, 15 March 2009.

[139] I have placed 'moderate' in inverted commas to acknowledge the fact that moderation in alcohol is a relative concept, which is variably defined by different groups. See: Yeomans, Henry, 'Blurred Visions: Experts, Evidence and Alcohol Policy', in Holmwood, John, and Smith, Alex T. (eds) *Sociologies of Moderation*, Oxford: Wiley, 2013.

[140] 'Alcohol Warnings Could Become Compulsory', *The Guardian*, 15 February 2010. Such warnings were part of the voluntary code of measures that the government agreed with drinks industry groups in 2007, although was not universally implemented.

[141] Hunt, *Governing Morals*.

[142] Whitehead, Tom, 'Alcohol-fuelled Crime Costs UK £13bn a Year', *Daily Telegraph*, 26 December 2009.

[143] 'A Drink Sodden Law that No One Wants', *Daily Mail*, 12 January 2005.

[144] Kettle, Martin, 'My Name is Britain and I Have a Drink Problem', *The Guardian*, 31 May 2003.

[145] UK Government, *Safe, Sensible, Social*, London: Department of Health, 2007. 'Harmful drinkers' are defined as women who drink more than 35 units of alcohol per week and men who drink more than 50 units per week.

[146] Critcher, Chas, 'Moral Panics: A Case Study of Binge Drinking', in Franklin, Bob (ed) *Pulling Newspapers Apart*, Abingdon: Routledge, 2008, pp 154-162.

[147] The challenge that health professionals have posed to this dominant position will be explored in the next chapter.

[148] Corrigan and Sayer, *The Great Arch*.

[149] Ruonavaara, 'Moral Regulation'.

[150] 'Drink Campaign to Target Parents', *BBC News*, 1 June 2008.

[151] 'That portion of the British public...', *The Times*, 9 August 1872.

[152] 'Conservatism in Lancashire', *Reynolds's Daily Newspaper*, 8 September 1872.

[153] UK Government, *Safe, Sensible, Social*.

[154] 'Alcohol the "New British Disease"', *BBC News*, 20 May 2004.

[155] Roberts, Bob, 'Gordon Brown Exclusive: Any Shop Twice Caught Selling Alcohol to U18s Should Lose its Licence', *Daily Mirror*, 3 October 2008.

[156] O'Malley, Pat, and Valverde, Mariana, 'Pleasure, Freedom and Drugs: The Uses of Pleasure in Liberal Governance of Drug and Alcohol Consumption', *Sociology*, 2004, vol 38 (1), pp 27-28.

[157] Rose and Miller, 'Political Power Beyond the State'.

SEVEN

Health, harm and risk

Introduction

Chapter Six identified efforts to morally regulate drinking within law and public discourse relating to crime and disorder in the late 20th and early 21st centuries, and found that these efforts were/are, to some degree, shaped by Victorian temperance attitudes. Along with crime and disorder, the other major social problem associated with alcohol in contemporary society is ill-health. Alcohol is consistently connected to a variety of health problems, including liver disease, heart disease, pancreatitis, foetal alcohol spectrum disorder (FASD) and certain types of cancer. Such forms of harm are associated with any forms of excessive consumption but especially with alcoholism, whose sufferers are usually defined by their habitual, compulsive or uncontrolled drinking. To deal with some of these problems, there has been: a promotion of abstinence from alcohol for young people under the age of 15;[1] experiments with bans on super-strength beer and cider;[2] demands for forceful clampdowns on the number of licensed premises entirely in so-called 'binge towns';[3] calls for a total ban on all alcohol advertising and sponsorship;[4] enhanced monitoring of patients' drinking by GPs;[5] and most prominently, persistent campaigns for the imposition of a minimum unit price to reduce the affordability of alcoholic drinks.

The significance and prevalence of alcohol-related health problems has been a magnetic topic for public debate and regulatory projects in recent years. Interestingly, public discourse on alcohol and health has been increasingly shaped by a variety of campaign groups, including public health organisations and professional medical bodies. Minimum unit pricing (MUP), in particular, has been tirelessly promoted by such groups.[6] The prominence of doctors, surgeons and epidemiologists within this health-focused discourse might imply that a more evidence-based approach to the social problem of alcohol, disconnected from the moralistic attitudes of the past, is emerging. Such a transformation would be consistent with the apparent triumph of the harm-based libertarianism of Hart over the legal moralism of Devlin in the 1960s, described in Chapter Five. It would also resonate with the macro picture of social change painted by sociologists Ulrich Beck and Anthony

Giddens, in which the rise of a social order dominated by rational, secular assessments of catastrophic risk serves to sideline more traditional moral considerations.[7] In regards to alcohol, to what extent is this accurate? Does this new public health coalition espouse a historically novel, scientific approach to alcohol? Have projects to morally regulate drinking been altered by these issues of health, harm and risk?

This chapter examines the development of drinking as a health problem from the 18th century onwards. It includes sections on health broadly as well as alcoholism specifically. Although sometimes characterised as a moral, social or psychological condition, it is usual in current parlance to frame alcoholism as ostensibly a health problem of some form. Its discursive development also tends to run parallel to the construction of wider alcohol-related health problems in the sense that two significant shifts have been identified in their recent histories. These are, first, the replacement of traditional and explicitly moral understandings of drink problems with medical ideas in the mid-20th century and, second, the emergence of a public health-oriented approach to governing drink in the late 20th century, which concentrated on total per capita consumption.[8] With an intensive concern for developments in the 1960s and 2000s, this chapter examines the changing construction of alcohol as a health problem through time.[9]

Drink, health and moral health until the 1960s

Historians and social scientists studying health discourse related to alcohol tend to identify a new approach that has developed since the mid-20th century. The 'value-based morality' of the temperance movement is seen to have been replaced by medical or scientific understandings of alcohol-related health problems.[10] Thom examines how the medically inspired 'disease model' of alcoholism attained dominance over the older 'moral model' during this period.[11] Nicholls further describes how 'the moral argumentation' of temperance activists was replaced by the apparently 'morally neutral language of science' in which the consequences of drinking are awarded primary importance.[12] Sulkunen argues that consensus on what constitutes the moral 'good life', as well as the legitimacy to promote this through public regulation, has been overridden by a process of 'normative neutralization'.[13] He claims that the saturation of contemporary Western societies with the principle of universal individuality has fatally weakened efforts to impose morals, including healthier lifestyles, on others. Do these developments indicate that, by the 1960s, the projects to morally regulate drinking had weakened?

The emergence of public health

The 'ulcer in the social body'

For much of history, alcoholic drinks were regarded as healthy. In part, this was because beer provided a safer alternative to water. The reasons water was often unsafe only began to be understood when Dr John Snow linked the outbreak of cholera in London in 1848–49 to the contaminated water supplied by the Broad Street Pump. But, as Barr describes, people all over the world had been aware that drinking water was potentially hazardous long before Snow's research.[14] Alcoholic drinks were not just safer beverages, they were also widely regarded as possessing certain health too. Whisky, for example, was believed by many to ward off influenza until at least the early 20th century[15] and beer was seen as an 'article of diet',[16] a normal foodstuff, for much of the 19th century. Burnett provides some support for the latter idea by calculating that, in the 17th century at least, beer provided 20 to 25% of an average person's required calorie intake.[17] Alcohol, beer particularly, was healthy and nutritious; the brewers were not, therefore, discordant with many people's opinions when they claimed that beer is a 'food beverage' and 'part of the strength of Britain'[18] during the First World War. Chapter Four noted that it became common to refer to teetotallers as 'pussyfoots' after the visit to Britain of US prohibitionist William 'Pussyfoot' Johnson in 1919. While the term might literally mean cautious or stealthy, it was commonly used pejoratively to imply indecision, timidity or fear.[19] Drinkers, by implication, were strong, brave and decisive.

Nevertheless, alcohol has also been connected to a variety of health problems since at least the 18th century. In 1729, the *London Journal* discussed how excessive consumption of meat or drink was 'pernicious to the Health and Vigour of any Person, in the Discharge of the Offices of Life'.[20] Later in the century, a letter from 'Setaymot' in the *Public Advertiser* reiterated these beliefs, stating that health of the body and mind could be improved with 'sobriety, gentleness, and temperance in meats, drinks, and exercises'.[21] These habits of cleanliness and sobriety, Setaymot continued, bestow virtue upon the observer; it is through this 'inward principle' that such persons 'are not subject to indispositions, nor molested with fevers; their heads are not dulled with fumes, nor their stomachs oppressed with fainting fits, or windy gripping humours; they rise fresh as the morning sun'.[22] It was common for excessive drinking to be connected to such broad, ill-defined health complaints, although some commentators were more specific about the ailments they associated with alcohol. On the subject of drink in 1710, the *Athenian News* asked: 'How many Diseases flow from that vitious [sic] fountain? How many are fed and nourished by it?', before specifically identifying gout, which can 'bring Pain enough with it, so as to make a few Years seem an Age', as one such disease.[23] The *Athenian News*, however, pointed out that gout was a 'Danger of Drunkenness' and a product of intemperance. The good and bad properties of alcohol were thus mediated by the concept of 'temperance', defined as restraint or balance in personal diet and lifestyle.

In 1754, the *Public Advertiser* noted that 'health is, more than is commonly thought, in a Man's own Power' and the reward of temperance is that 'one immediately feels its good Effects'.[24] If general personal restraint improves wellbeing, then health (and ill-health) is in the hands of the individual. Writing in *World*, 'Academicus' elaborated further:

> The thinking part of man being allowed to be a modification of matter, it must be supposed to be a part of the body.... Hence it will indisputably follow, that all powers of the mind, even the moral faculties, are inseparably connected with the temperament and habit of that body, of which she is part. Insomuch that prudence (the foundation of all morality) as well as justice, fortitude and temperance (the other cardinal virtues) and their opposites entirely depend upon the constitution. It will therefore become the province of the physician to extirpate the vicious habits of mankind, and introduce the contrary; to suppress luxury, and create chastity; to make the foolish prudent; the proud humble.... And all this is easy to be done, by the assistance of alternative medicines, and by a properly adapted regimen, that shall be perfective of each virtue, and repugnant to each vice.[25]

The body and mind were inseparable and morality of the body, expressed through the 'properly adapted regimen', was believed to improve the virtuosity of the mind. Individuals were responsible for their own physical and mental wellbeing; a virtuous life led to good health and, by inference, an intemperate life led to ill-health. Either way, health was fused to moral health.

The virtuous practice of temperance mediated between the purported good and bad effects of alcohol in the 18th century. To an extent, this approach continued to be evident in the 19th century. In 1830, the *Derby Mercury* recognised alcohol's two faces by attacking the Beer Act on the grounds that it would discourage working men from taking beverages home to their families where they would be consumed as a 'bodily nutrient, and not a moral poison'.[26] But the rise of the temperance movement and the turn to teetotalism in the 1830s signified a hardening in attitudes as alcohol became associated with a larger number of often serious conditions. Some of these aetiological connections, such as the *Morning Chronicle*'s statement that a man's consumption of spirits would 'ruin his health by destroying his liver',[27] are now clinically established. Others have been discredited, as Barr highlights by describing how in the 1830s and 1840s temperance supporters blamed alcohol for the cholera epidemics.[28] In addition to highlighting alcohol's negative effects, teetotal pioneer Joseph Livesey sought to repudiate the positive nutritional value of beer. In his famous 'Malt Lecture', Livesey endeavoured to extract the 'spirit' from beer and then burn it in order to show its lack of value. He argued that the brewing process removed nutrients from beer, leaving only one penny's worth of nutrition in a gallon of beer worth one shilling and four pence.[29] Although faith in alcohol's positive effects survived, they were increasingly challenged in the 19th century with the negative effects conversely emphasised.

For Victorian teetotallers, a temperate lifestyle was still a route to health and virtue as it had been for the Georgians. But as Livesey and others dismissed the merits of moderate drinking or beer drinking, temperance was redefined as abstinence from all forms of alcohol. In 1841, W. Hunt claimed that alcohol was a poison that could not be digested; it remained in the body and, in a twist on the temperance preoccupation with 'the struggle', became engaged in a 'war of extermination' with capillaries.[30] Lawrence Heyworth echoed these points in *The Times* in 1856, stating that alcohol was an indigestible and 'virulent poison'.[31] This characterisation of alcohol problematised any form of consumption; W. Hunt quoted Dr Charles A. Lee's claim that even 'the moderate use of, so called, alcoholic drinks tends directly to debilitate the digestive organs, to cloud the understanding, weaken the memory, unfix the attention, and confuse all the mental operations, besides inducing a host of nervous maladies'.[32] As Geo A. Smith explained, all drinking was poisonous and so moderate drinking was simply 'moderated indulgence in a narcotic–acrid poison'.[33] Interestingly, these medical or scientific claims mirrored the moral discourse of the time. Chapter Two described how, as drinking was constructed as a slippery slope to intemperance, all drinking became tantamount to intemperance and therefore sinful. Equally, as alcohol became understood as an indigestible poison, so even moderate consumption was seen as damaging to individual health.

As well as an individual problem, the effect of drinking on health soon became viewed as a social problem. It was in the Victorian period that public health became a major concern for government. In 1842, Edwin Chadwick presented his *Report on the Sanitary Condition of the Labouring Population of Great Britain* to Parliament and called for much greater state involvement in the improvement of sanitary conditions in towns and cities.[34] The subsequent Public Health Act 1848 authorised the formation of local boards in certain areas, which would be tasked with improving facilities such as sewage systems, but it was not until the passage of the Public Health Act 1875 that more robust requirements for authorities to provide drainage and water supply were implemented. In the wake of work by Snow as well as Louis Pasteur, diseases became increasingly recognised as either contagious or connected to the social environment. So the new approach to public health could be justified in utilitarian terms as compromising the autonomy of some for the benefit of many.[35] Many people, however, were distinctly displeased at the transformation of their bodies into a political subject to be shaped and governed; the Anti-Compulsory Vaccination League campaigned against the tendency for governments, as demonstrated by the Vaccination Acts 1853 and 1867, to engage in what Rowbotham calls 'legislating for your own good'.[36] It has already been described how temperance advocates promoted the idea that alcohol was a purely negative influence on health in this period. Given the emerging eminence of what Foucault calls 'bio-politics',[37] alcohol increasingly became a public health problem as well as a threat to the individual.

This new biopolitics was partially expressed in the language used to describe drink problems. Kneale examines how, in Victorian temperance discourse, 'the wider context is reproduced as a dangerous space of seduction … as an environment contaminated by drink'[38] and his research found further evidence to suggest that, by the early 20th century, the semantics of contamination were used more widely. Chapter Five examined how, in the early 20th century, concerns for maternal behaviour were articulated in reference to the need, as expressed at a meeting of the Women's Total Abstinence Union, 'to protect the child life of the nation against the contamination of the public-house bar'.[39] In the inter-war years, demands for restrictions on youth drinking were justified in reference to medical evidence showing that alcohol use by adolescents harmed their brains and nerves. These specific claims were made by a group of teachers who were not identified as temperance supporting but argued that without legal intervention 'the lure of drink and the contamination of the tap-room' would undo the good effects of expanding education.[40] Worryingly, the contaminating potency of drink was not believed to be limited to the drinker and constituted a threat to the drinker's children and grandchildren. Fred Mackenzie claimed that the great-grandsons of 'three-bottle men' were now paying for their forebears' excesses in 'hereditary gout'.[41] Public houses were no longer just a 'terrible temptation'[42] to the individual drinker, but also posed the threat of contamination to present and future generations.

The dominance of the Classical or Christian concept of 'temperance' in the Georgian discussions of health shows that alcohol consumption was positioned within a moral context. But the emphasis on alcohol's negative properties propagated by teetotallers, and the conception of the issue in public health terms, led to the decline of temperance as an individual mediator of alcohol's apparent advantages and disadvantages. By the early 20th century, individuals' bodies had been positioned within a legal or political context and redefined as potential sites for government intervention. Drink became, as *Lloyd's Daily Newspaper* put it, 'the ulcer in the social body'.[43]

The spreading 'social disease'

In the early 1960s, the expansion of health conditions with which alcohol was linked was noticeable. The *Daily Express* connected alcohol consumption with heart disease,[44] and *The Times* reported on research by the World Health Organization, which linked drinking to cancers of the mouth, larynx and oesophagus.[45] In 1963, *The Guardian* described alcohol, malnutrition and syphilis as the 'major known environmental causes' of mental illness[46] and, in 1965, the same newspaper reported that alcoholism was, in some degree, a product of 'mental disturbances'.[47] *The Times* reported on a lecture by Dr B.G.B. Lucas at the Royal Institute of Public Health and Hygiene in which he claimed that drinking 'was a form of escapism' that, by allowing man 'to climb down his genealogical tree occasionally', enabled some form of temporary evolutionary regression.[48] As well as these direct effects of personal harm and temporary de-civilisation, drinking and alcoholism particularly were also connected to wider, indirect harm inflicted on people other than the drinker. *The Times* claimed that alcoholism was an 'industrial liability' that cost the economy between £30 million and £40 million per year in absence from work[49] and, speaking at the General Medical Council, Lord Cohen claimed that 'the victim of alcoholism gradually loses his efficiency as a worker and a spouse'.[50] Cohen said that this loss of efficiency led to family breakdown, which in turn produced juvenile delinquency. Partially supporting this point, Edgar Myers wrote in *The Observer* that wives therefore had to play a part in supporting alcoholic husbands and encouraging them to change their behaviour.[51] Alcohol was linked to a variety of direct and indirect harms.

Alcohol also featured heavily in an emerging topic of diet and fitness. In 1963, the *Daily Express* quoted Russian distance runner Vladimir Kuc warning that 'even the smallest dose of vodka or wine taken before a competition becomes the long-distance runner's deadliest foe'.[52] But it was not just elite athletes who were to use alcohol warily; the *Daily Express* claimed that alcohol slowed the rate at which the body burned surplus fat[53] and another article stressed the impact on bodily weight of the calorie content of most alcoholic drinks.[54] There appears to have been a growing recognition that regular drinking may compromise both fitness and figure. The *Daily Mirror* reported on an exclusive Texan 'beauty farm' where rich women paid to be transformed through, among other things, abstinence from alcohol.[55] In 1964 and 1965, the *Daily Express* repeatedly insisted that moderation or abstinence from alcohol was necessary to lose weight and acquire 'a perfect body'.[56] A column by a 'family doctor' also advised husbands that 'if a woman's plump and jolly put her on a diet', which included decreased drinking.[57] Alcohol was seen to contribute to excess weight and lack of fitness and, concomitantly, reduced alcohol intake was repackaged as part of a regime of physical wellbeing, which particularly concentrated on women.

As with crime and disorder, many of the health problems connected to alcohol were specifically associated with young people. A report published by the British Medical Association in 1961 described the situation: 'With their scooters, motor cycles, and even cars, well-lined wage packets and sense of liberation from the constricting discipline of school, today's young people saw themselves as able to enjoy their youth for a few brief years before being submitted to the maturer discipline of marriage.'[58] But this newfound freedom bore consequences; Dr N.A. Ross blamed an increase in venereal disease (VD) among teenagers on 'American servicemen, too much money, alcohol and lack of sex education'.[59] Other articles expanded on the 'well known relationship'[60] of drink to VD, which was encapsulated by the story of Joan. Featured in the *Daily Mirror*, Joan was 'a lively and jolly secretary who passed her GCE and left school only a few months ago'. Joan had never had sex and 'had never touched alcohol before' but, after having a few drinks at a party, ended up having sex and contracting VD.[61] A rise in illegitimate births was also seen as a problem growing from teenage sexual promiscuity; Dr H. Mackenzie-Wintle blamed high wages paid to under-educated teenagers for this trend.[62] The concentration of moral discourse on young people, particularly women, was identified within wider debates around alcohol in Chapter Five. Discourse on drink as a health problem was similarly related to the emerging demographic category of youth and the broader moral crisis, exacerbated by affluence, seen to be affecting this group.

As well as affluence and lack of education, Mackenzie-Wintle attributed these problems to teenagers being 'ceaselessly bombarded by pornographic literature and films, and shouted at from every hoarding to drink more alcohol'.[63] In a letter to *The Guardian*, Wilfrid Winterton similarly attacked 'the continuous high-pressure salesmanship to promote social drinking'[64] and the influence of advertising was discussed in a House of Lords debate on why young people become alcoholics.[65] This comment has some resonance given the positive messages described in Chapter Six, such as 'Don't you feel marvellous? People who drink Cossack Vodka do', which suffused drink advertising during this period. A page of the *Daily Mirror* in 1963 captured this point aptly by featuring an article connecting alcohol to heart disease, 'the greatest killer in Britain today', directly adjacent to an advert for Gaymer's cider, which read: 'Have Gaymer's, Have Fun.... For a quick trip to feeling on top of the world – have Gaymer's!'.[66] This odd juxtaposition reflected the flat contradiction between discourse on health, which increasingly connected alcohol to a variety of direct and indirect harms, and adverts that featured brazenly positive representations of specific products and the effect they would purportedly have on one's life. Furthermore, the salience of concern about this type of advertising constructed the individual drinker or the troublesome teenager as something of a victim; the product of a failure to reign in problematic economic forces.

In 1961, *The Times* discussed a report by the British Medical Association, which argued that young people were not to blame for the 'moral climate of our day'. Churches had ceased to be attractive to young people and so the report stressed 'a great need to encourage the development of a higher standard of morality and a greater reward for spiritual values in the home'. Parents, as well as schools and doctors, were therefore called upon to ensure that 'alcohol and drinking at an early age were to be deprecated'.[67] Speaking at a British Medical Association conference in 1964, adviser to the Ministry of Health, Dr Ambrose King, argued that problems such as increasing VD among young people were symptomatic of a deeper moral problem:

> If we fail to provide some substitute for religion we must be prepared to face the fact that in spite of material prosperity,

the numbers in our midst of those with inadequate personalities, the unloved and unloving, the anti-social and the delinquents will continue to increase.... Apart from venereal disease and illegitimacy the results are to be seen in aggressive and antisocial behaviour, criminal abortions, broken marriages, neglected children, alcoholism and drug addiction. This is the spreading social disease.... which leads to the denial of rights to others and to the decay and destruction of our society.[68]

Health problems among young people were vividly connected to an apparent moral vacuum at the heart of an increasingly secular society and, in an echo of the temperance mentality of 'the struggle', King further argued that it is 'personal duty' of everyone 'to consider what could be done to combat these evil forces in our society'.[69] King's views clearly resonated with the legal moralism of his contemporary Lord Devlin, who argued that shared values must be enforced to prevent social disintegration, as well as the theoretical position of Durkheim, who saw moral regulation as functionally necessary to prevent society from becoming anomic.

In the early 1960s, alcohol was therefore connected to a variety of health problems, from terminal illness to (women) being 'plump and jolly', which affected the individual drinker as well as their family and employers. The consistent connection of alcohol to youth also positioned the issue within a broader discourse relating to a perceived crisis of declining social morals. Through indirect harm as well as the influence of a culture of moral laxity over a specific generation, drinking in the 1960s was constructed as a problem for the whole of society. Alcohol remained the 'ulcer in the social body' or, to quote Ambrose King, the 'spreading social disease'.

The disease model of alcoholism

This biopolitics of public health indicates the endurance of moral concerns for public behaviour. But are discourses relating to alcoholism equally permeated by both moral and medical ideas?

The marriage of medicine and morality

The relationship between the moral and the medical is significant in understanding discursive developments relating to alcoholism. Alcoholism is usually defined with reference to compulsive or uncontrolled consumption driven by alcohol's 'habit-forming' properties.[70] Room describes how, despite severely limiting people's ability to fulfil various social roles, regular drinking was so intertwined with work and social life that habitual consumption was barely confronted until the 19th century.[71] Even during the 19th century, Kneale notes that alcoholism was recognised as a disease in Britain only after many other European countries had already acknowledged it as such.[72] Harrison explains that the Victorians had difficulty separating alcoholism from drunkenness and the word 'alcoholism', although coined in the 1860s, was not widely used in Britain until the 20th century.[73] The condition of alcoholism has, at various points in time, been attributed to moral frailty, been connected to 'diseases' such as inebriety or viewed in criminal terms.[74] Furthermore, there have been debates over whether alcoholism is a disease in itself or a symptom of another affliction such as monomania or dipsomania.[75] Nowadays, it tends to be understood as a disease or physiological or psychological dependence that usually requires some form of medical intervention. The discourse surrounding the emergence of alcoholism is a key site in which the medical ideas about drinking have been advanced.

W. Hunt and Heyworth's depiction of alcohol as an indigestible poison show that, as long ago as the 1840s, temperance supporters sought to justify their views with reference to physiological science (even if the medical evidence presented is questionable by modern standards). But from the mid-19th century onwards, a more developed medical strand of campaigning began to emerge. The rise of prohibitionism in the 1850s and 1860s had made it common to relate drinking to causes other than individual weakness, and Donald Dalrymple MP and others shifted the focus from a permissive sociolegal environment to the medical arena. Dalrymple was involved in the 1872 Select Committee that recognised habitual drunkenness as a disease, a product of physical pathology rather than moral frailty. Subsequently, the Habitual Drunkards Act 1879 allowed for the detention of drunkard criminals in specialised facilities but only if they agreed to such a sentence. The Inebriates Act 1898 strengthened these powers by enabling the compulsory detention of such persons.[76] Valverde examines the facilities where inebriate criminals were detained and finds that they varied in form; there were pastoral private retreats that catered for aristocratic men whose drinking was viewed as characteristic of excess virility, as well as more punitive state reformatories for working-class men seen as degenerate or women found guilty of prostitution offences.[77] The differing facilities and divergent models of the problem drinker reveal that medical definitions of compulsive drinking remained structured by class, gender and moral concerns.

Due to its punitiveness, the use of inebriate reformatories to regulate the behaviour of certain groups undermined the potentially destigmatising effects of the disease model. This potential, housed in the disease model's removal of habitual drunkenness from the ambit of individual culpability, was further undermined by the hybrid nature of most treatment programmes. In 1901–02, for example, Canon Fleming told the *Windsor Magazine* about the Keeley method of treating drunkenness as a disease, administering a 'cure' that produces aversion to alcohol.[78] But this instance seems to be a rare example of a treatment programme that was decidedly medical; most treatments were only partly medical. In 1914, Sir Owen Seaman lambasted the Church of England Temperance Society as its own treatment failed to acknowledge 'the fact that alcoholism is a physical disease that often renders its victim unamenable to religious influences'. Seaman went on to describe his preference for the Normyl Treatment, which involved the patient taking a vegetable-based medicine that 'renews the will power, and so restores the patient so that he should not therefore be liable to relapse through sudden temptation'.[79] Treatments based on the disease model still drew on older understandings of drink as a temptation and often possessed distinctly moral components, such as the fostering of willpower.

Valverde uses this juxtaposition of medical and moral as evidence of the continuing relationship of habits of consumption to morality. She describes how the *British Journal of Inebriety* allowed adverts for non-alcoholic drinks in its pages 'as if by drinking Cadbury's cocoa one directly imbibed moral resolve along with nutritious matter'.[80] This point is reminiscent of the 1880 *F. Allen & Sons Cocoa Chocolate* advert cited in Chapter Three; whether it was through the alleged properties of the drink or simply its substitution for beer, non-alcoholic beverages were often claimed to improve morality. Valverde's most striking elaboration of the moral/medical overlap is provided by Alcoholics Anonymous (AA), which espouses the belief that alcoholism is a disease at the same time as prescribing the profoundly religious 'Twelve Steps' treatment. This programme, written in the 1930s, includes such steps as making 'a decision to turn our will and our lives over to the care of God as we understood him' and humbly asking 'Him to remove our shortcomings'.[81] AA is now a respected, multinational organisation, regarded as possessing considerable authority on the subject of addiction. Its popularity is testament to the survival of the idea that alcoholism is at least partially a 'disease of the will',[82] an issue of personal fortitude as well as a physiological affliction.

By the 1930s, habitual heavy drinking was beginning to be seen as separate from mere drunkenness and commonly defined as alcoholism. But, as Valverde argues, alcoholism was never fully medicalised and remained at least partially constructed by distinctly moral discourses. This confused diagnosis reflects a broader social context in which, in the 18th, 19th and early 20th centuries, the idea of mental or physical health was inseparable from the notion of moral health. Although the temperance movement redefined virtuous self-restraint as teetotalism, the inseparability of mind and body so apparent in the Georgian period continued to ensure that medical and moral understandings of alcohol were entirely fused until at least the 20th century.

Separating the medical and the moral?

The classification of alcoholism became more widespread and more refined in the 1960s. Of particular influence was the work of American academic E.M. Jellinek, who drew on earlier knowledge of habitual or compulsive drinking to devise a five-part classification of alcoholism. This taxonomy consisted of:

- *alpha alcoholism*, which is caused by an underlying personality disorder;
- *beta alcoholism*, which is not a disease but can produce health problems;
- *gamma alcoholism*, in which the drinker is addicted, although able to abstain for periods, and loses control when drinking;
- *delta alcoholism*, where an addicted person tipples constantly but remains in control of himself;
- *epsilon alcoholism*, characterised by heavy bouts of drinking.[83]

Valverde comments that Jellinek's typology is eclectic and sometimes contradictory, incorporating a harm-based focus (*beta*), the disease model (*gamma, delta* and *epsilon*), the older idea that alcoholism may be a symptom of another condition (*alpha*), as well as a crucial concern for the notion of self-control (*gamma* and *delta*) popular with temperance movements and AA.[84] Despite these ambiguities, Jellinek's work coincided with an advancement of the disease model of alcoholism. It became more common to claim, as the medical correspondent for *The Times* did in 1964, that 'alcoholism is a disease, just as much as diabetes or tuberculosis'.[85]

Delta alcoholism where men tipple for most of the day was seen as typical of France whereas *gamma alcoholism*, involving the loss of control during heavy bouts of drinking, was seen to characterise North American and British problem drinking.[86] Some commentators, such as Edgar Myers, complained that the social extent of this habitual loss of control was obscured by the 'moralistic atmosphere we have created'.[87] The alcoholic was until recently 'regarded as a sinner'[88] and, according to the Bishop of Chester, the issue was still 'bedevilled' by moralistic attitudes.[89] The Bishop further argued that, once alcoholism is recognised as a disease, the drunkard can be treated and become a 'respectable citizen'. He must have been encouraged by Lord Cohen's words, later in 1964, when he spoke of a recent survey that 'had shown that alcoholism was widely regarded as distinct from drunkenness, a disease in which psychological, physical and possibly genetic factors were involved'.[90] With the increasing eminence of the concept that compulsive or habitual drinking is separate from drunkenness and more problematic, the possibility of bringing these diseased *gamma alcoholics* back into the fold of respectability arose.

Consistent with the increased profile of alcoholism, there were a number of new initiatives in the 1960s aiming to tackle this problem. Thom documents how these initiatives often involved the combined efforts of government, professional bodies and voluntary groups.[91] In 1964, AA was reported to be expanding its operations in Britain[92] and sometimes worked in conjunction with the newly formed voluntary group the National Council on Alcoholism (NCA). NCA advice centres, mentioned in Chapter Five, opened in Liverpool,[93] Leeds, Brighton and Gloucester.[94] The Department of Health's planned new treatment units also reflected the new impetus behind addressing alcoholism and, seemingly accepting alcoholism's classification as a disease, were oriented towards the 'treatment of alcoholism as a chronic disease'.[95] These initiatives were deemed inadequate by many and there were calls for further interventions: writing in the *Daily Express*, Wilfred Winterton called for schoolchildren to be given 'scientific guidance' on alcohol;[96] putting warning posters in pubs was discussed in the House of Commons;[97] *The Times* reported on the possibility of banning alcohol and tobacco advertising;[98] and at the Royal Society of Health Congress, Dr Griffith Edwards called for courts to treat rather than punish alcoholics who came before them.[99]

The spread of advice and treatment facilities as well as, to a fair extent, the calls for greater legal intervention testify to the growing influence that the disease model of alcoholism had over how alcohol was governed.

So, did the rise of the disease model signify the advent of a new value-free, scientific approach to drinking? First, the issue of agency must be addressed. Writing in *The Guardian*, the Administrative Officer of the NCA, P. Perfect, was at pains to highlight that 'this council is not a temperance organisation' and is 'not against the alcohol'.[100] Nevertheless, the NCA was reportedly established on the instigation of the Church of England Temperance Society.[101] The Director of the NCA from 1972 to 1980 was Derek Rutherford. Rutherford was a temperance activist with a professed interest in the 'spiritual aspect of alcohol dependence'[102] and later became chief executive of the United Kingdom Temperance Alliance.[103] Furthermore, *The Guardian* reported in 1963 that local churches were a constituent part of the Merseyside council running the new advice centre,[104] and were working nationwide with the NCA and AA. In terms of agency, the medical drive to treat alcoholism as a disease and its accompanying policy initiatives (both government and voluntary) were at least partly undertaken by members of groups who had long been involved in moralising the consumption of alcohol.

Perfect also argued that 'alcoholism is a disease, like any other disease, and not a moral failure';[105] yet much of the discourse surrounding alcoholism undermined Perfect's position. It is worth reiterating that while rejecting the idea of alcoholism as sinful, the Bishop of Chester nonetheless linked recovery to the normative code of social respectability. It has also been noted that Jellinek's taxonomy of alcoholism drew on the temperance movement's preoccupation with individual self-control, which, it was suggested in Chapter Two, owes some formative debt to the absolute morals of evangelical Protestantism. This valuation of individual ethical conduct seems at odds with Perfect's attempts to absolve the individual alcoholic of culpability for their condition. Winterton's comments further elucidate this peculiar hybrid discourse by calling for schools to provide children with 'scientific guidance' about 'the effects of alcohol upon the human body, mind, and spirit'.[106] The notion that science may provide spiritual guidance was not inconsistent with the broader frameworks within which debate was constructed; in 1963, delegates at the Church Assembly spoke of the need to tackle alcoholism, which was described as 'a social and moral – as well as a medical problem'.[107] The medical and moral were still fused, revealing that, in terms of both agency and discourse, the newfound eminence of the disease model of alcoholism did not overwhelm older understandings of alcohol.

Although the Victorians struggled to differentiate alcoholism from drunkenness, it is clear that by the 1960s a more refined understanding of alcoholism as a disease was being advanced and used as a basis for certain interventions. However, at least two centuries of public attitudes had fused notions of mental and physical health with the normative category of moral health. And what history had brought together, the disease model could not or would not tear asunder.

Reflections

Despite the weakening of the organised temperance movement and the reduction of state intrusion into personal affairs, individual drinking habits remained morally charged. The increased prominence of the disease model of alcoholism in the 1960s indicates a degree of discursive change since the earlier time periods studied. But exponents of the disease model did not manage to completely medicalise alcoholism and, as Valverde argues, the condition remained mired in normative issues of individual culpability and respectability. Based on the sources and time period studied, public discussion addressed not just the harmful potential consequences of drinking (such as alcoholism) but also the behaviour of specific social groups. Wider health discourse in the 1960s, as with discourse on law and order, continued to show a preoccupation with the regulation of the behaviour of young people who were apparently affected by a moral vacuum left by the demise of organised religion. So the manner in which drinking was connected to various health problems continued to be infused with issues of blame, valuations of self-control and the perception of declining ethical standards (as a precursor to social disintegration). The emerging medical discourse on alcohol did not engender a clean break with the past. Health was still inextricably linked to the moral health of the individual and society.

Debates about alcohol and health, 2003–10

The apple and the tree

Drawing on this chapter and Chapters Five and Six, it is apparent that discourse on alcohol in the mid-20th century was dominated by a focus on crime and disorder, drink-driving and alcoholism. Debates differed from earlier periods studied in that they did not focus on the evil of alcohol as such but largely concentrated on the specific social evils that alcohol was seen to cause. Public attitudes and regulation were not completely remade. It is clear from the continued activities of various temperance groups, the moralising tone of much public discourse relating to alcohol and the particular identification of social problems within the consumptive practices of young people, and especially young women, that alcohol consumption was still widely moralised. Nevertheless, regulation did become targeted and the ban on alcohol sales to young people under the age of 18, the toughening-up of drink-driving laws and the expansion of treatment facilities all demonstrate the targeting of interventions on specific social groups or behaviours deemed problematic or harmful in some way. Despite this shift in discursive and governmental focus, the fundamental elements of the existing system of regulation, bequeathed primarily by the Licensing Act 1872, remained in place. As earlier in this chapter showed, legal restrictions and moral compulsion just became targeted more rigorously at certain groups and forms of conduct.

Since the 1960s, this model of governance has consistently been challenged by exponents of public health-oriented 'total consumption theory' (TCT).[108] The 1956 research of demographer Sully Ledermann seemed to show a strong relationship between total per capita alcohol consumption of the population and the number of heavy drinkers. Overall alcohol consumption was thus regarded as the most important factor determining the quantity of problem drinkers in society.[109] Following Ledermann, it was apparent to many that focusing interventions on the few 'bad apples' who have become alcoholics or criminals would be markedly less effective than concentrating on the social tree that produces these problem drinkers. This position grew in popularity internationally in the 1960s and, in 1967, the World Health Organization began to emphasise the importance of prevention.[110] It was slower to catch on in Britain perhaps, to borrow from Nicholls, due to the salience of 'the classic liberal argument in which moral responsibility is tied to individual freedom'.[111] Nevertheless, in 1979, TCT was endorsed by the Royal College of Psychiatrists which argued for government interventions to prevent the consumption of alcohol increasing above its existing level.[112] More notably, Thom argues that the focus on consumption and harm within the 1982 government report *Drinking Sensibly* showed the growing potency of TCT.

TCT began to make inroads into policy in the 1980s, especially through the issuing of units guidance. In 1987, the Department of Health, acting on the advice of the Royal College of Physicians, instituted official guidance, which advised that a 'safe' level of consumption should not exceed 21 units per week for men and 14 for women. These recommended limits, which were divided into daily unit allowances in 1995, show an enhanced governmental focus on all drinkers rather than just alcoholics, drivers or deviant youths. Thom argues that espousal of units-based advice meant that all drinkers could be more easily 'located along a continuum from non-harmful to harmful drinking and the size and degree of problem in the population more precisely calculated'.[113] The issuing of units guidance therefore allowed professional medical groups to define the 'drink problem' in epidemiological or public health terms. The regulatory gaze of government and health professionals began to stretch beyond the specific groups or activities that had been targeted in the mid-20th century.[114]

The rise of TCT means that current discourse on alcohol is underwritten by conflicts of treatment versus prevention, cause versus symptom and individual problem versus social problem. But does this new public health approach engender new governmental dilemmas? How, if at all, does it relate to older efforts to morally regulate the use of alcohol?

Passive drinking

Chapter Six investigated how public alarm about drinking did not disappear after the widely predicted disastrous effects of the Licensing Act 2003 failed to materialise. Public discourse continued to feature regular references to the 'national epidemic'[115] of heavy drinking, which was apparently 'getting worse'.[116] In 2008, Penny Cook of the Centre for Public Health stressed that the cost of drinking was 'violence and other disturbances' as well as 'increased short and long term risks to the health of young people'.[117] Alcohol was connected to teenage underperformance at school,[118] mental health disturbances in children[119] and suicide.[120] These were all part, as the *Daily Mirror* described, of 'the crime and health issues linked to reckless boozing' in 2009.[121] Compared with debates around drink in 2004–05 (which were examined more fully in Chapter Six), the subsequent years saw an increased recognition of the health problems associated with drink. This discursive shift reflects the increased prominence of TCT and its preventative, population-based programmes of reform.

Among the keenest exponents of this approach has been Sir Liam Donaldson, who has expressed his desire to change public attitudes to drinking in the same way that attitudes to smoking have, apparently, been altered in recent years. Donaldson served as Chief Medical Officer for England from 1998 until 2010 during which time he used the *Annual Report of the Chief Medical Officer 2008* to highlight the significance of 'passive drinking',[122] which he defines as the 'collateral damage' of alcohol consumption:

> The many people who drink regularly to excess cause damage far beyond their own bodies. Directly and indirectly they affect the well-being and way of life of millions of others.... They include harm to the unborn foetus, acts of drunken violence, vandalism, sexual assault, and a huge health burden carried by both the NHS and friends and family who care for those damaged by alcohol.[123]

Alcohol consumption has been connected to harm inflicted on individual health since at least the 18th century. But Donaldson argues that the effects of drinking go beyond damage to the health and wellbeing of the individual drinker; this is 'a problem for everybody', which affects 'many spheres of life and leaves no communities untouched'.[124] Drinking should be understood in the same way as smoking increasingly is, as a practice that is not socially insulated and has a powerful negative effect on the rest of society.

Donaldson's argument is immediately reminiscent of that articulated by the Victorian temperance movement, especially its prohibitionist strand. Prohibitionists equally highlighted that the consequences of alcohol consumption were social, rather than individual, problems. In 1856, Secretary of the UK Alliance, Samuel Pope, explained how the drinking of others:

> ... destroys my primary right of security by constantly creating and stimulating social disorder. It invades my right of equality by deriving a profit from the creation of misery I am taxed to support. It impedes my right to free moral and intellectual development by surrounding my path with dangers, and by weakening and demoralising society, from which I have a right to claim mutual aid and intercourse.[125]

Likewise, the preamble to Sir Wilfrid Lawson's Local Veto Bill, presented to Parliament regularly between the 1860s and 1880s, read:

> The common sale of intoxicating liquors is a fruitful source of crime, immorality, pauperism, disease and premature death, whereby not only the individuals who give way to drinking are plunged into misery, but grievous wrong is done to the persons and property of Her Majesty's subjects at large, and the public rates and taxes are greatly augmented.[126]

In all three examples, the extent of the harm and its effects, which stretch far beyond harm to the individual drinker, is paramount. Some of the central tenets of prohibitionism are evident in Donaldson's rhetoric.

It must be stressed that Donaldson and other exponents of this population-based approach do not consider harm to the whole of society to result only from the actions of problem drinkers. Liver specialist Ian Gilmore, Professor Jon Rhodes of the British Society of Gastroenterology and Dr Nick Sheron of the Royal College of Physicians wrote to *The Times* in 2010 criticising the government's concentration purely on binge drinking and urging a wider appraisal of drinking habits.[127] Donaldson corroborates this position, explaining how drinking above the recommended weekly limits increases the risk of heart disease and stroke, how any amount of drinking is linked to osteoporosis and reduced fertility and, in regard to the risk of cancer, 'there is no safe alcohol limit'.[128] This message has been repeated by David Nutt, former member of the Advisory Council on the Misuse of Drugs, who stressed the toxic and addictive properties of even small amounts of alcohol in an attempt to dispel 'the myth of a safe alcohol dose'.[129] Various groups have urged drinkers to restrict their consumption to significantly less than the Department of Health's official advice of three or four units per day maximum. The Royal College of Psychiatry has urged the over-65s to consume no more than 1.5 units of alcohol per day and the Science and Technology Committee has advised drinkers to have at least two alcohol-free days per week.[130] Even moderate drinking can therefore produce the 'health burden' to friends, families and the NHS that Donaldson highlights. This medical discourse does not overtly promote abstinence as a solution but, like the Victorian prohibitionists, it is evident that all consumption of alcohol is regarded as inherently problematic.[131]

Donaldson, Gilmore and others tend to combine TCT with the availability theory (outlined in Chapter Six). Derek Rutherford expounds that this public health approach to drink, following Ledermann, is based on the premise that 'the problem is actually all to do with alcohol, and that if consumption increases then so will the level of harm. Hence the importance the movement placed on factors such as price and availability'.[132] In the *Daily Mirror*, for example, Donaldson was reported claiming that alcohol is now 60% cheaper in real terms than in 1980 and associating this increased affordability with an apparent doubling of alcohol-related mortality since 1990.[133] Former Home Secretary, Jacqui Smith, spoke of her 'duty to crack down on irresponsible promotions that can fuel excessive drinking'[134] and Prime Minister David Cameron has complained that 'when beer is cheaper than water, it's just too easy for people to get drunk on cheap alcohol'.[135] The availability of cheap alcohol is constructed as a temptation to excess, an environmental cause of alcohol-related problems, inferring that people lack the requisite self-control to resist such offers. While prohibitionists worried about the 'legalised system of temptation' that permitted the trade in alcohol, recent public health discourse shows a preoccupation with a legalised system of temptingly cheap drinks.

Following TCT and the availability theory, this public health approach situates greater restrictions as the best means to tackle drink problems. It is believed that, if alcohol is made less affordable (and hence less available), consumption and its corollary harm will decrease. On these grounds, the public health lobby advocate a minimum price per unit of alcohol (usually 50 pence). Donaldson proposed this idea in his *Annual Report 2008*[136] and it was subsequently endorsed by groups including the National Institute of Clinical Excellence,[137] the Parliamentary Select Committee on Health,[138] the Scottish National Party and the Coalition Government. Variants of MUP are thus espoused as policy by the Scottish and British governments.[139] After the zenith of its international popularity in the period 1914–21, prohibition was abandoned by the USSR in 1924, Finland in 1932 and the US in 1933. Although there are still 'dry counties' in the US, it is only in Islamic countries, such as Iran and Saudi Arabia, that prohibition continues to be a viable national policy option. That said, the idea that all forms of drinking harm the rest of society and that only strong legal intervention can reduce this harm shows clear affinities between the beliefs of Victorian prohibitionists and public health groups who have shaped recent discourse on alcohol.[140]

The slippery slope of risk

The qualitative affinities between past and present campaigns for greater legal controls on alcohol are not simple coincidence. Rutherford has spoken of how he welcomed TCT and the new public health approach in the 1960s and 1970s because they rejected the disease model's 'view that alcoholism comes in people, not in bottles' and marked 'a return to the temperance perspective', which he had avidly espoused since childhood.[141] The view that even moderate consumption is linked with a variety of health problems that affect the individual drinker and society at large has roots in older discursive frameworks. This subsection examines the contemporary eminence of risk, as the mechanism through which the relationship of alcohol to these harms is expressed, and consider its precedents in Victorian prohibitionism.

For the Victorians, alcohol was understood as predisposing people to inflict harm on either themselves or others. Pope claimed that drinking 'tempts to crime' and others linked it to 'the worst cases of murder, street robbery, housebreaking, seduction, and suicide'.[142] Through either provision of opportunity or weakening of moral resolve, drinking entailed the 'temptation' to do wrong'.[143] An equivalent notion, regarding the propensity of drink to predispose towards harm, is identifiable in contemporary discourse. It is claimed by campaigners that binge drinking or other forms of excessive consumption increase the likelihood that a person will become a victim of crime, require emergency treatment or harm their health in the long term.[144] Government alcohol strategies have articulated similar messages; in 2004, the national *Alcohol Harm Reduction Strategy for England* reported that binge drinking increases the risk of accidents, alcohol poisoning and sexual assault. Binge drinking has also been connected to an enhanced likelihood of both suffering and committing violent crime.[145] Excessive consumption also enhances the threat that drinkers' face from liver disease, heart disease, various types of cancer and suicide, while simultaneously increasing the risk that they will commit drink-driving or domestic violence.[146] In modern parlance, it is the *risks* rather than *temptations* to which alcohol exposes its consumers that is troubling. While the vocabulary has been modified, the discursive structure that connects alcohol to heightened vulnerability of various harms is still intact.

As well as increasing the risks of certain harms, alcohol is also conceived as a risk in itself by prohibitionists and the new public health lobby alike. Dawson Burns and other prohibitionists believed that drinking was a slippery slope; it may begin as a moderate habit, but eventually a person will become intemperate. This position is echoed by the rhetoric of the NHS's recent 'Change4Life' campaign:

> After a long day, many of us like to unwind with a nice glass of something. But it's funny how drink can sneak up on us. The odd glass in the evening can quickly become two or three regular glasses, most evenings. The trouble is that drink sneaks up on bodies too – it can give our organs a hard time. Regularly drinking over the guidelines can lead to serious health problems, from liver damage to a greater risk of getting cancer or having a heart attack.[147]

Moderate drinking is therefore constructed as a volatile or precarious state, liable to morph into excessive consumption at any time. Even if a drinker is able to keep within the official consumption limits, risk is not eliminated. The 'Change4Life' campaign adds: 'don't forget that alcohol also contains calories, so it can help to give you a bit of a spare tyre'.[148] This reminder that no form of drinking is free of negative potential mirrors the problematisation of all consumptive practices inherent the growing insistence from some groups that there is no safe alcohol limit. Drinkaware, an industry-funded group, has an alcohol self-assessment feature on its website, which, even if an individual records consumption as considerably lower than the Department of Health's recommended limits, advises: 'Your current drinking is likely to be harmful to your health.'[149] For Victorian teetotallers, intemperance was considered sinful and so, if all drinking led to intemperance, all drinking was sinful.[150] Similarly, alcohol is now constructed as a dangerous substance; it no longer endangers the mortal soul but even moderate drinking threatens long-term wellbeing by exposing the drinker to harmful eventualities.

The wording of the phrases that alcohol '*can* lead to serious health problems' or 'is *likely to be* harmful to your health' alludes to some ambiguity within the medical problematisation of alcohol. Alcohol has been clinically connected to a variety of problems but knowledge about what level or form of consumption will produce these problems in any one person is limited. This is partly because many such conditions are chronic or 'lifestyle' illnesses, such as heart disease or liver disease, which can be caused by a variety of factors, including obesity, other drugs and viral infections. It is not often possible to isolate the precise aetiological influence of alcohol. Moreover, the issue of harm causality is complicated by evidence that abstinence from alcohol may be less healthy than low-levels of consumption.[151] Given this scientific uncertainty, it is unsurprising that official recommendations on advisable levels of consumption vary considerably between countries. The current UK guidance is based on the Royal College of Physicians' 1987 report *A Great and Growing Evil*.[152] One of the authors of this report told *The Times* in 2007 that the recommendations had been 'plucked out of the air' as there was very limited evidence available on what was and was not safe.[153] Similarly, in 2007 the Department of Health changed the official alcohol guidance given to pregnant women from suggesting that one or two units once or twice per week was safe to advising teetotalism. Lowe and Lee explain that the change in guidelines was not driven by any new knowledge; instead, uncertainty about the probability of harm was re-interpreted as danger.[154] Associating any alcohol consumption with harm is used to circumvent scientific uncertainty about what is and is not a 'safe' level of alcohol consumption.[155]

It appears that risk has ceased to be understood as a probabilistic assessment about the likelihood of harm and has become something understood as dangerous in itself. Risk is the discursive legacy of temptation and contamination, a malevolent external force that continually threatens the individual.[156] Chapter Two found the conflation of drink with harm to be a crucial reason why the temperance movement turned teetotal in the 1830s and, now risk is understood to mean danger, the usage of alcohol once again leads inevitably to a variety of personal and social harms. Just as temperance campaigners focused on all consumption because moderate drinking was the start of the 'highway to drunkenness' and sin, so any drinking now entails the risk of developing cancer, requiring emergency treatment or becoming a victim of crime. Armstrong argued that contemporary understandings of health attribute huge importance to the long-term formative impact of lifestyle; an individual's physical and mental wellbeing, both present and future, is in a state of 'perpetual becoming', constantly affected by daily decisions about alcohol, food, exercise and other factors.[157] This emergent understanding demonstrates a shift away from the targeted alcohol discourse and regulation that became prominent in the era of partial permissiveness and relates to the emergence of lifestyle as the primary determinant of long-term health. In this temporal spectrum of risky uncertainty, we no longer have a healthy moderate drinker, only a potential liver disease patient. Hence, everyone's alcohol consumption, not just that of young people and those dependent on alcohol, is seen as problematic.

This new paradigm is a secular rendering of the religious struggle to lead a virtuous life, which, for the largely Protestant pioneers of temperance, involved the opposition of sinful indulgence and individual self-control. The slippery moral slope, which the Victorian temperance movement believed resulted from lapses in self-control, is now a continuum of risk within which harm becomes more real with every sip of an alcoholic drink. In alcohol discourse, risk is constructed within older heuristic frameworks, shaped by the public attitudes of previous eras.[158]

New regulatory directions

Chapter Six described how both legal and moral frameworks govern the choices that people make about alcohol. In what many people call a 'neoliberal' society, individuals are also required to manage the risks that they personally face by making choices that are informed by available evidence regarding the risks that alcohol consumption entails.[159] This wider social context makes the slippery slope of risk, described in the previous subsection and embodied in a broader public health paradigm, increasingly significant. Notably, the Alcohol Health Alliance (AHA) was formed in 2007 from a plethora of professional medical or health bodies and other groups and, articulating the renewed problematisation of all forms of drinking, has begun to extend the regulatory gaze beyond the issue of binge drinking by young people. The AHA and affiliated groups have consistently stressed that the consumption habits of older people and the middle classes can also be harmful[160] and, echoing this, the House of Commons Health Committee criticised government policy in 2012 for neglecting 'wider long-term alcohol misuse issues'.[161] Has this new public health paradigm, spearheaded by the AHA, influenced the governance of drinking in England and Wales? This subsection will investigate how choices about drinking have been structured from 2007 onwards.

While individuals are required to manage the risks they personally face from alcohol, the available evidence on risk is often articulated in a selective or inflammatory fashion. In November 2007, newspapers reported on an apparent increase of 'exploding bladders' among female binge drinkers. On closer inspection, this news story was based entirely on a short piece published in the *British Medical Journal* in which only three cases of this condition were discussed.[162] Lowe and Lee describe how, in the same year, the Department of Health borrowed the highly questionable statistic that 6,000 babies per year are born with FASD from an American lobby group.[163] Similarly, a 2011 article in *The Lancet* by Sheron et al arguing that up to 250,000 people could die as a result of drinking in the next 20 years was widely reported in the press. But the authors made little attempt to actually predict future deaths from liver disease; their projection was based simply on a scenario in which recent increases in liver disease mortality continue unabated.[164] Considering that both survey data and HM Revenue & Customs data show a sustained decline in alcohol consumption 2002–04 onwards it might be feasible to consider whether this will, in time, produce a related decline in liver disease mortality.[165] But recognition of the downward trend in alcohol consumption, along with Britain's middling consumption level in European terms, are rarely acknowledged in public discourse. It is more typical to read journalists' alarming commentaries on 'out of control'[166] drinking or hear 'experts' claim that Britain's alcohol problem is 'pre-eminent in Europe'.[167]

Sheron et al's use of an epidemiological worst-case scenario is mirrored in advice given to individuals regarding personal risk management. In 2008, social scientist Andrew Bengry-Howell criticised the government's 'Alcohol: Know Your Limits' campaign. The campaign's website highlights the disastrous potential of drinking by allowing people to go on a virtual night-out. 'In one scenario,' Bengry-Howell explains, 'after drinking four shots a woman gets into an unlicensed taxi and is sexually assaulted.'[168] By singling out drinking as a factor in victimisation, this virtual night-out responsibilises drinkers and advances the paramount need for preventative action by potential victims above, say, the need for better policing of taxi licensing. Additionally, while promoting knowledge of risks attached to alcohol consumption, the campaign also clearly ignores the majority of cases in which drunk people make their way home safely. As the previous subsection argued, risk is not being constructed as a matter of probability to be calculated in relation to personal behaviour; this simulation highlights the terrible yet fairly unusual consequences above the more routine. Elucidating a similar point in relation to personal security, Haggerty describes how decisions are rarely made in reference to a probabilistic notion of risk and are more often based on a situational rationality of precaution that prioritises the need to avoid the worst-case scenario.[169] The example of the 'Alcohol: Know Your Limits' campaign shows that government policy can promote this worst-case-scenario, precautionary logic above probabilistic assessments of the likelihood of harm.

Burgess stresses that this precautionary risk logic, as well as other information and expert opinion that informs individual decisions, may be supplied by individuals or groups whose motives are not straightforward. Some important agents are government funded; this applied to Donaldson, when he served as Chief Medical Officer, and Alcohol Concern, which was formed to replace the NCA in 1983 and receives funding from the Department of Health.[170] Moreover, the authors of the fatalistic projection of liver disease deaths published in *The Lancet* are heavily involved in the AHA and the campaign for MUP.[171] As I have argued elsewhere, their projection thus appears as something of a scarecrow positioned to warn governments away from their current path and direct them towards the development of new policies.[172] Moreover, earlier discussion showed that some influential actors in public health approaches to drinking, such as Rutherford, have strong links with the temperance movement. The Institute of Alcohol Studies (IAS), an AHA member, proudly describes itself as 'an independent voice on alcohol policy'.[173] But, the IAS was formed in 1983 by the Alliance House Foundation, which itself was established in the mid-20th century by the UK Alliance – the prohibitionist behemoth of Victorian society. The Alliance House Foundation remains publicly committed to spreading the principle of total abstinence from alcohol[174] and continues to supply the majority of the IAS's funding. Similarly, the Band of Hope temperance society now exists under the new moniker Hope UK and defines its mission as educating children and helping them to make 'drug free choices'.[175] The impartiality of the 'informed choices' or 'evidence-based' policies that these groups champion might be questioned. Choices about drinking are, therefore, partly structured by discursive agents with clear links to government, prominent lobby groups or Victorian temperance societies.

A future-oriented focus on reducing total consumption, promoted by the AHA and consistent with a wider public health paradigm, has become a visible trope within some government policies. The promotion of the recommended levels of consumption has already been mentioned as an example of policy that targets general drinking habits rather than problem drinkers. Furthermore, Chancellor Alistair Darling's 2009 Budget implemented a tax escalator, which ensures that all drinkers are affected by annual increases in the duty on alcohol of 2% above the rate of inflation.[176] These measures correspond to a shift in policy focus in the last decade. In the foreword to the government's *Alcohol Harm Reduction Strategy 2004*, Tony Blair supports the idea that most drinking is harmless by stating that 'most of us enjoy drinking with few, if any, ill effects. Indeed moderate drinking can bring some health benefits'.[177] But in a context of ongoing anxieties about alcohol-related crime and disorder and increasing alarmist discourse about the impact of drink on health, the foreword to 2007's *Safe. Sensible. Social* was rather different. Public Health Minister, Caroline Flint, stated that 'our relationship with drink in this country is complicated.... Most of us do drink sensibly (although we may drink more than we think we do at times)'.[178] As well as reinforcing the old idea that British drinking culture is peculiar, Flint replaces the idea of harmless drinking with sensible drinking. The document explicitly acknowledges that 'the risk of harm ... increases the more alcohol you drink'[179] and that 'alcohol misuse may not only harm the drinker'.[180] The shifting policy context thus incorporates an intensified focus on all drinkers and all forms of drinking.

These changes in governmental attitudes were vividly articulated in the Coalition Government's *Alcohol Strategy 2012*.[181] In 2009, both the Conservative and Labour Parties backed 'targeted' action against binge drinking and youth drinking and rejected MUP on the grounds that it would penalise the majority of responsible, sensible drinkers.[182] But, since 2009, political faith in the 'responsible majority' to drink sensibly has increasingly been countered by the public health lobby's argument that even apparently sensible, moderate consumption entails risk. The Coalition Government's alcohol strategy lists figures relating to the harms associated with alcohol before asserting that '[t]hese statistics highlight the urgent and unquestionable need for all those who drink alcohol – no matter who they are or what they do – to take responsibility for their drinking behaviour and establish a less risky approach to drinking as the norm'.[183] This statement embodies the public health movement's insistence that problem drinking is a societal, not individual, issue. All forms of drinking are problematic and thus everyone, conceivably even non-drinkers, are tasked with addressing the ubiquitous risks of drink. The main policy advocated by this strategy was MUP, the primary demand of the AHA and other groups. Following TCT and the availability theory, the government envisages that a higher price for alcohol will cause total consumption and alcohol-related harm, its corollary, to decline.

It must be stressed, however, that the conversion to the AHA's agenda has been far from total. Opinion polls and focus groups have found strong public opposition to MUP.[184] Letters in the *Daily Telegraph* have expressed anger about the proposed policy as it would allegedly punish poor people more than rich people, young people above older people, and the responsible majority for the actions of the irresponsible minority.[185] Perhaps affected by such opposition, David Cameron has insisted that MUP 'isn't about stopping responsible drinking' and will not financially damage pubs.[186] The measure is depicted by the government as designed to target the disorder, the 'scourge of violence' and the burden on the health service created *specifically* by binge drinking and particularly binge drinking by young people.[187] In a sense, this is consistent with public health arguments that, more latterly, have stressed that MUP would affect heavy drinkers more than moderate drinkers.[188] Nevertheless, it results in a peculiar situation where a government argues that a policy initially mooted as a future-oriented means of reducing harm by lowering total consumption is actually a targeted means of addressing undesirable drinking that will leave responsible, older drinkers unaffected.

Particularly from 2007 onwards, the dominance of targeted regulation has been threatened by the accelerated momentum of TCT-inspired public health approaches to governing alcohol. At the time of writing, the two appear to co-exist as uncomfortably entwined influences over the manner in which alcohol is understood and regulated. A discernible trend within this rather confused picture is that governance is increasingly distanced from the libertarian ideals of J.S. Mill and Hart, which were cemented as significant governmental principles in the mid-20th century. The issue is not that the harm principle has lost its pertinence; rather, it is being redefined along distinctly less libertarian lines. Von Hirsch describes how immediate harm has become less common as a justification for legal intervention and 'remote harms', such as long-term harm or potential harm to others, have become more salient.[189] Similarly, Harcourt has argued that in recent years legal discourse has been characterised by a 'cacophony of competing harm arguments' as a multiplicity of cases for legal intervention are re-articulated in reference to some notion of harm.[190] Analysis of the rhetoric of public health groups presented here is supportive of these conclusions; arguments for alcohol regulation that used to be made with reference to more explicitly moral ideas are now articulated in reference to extensive, pervasive and sometimes passive forms of harm that alcohol inflicts upon the drinker and others. Groups such as the AHA have, as Von Hirsch argued in regard to wider legal issues, co-opted the harm principle and used it to advance the case for greater legal interventions. The libertarian harm principle, which delimited the functions of the state, is thus being superseded by a public health-inspired harm principle that necessitates the expansion of regulation in order to better facilitate the governance of behaviours deemed risky.[191]

So, in the context of uncertainty becoming understood as risk and risk being conceived as danger, efforts to regulate alcohol have moved in new directions, which entail both efforts to 'govern through choice' as well as attempts to limit choice. Government rhetoric and public health campaigns seek to direct behavioural choices by highlighting various risks associated with drinking and obliging evasive, precautionary action to be taken by individuals. Simultaneously, many actors are pursuing legal changes that would reduce the scope for individual decisions about alcohol, for example through pricing controls. The latter agenda, based on TCT and the availability theory, has been actively promoted by the AHA and others, and policy changes discussed show that successive governments have looked more favourably on these ideas. It is too early to say whether these alterations amount to a decisive paradigm shift in governance, from focusing on bad apples such as problem drinkers to problematising all forms of alcohol consumption. It certainly appears, nonetheless, that current public attitudes are increasingly animated by a perceived need to reduce drinking among the whole population and a faith in the power of legal rules to achieve this.

Good health!

The salience of health, harm and risk in contemporary society has not, in reference to drinking, forced a clean governmental break with the past. Understandings of personal health were entwined with conceptions of good moral conduct in the 18th and 19th centuries, and public health, during its emergence as a social issue in the mid-19th and early 20th centuries, was intimately connected to anxieties about national moral health. Drawing on Valverde and others, this chapter has examined how, beneath its veneer of neutral science, the disease model of alcoholism continued to embody older, moralistic preoccupations with individual conduct, self-control and social respectability. This point parallels Chapter Five's conclusion that targeted regulatory innovations in the mid-20th century refocused moralising energies at certain groups or activities rather than abolishing them. Equally, this chapter has found that the slow rise of drink as a public health problem, tied to the emergence of TCT and the availability theory, has engendered attempts to morally regulate drinking. Public health groups and campaigns publicise the dangers of drink and, spurred on by a risk-based conception of all drinking as entailing social problems, urge all drinkers to adopt 'responsible' consumptive practices. These discursive forms sharpen the boundaries between desirable and undesirable behaviour and widen the scope of moral regulation beyond individual 'problem drinkers' or deviant groups.

In regulatory terms, the result is an increased normative burden placed on individual choices. Chapter Six described how individual decisions about alcohol are made within restrictive legal parameters and guided by explicit moral directions, often from politicians, regarding the acceptability of certain courses of action. This chapter has examined how discourse and regulation relating to health further weight these choices. As well as this 'governance through choice', a concerted effort has been made since 2007 to redraw the legal parameters of individual choices, especially through the creation of pricing controls. A fault-line that separated Victorian suasionists and prohibitionists is visible once again between those who wish to address the problem of alcohol by helping and persuading individuals into making 'responsible' choices about drinking and those seeking to regulate the social environment (in this case, price) in order to force behavioural change upon people. While Chapter Six argued that the established model of governing drink through legal restriction and moral compulsion owes a formative debt to Victorian moral suasionism, its principal current challenge comes from the AHA and other similarly minded groups who have discursive and, in some cases, organisational roots in prohibitionism. Once again, disputes about how to regulate alcohol rest on conflicting attitudes towards the virtue and efficacy of either the individual or the state to reform behaviour.

Of course, there are differences between Victorian temperance and contemporary discourses on alcohol. For example, binge drinking by young people is a more recent preoccupation and abstinence is no longer insisted upon, although any other consumption habit is deemed risky. Additionally, the language in which the problematisation of alcohol is reproduced differs, with the new semantics of risk replacing the explicitly moral frameworks of temptation and sin. But the broader discursive frameworks are similar; just as the prohibitionists Pope and Lawson used utilitarian discussions of harm to advocate a coerced form of abstinence, so the public health lobby uses the rhetoric of risk to posit government intervention as the best vaccination against the wholly problematic substance alcohol. Such interventions will act as a substitute for self-control, vastly reducing the temptation or risk posed by alcohol and allowing individuals to lead more virtuous, harm-free lives. This chapter thus rejects any suggestion that the rise of medical and secular notions of risk displaced moral considerations. As Hunt, Burgess and others have argued, risk is subsumed within older, more explicitly moral discourses.[192] Health discourse on alcohol is not based on a 'scientific' or value-neutral expression of risk as a probability of harm. Risk reproduces the historical fusion of health and morality; it is a normatively charged concept that differentiates the desirable from the undesirable and supports efforts to reform the behaviour of those whose conduct is judged to be the latter. It is, therefore, a crucial component of contemporary efforts to morally regulate the consumption of alcohol.

Notes

[1]   Donaldson, Sir Liam, *Guidance on the Consumption of Alcohol by Children and Young People*, London: Department of Health, 2009.

[2]   'Police Plan for Norfolk Ban of Super-Strength Alcohol', *BBC News*, 11 April 2013.

[3]   Johnston, Lucy, 'Ban Alcohol in Binge Towns', *Sunday Express*, 22 March 2009.

[4]   Campbell, Denis, 'Doctors: Urgent Action of Alcohol Needed', *The Guardian*, 1 March 2013.

[5]   Boffey, Daniel, 'Patients to be Quizzed by GPs about Drinking under New Alcohol Strategy', *The Guardian*, 24 March 2012.

[6]   At the time of writing, MUP has been adopted as policy by both the British and Scottish Governments although not yet implemented by either.

[7]   See: Ericsson, Richard V., and Doyle, Aaron, *Risk and Morality*, Toronto: University of Toronto Press, 2003.

8   Thom, *Dealing with Drink*; Sulkunen, Pekka, 'Ethics of Alcohol Policy in a Saturated Society', *Addiction*, 1997, vol 92 (9); Nicholls, *The Politics of Drink*.

9   Systematic searches of the newspaper archives returned 840 items, which were read and analysed with respect to the issues discussed in this chapter. It is worth mentioning that 333 of these items were identified using searches for 'licensing act/bill' in 1961 and 1963-65 and hence have already been utilised in Chapter Six. A number of newspaper clippings gathered by the author over recent years have been used in this chapter.

10 Sulkunen, 'Ethics of Alcohol Policy', p 1120.

11 Thom, *Dealing with Drink*.

12 Nicholls, *The Politics of Alcohol*, p 206.

13 Sulkunen, 'Ethics of Alcohol Policy', p 1120. See also: Sulkunen, *The Saturated Society*.

14 Barr, *Drink*, p 255.

15 Harford, Charles F., 'To the Editor of *The Times*: Alcohol for Medicine', *The Times*, 5 March 1919.

16 'The Licensing Bill was appointed for ...', *The Times*, 7 August 1872.

17 Burnett, *Liquid Pleasures*, pp 114-115.

18 'The Strength of Britain', *Daily Express*, 25 January 1917.

19 In a 1919 discussion of the question 'Do Women Prefer Pussyfoots?', the *Daily Mirror* defended the achievements of drinkers, and vilified teetotallers: 'In the past our great battles on land and sea were won, and our Colonies were acquired, by men who were by no means teetotallers. In the late war not one successful admiral or general denied himself a glass of wine, and doesn't today. The fact is a man who is unable to command himself cannot command others.' See: 'Pussyfoot', *Daily Mirror*, 16 September 1919.

20 'To the Author of the *London Journal*: Privates Vices, not Publick Benefits', *London Journal*, 14 June 1729.

21 Setaymot, 'To the Printer of the *Public Advertiser*', *Public Advertiser*, 18 July 1789.

22 Ibid.

23 'The Drunken Post', *Athenian News or Dunton's Oracle*, 23 May 1710.

24 'London', *Public Advertiser*, 2 January 1754.

25 Academicus, 'To Mr Fitz-Adam', *World*, 18 March 1756.

26 'The Beer Bill', *Derby Mercury*, 14 July 1830.

27 'Sale of Beer Bill', *Morning Chronicle*, 22 May 1830.

28 Barr, *Drink*, p 255.

29 'Lecture on Temperance', *Preston Chronicle*, 8 March 1834.

30 Hunt, *History of Teetotalism in Devon*, pp 7-9.

31 Heyworth, Lawrence, 'The Temperance Movement: To the Editor of *The Times*', *The Times*, 18 October 1856.

32 Hunt, *History of Teetotalism in Devon*, p 12.

33 Smith, Geo. A., 'To the Editor of *The Times*', *The Times*, 25 September 1891.

34 Chadwick, Edwin, *Report on the Sanitary Condition of the Labouring Population of Great Britain*, Edinburgh: Edinburgh University Press, 1965.

35 Fulton Phin, Nicholas, 'The Historical Development of Public Health', in Wilson, Frances, and Mabhala, Mzwandile (eds) *Key Concepts in Public Health*, London: Sage Publications, 2008, pp 5-10.

36 Rowbotham, Judith, 'Legislating For Your Own Good: Criminalising Moral Choice. The Echoes of the Victorian Vaccination Act', *Liverpool Law Review*, 2009, vol 30, pp 13-33.

37 Foucault, Michel, *Security, Territory, Population: Lectures at the College de France 1977-78*, Palgrave: Basingstoke, 2007, p 120.

38 Kneale, James, 'The Place of Drink: Temperance and the Public 1856-1914', *Social and Cultural Geography*, 2001, vol 2 (1), p 52.

39 'Women's Total Abstinence Union', *Manchester Guardian*, 8 May 1914.

40 'Adolescents and Peril of Alcohol', *Manchester Guardian*, 16 April 1921.

41 Mackenzie, Fred A., 'Is there a Cure for Drunkenness? An Interview with Canon Fleming', *Windsor Magazine*, 1901-02.

42 Burns, Dawson, 'Dawson Burns and the Permissive Bill', *Preston Guardian*, 26 July 1873.

43 'Questions for the Recess', *Lloyd's Daily Newspaper*, 25 August 1872.

44 Grosvenor, Peter, 'Walk Further ... Live Longer!', *Daily Express*, 20 May 1965.

45 'Lipstick Warning in Cancer Survey', *The Times*, 10 December 1963.

46 'Disorders of Mind', *The Guardian*, 14 February 1963.

47 'Average Stay in Mental Hospital Six Weeks', *The Guardian*, 6 September 1965.

48 'Drink and Drugs "Necessary"', *The Times*, 11 April 1961.

49 'New Approach to Alcoholism', *The Times*, 13 November 1964.

50 'Back to the Hard Stuff – Like 40 Years Ago', *The Guardian*, 11 August 1964.

51 Myers, Edgar, 'Alcoholics', *The Observer*, 14 June 1964. The strongly gendered nature of Myers' comments were criticised by correspondents in subsequent issues of the newspaper who emphasised the problem of female alcoholism. See: 'Alcoholics', *The Observer*, 28 June 1964.

52 'Kuc Talks', *Daily Express*, 10 July 1963.

53 Pincher, Chapman, 'Careful All You Carboholics', *Daily Express*, 28 December 1965.

54 'How Not to Kill Your Wife', *Daily Express*, 7 October 1964.

55 Delano, Tony, 'Welcome, Girls, to the Platinum-Plated Beauty Greenhouse', *Daily Mirror*, 7 October 1965.

56 Hickey, William, 'Now it's Boom Time Among the Body Shrinkers', *Daily Express*, 31 August 1964; 'Wanted: A Perfect Body', *Daily Express*, 3 September 1964.

57 'How Not to Kill Your Wife', *Daily Express*, 7 October 1964.

[58] 'BMA Urged to Start Training Courses for Parents', *The Times*, 24 March 1961.

[59] 'Mums Rush to Send Girls to Sex Talks', *Daily Mirror*, 29 September 1961.

[60] Marcus, Abraham, 'Syphilis Increase Shock', *The Observer*, 27 December 1964.

[61] 'What Can We Do or Say to Protect Our Children?', *Daily Mirror*, 4 September 1963.

[62] 'Tempting for Teenagers', *Daily Mirror*, 3 October 1961.

[63] Ibid.

[64] Winterton, Wilfrid, 'Letters to the Editor: Alcoholics', *The Guardian*, 29 April 1963.

[65] '£300m Lost Through Alcoholism', *The Guardian*, 3 December 1965.

[66] 'The Human Heart', *Daily Mirror*, 13 June 1963; 'Gaymer's Cider, *Daily Mirror*, 13 June 1963.

[67] 'B.M.A. Urged to Start Training Courses for Parents', *The Times*, 24 March 1961.

[68] 'Sex Education Urged as Part of School Syllabus', *The Guardian*, 9 November 1964.

[69] Ibid.

[70] Room, 'Addiction and Personal Responsibility', p 50; Nicholls, *The Politics of Alcohol*, p 161; Valverde, *Diseases of the Will*, pp 23-42.

[71] Room, 'Addiction and Personal Responsibility'.

[72] Kneale, 'The Place of Drink', p 52.

[73] Harrison, *Drink and the Victorians*, pp 21-22.

[74] Thom, *Dealing with Drink*.

[75] Valverde, *Diseases of the Will*.

[76] See: Nicholls, *The Politics of Alcohol*, pp 161-179.

[77] Valverde, Mariana, 'Slavery from Within: The Invention of Alcoholism and the Question of Free Will', *Social History*, 1997 vol 22 (3), pp 251-268.

[78] Mackenzie, 'Is there a Cure for Drunkenness?'.

[79] Seaman, Owen, 'The Curse of Drink', *Daily Express*, 27 February 1914.

[80] Valverde, *Diseases of the Will*, pp 63-64.

[81] Alcoholics Anonymous, 'The Twelve Steps of Alcoholics Anonymous', www.aa.org/en_pdfs/smf-121_en.pdf

[82] Valverde, *Diseases of the Will*.

[83] Glatt, Dr M.M., 'Alcoholism Redefined', *The Observer*, 12 March 1961.

[84] Valverde, *Diseases of the Will*, pp 110-115.

[85] 'New Approach to Alcoholism', *The Times*, 13 November 1964.

[86] Glatt, Dr M.M., 'Alcoholism Redefined', *The Observer*, 12 March 1961.

[87] Myers, Edgar, 'Alcoholics', *The Observer*, 14 June 1964.

[88] Ibid.

89 'Call for Reappraisal of the Welfare Services', *The Guardian*, 23 April 1964.

90 'Liverpool Unit for Alcoholics Praised', *The Times*, 11 August 1964.

91 Thom, *Dealing with Drink*, pp 67-84.

92 'Sober Facts about Alcohol', *The Times*, 28 December 1964.

93 'New Centre for Advice to Alcoholics', *The Guardian*, 23 July 1963.

94 Perfect, P., 'Letters to the Editor: Help for Alcoholics', *The Guardian*, 20 April 1965.

95 'Special Units for Treating Alcoholics', *The Guardian*, 10 December 1963.

96 Winterton, Wilfrid, 'Letters to the Editor: Alcoholics', *The Guardian*, 29 April 1963.

97 'Warning Smokers of the Risks', *The Times*, 9 May 1964.

98 Platt, Robert, and Fletcher, Charles, 'To the Editor of *The Times*: Why Advertising is Harmful', *The Times*, 1 December 1964.

99 'Force and Persuasion in Curing Addictions', *The Guardian*, 30 April 1964.

100 Perfect, P., 'Letters to the Editor: Help for Alcoholics', *The Guardian*, 20 April 1965.

101 'Alcoholics Still in Need of Help', *The Guardian*, 9 November 1963.

102 'Conversation with Derek Rutherford', *Addiction* vol 107 (5), p 893.

103 See 'Institute of Alcohol Studies' and other entries in: Blocker et al, *Alcohol and Temperance in Modern History*.

104 'New Centre for Advice to Alcoholics', *The Guardian*, 23 July 1963.

105 Perfect, P., 'Letters to the Editor: Help for Alcoholics', *The Guardian*, 20 April 1965.

106 Winterton, Wilfrid, 'Letters to the Editor: Alcoholics', *The Guardian*, 29 April 1963.

107 'Alcoholics "Still in Need of Help"', *The Guardian*, 9 November 1963.

108 Sulkunen, 'Ethics of Alcohol Policy', p 1120. TCT is also referred to as the 'public health model' by Rutherford and the 'consumptionist perspective' by Thom. See: 'Conversation with Derek Rutherford', p 893; Thom, *Dealing with Drink*, p 110.

109 Nicholls, *The Politics of Alcohol*, pp 206-207.

110 Thom, *Dealing with Drink*, pp 110-111.

111 Nicholls, *The Politics of Alcohol*, p 209.

112 Ibid.

113 Thom, *Dealing with Drink*, p 130.

114 I have explored the relationship between evidence, expertise and the regulation of drinking in more detail elsewhere. See: Yeomans, 'Blurred Visions'.

115 Armstrong, Jeremy, 'All You Can Drink Offer Slammed by Experts', *Daily Mirror*, 28 January 2009.

116 Palmer, Alun, 'Should We Ban Cheap Booze?', *Daily Mirror*, 16 March 2009.

[117] Armstrong, Jeremy, 'All You Can Drink Offer Slammed by Experts', *Daily Mirror*, 28 January 2009.

[118] Stoppard, Miriam, 'Save Teens from Alcohol Tragedy', *Daily Mirror*, 22 July 2009.

[119] Hall, Sarah, 'Child Mental Health Disorders Have Soared', *The Guardian*, 21 June 2006.

[120] Bowcott, Owen, 'Recession Drives Suicide Rate up 6%', *The Guardian*, 29 January 2010.

[121] Palmer, Alun, 'Should We Ban Cheap Booze?', *Daily Mirror*, 16 March 2009.

[122] Donaldson, *Annual Report of the Chief Medical Officer 2008*.

[123] Ibid, p 17.

[124] Ibid, p 22.

[125] Pope, Samuel, 'To the Editor of *The Times*: Further Reply by the Hon. Secretary', *The Times*, 2 October 1856.

[126] Taken from: Farrar, F.W., 'Drink and Crime', *Fortnightly Review*, 1893, vol 3, p 789.

[127] Rhodes, Professor Jon, Gilmore, Professor Ian, Sheron, Dr Nick, 'Nation's Health At Risk from Cheap Alcohol', *The Times*, 24 May 2010.

[128] Donaldson, *Annual Report of the Chief Medical Officer 2008*, p 19.

[129] Nutt, David, 'There is No Such Thing as a Safe Level of Alcohol Consumption', *The Guardian*, 7 March 2011.

[130] Hughes, Dominic, 'People Over 65 Should Drink Less', *BBC News*, 22 June 2011; Science and Technology Committee, *Alcohol Guidelines*, London: UK Parliament, 2011.

[131] See: Yeomans, 'Blurred Visions'.

[132] 'Conversation with Derek Rutherford', p 893.

[133] Moss, Vincent, 'Can It!', *Sunday Mirror*, 15 March 2009.

[134] Rose, David, 'Alcohol Abuse Curbs Will End "Get One Free" Wine Deals', *The Times*, 4 December 2008.

[135] UK Government, *The Government's Alcohol Strategy*, London: The Stationery Office, 2012.

[136] Donaldson, *Annual Report of the Chief Medical Officer 2008*.

[137] Bowcott, Owen, and Campbell, Denis, 'NICE Backs Minimum Pricing on Alcohol to Cut Harmful Drinking', *The Guardian*, 14 October 2009.

[138] Campbell, Denis, 'MPs Back Alcohol Price Control to Curb Drinking', *The Guardian*, 12 December 2009.

[139] At the time of writing, there is some doubt about whether the coalition government will proceed with plans for a MUP in England and Wales. Scotland, however, appears close to implementing a MUP of 50 pence.

[140] I have also explored these affinities in: Yeomans, 'Theorising Alcohol in Public Discourse'.

[141] 'A Conversation with Derek Rutherford', p 893.

[142] Homo, 'Abuse of Spirituous Liquor', *The Times*, 4 January 1830.

[143] Burns, Dawson, 'The Permissive Bill Question', *Preston Guardian*, 23 August 1873.

[144] Sorensen, Nicolay, 'Should Alcohol Carry Health Warnings?', *The Times*, 28 November 2008.

[145] UK Government, *Alcohol Harm Reduction Strategy for England*, London: Strategy Unit, 2004; UK Government, *Government's Alcohol Strategy*.

[146] UK Government, *Alcohol Harm Reduction Strategy*; Drinkaware, 'Why Let the Good Times Turn Bad?', www.drinkaware.co.uk/good-times

[147] National Health Service, 'Cutting Down on Alcohol', *Change4Life*, http://www.nhs.uk/Change4Life/Pages/cutting-down-alcohol.aspx

[148] Ibid.

[149] Drinkaware, 'Alcohol Self-Assessment', https://www.drinkaware.co.uk/selfassessment

[150] See: Cook, *Alcohol, Addiction and Christian Ethics*.

[151] UK Government, *Sensible Drinking*, Wetherby: Department of Health, 1995; Anderson, Peter, and Baumberg, Ben, *Alcohol in Europe*, London: Institute of Alcohol Studies, 2006, p 165.

[152] Royal College of Physicians, *A Great and Growing Evil*, London: Tavistock, 1987.

[153] Norfolk, Andrew, 'Drink Limits "Useless"', *The Times*, 20 October 2007.

[154] Lowe, Pam K., and Lee, Ellie J., 'Advocating Alcohol Abstinence to Pregnant Women: Some Observations about British Policy', *Health, Risk and Society*, 2010, vol 12 (4), pp 301-311.

[155] Yeomans, 'Blurred Visions'.

[156] See: Burgess, Adam, 'Passive Drinking: A Good Lie too Far?', *Health, Risk & Society*, 2009, vol 11, pp 527-540.

[157] Armstrong, David, 'The Rise of Surveillance Medicine', *Sociology of Health and Illness*, 1995, vol 17 (3), pp 393-404.

[158] I have explored similar issues in: Yeomans, 'Theorising Alcohol in Public Discourse'.

[159] The AHA states its intention to 'highlight the rising levels of alcohol-related health harm' and Alcohol Concern describes its ideal world as one where 'people can manage the risks and make sense of alcohol'. See: Royal College of Physicians, 'AHA Welcomes Minimum Alcohol Unit Price Consultation and Calls for 50 Pence per Unit', *Royal College of Physicians Press Release*, 28 November 2012, www.rcplondon.ac.uk/press-releases/aha-welcomes-minimum-alcohol-unit-price-consultation-and-calls-50-pence-unit; Alcohol Concern, 'About Us', *Alcohol Concern: Making Sense of Alcohol*, www.alcoholconcern.org.uk/about-us. On neoliberalism and risk, see: Haggerty, Kevin D., 'From Risk to Precaution: The Rationalities of Personal Crime

Prevention', in Ericson, Richard V., and Doyle, Aaron (eds) *Risk and Morality*, Toronto: University of Toronto Press, 2003, pp 193-214.

[160] Triggle, Nick, 'Baby Boomer Alcohol Harm "More Likely than in Young"', *BBC News*, 12 October 2012.

[161] Triggle, Nick, 'Tougher Alcohol Marketing Rules "May Be Needed"', *BBC News*, 19 July 2012.

[162] Dooldeniya, M.D., Khafagy, R., Mashaly, H., Browning, A.J., Sundaram, S.K., Biyani, C.S., 'Lower Abdominal Pain in Women after Bring Drinking', *British Medical Journal*, 2007, vol 335, pp 992-993. See reaction in: Atkins, Lucy, 'If You Thought Your Hangover Was Bad ...', *The Guardian*, 20 November 2007; 'Women Drinkers Fit to Burst', *BBC News*, 9 November 2007.

[163] Lowe and Lee, 'Advocating Alcohol Abstinence'.

[164] Sheron et al, 'Projections of Alcohol Deaths'. See also: Campbell, Denis, 'Drink Deaths: Failure to Act Will Cost An Extra 250,000 Lives by 2031, say Doctors', *The Guardian*, 21 February 2011.

[165] Office for National Statistics, *General Lifestyle Survey*; Whalley, 'Drinking Alcohol'; 'Alcohol Consumption "Continues to Fall"', *BBC News*, 3 September 2010.

[166] Stoppard, Miriam, 'Save Teens From Alcohol Tragedy', *Daily Mirror*, 22 July 2009.

[167] Boseley, Sarah, 'Expert Blames UK Drink Culture for Youth Deaths', *The Guardian*, 11 September 2009. The 'expert' to which the article referred was co-author of a large comparative research project. However, the article in *The Lancet* on the findings of this project makes scant reference to alcohol. See: Patton, G.C., Coffey, C., Sawyer, S.M., Viner, R.M., Haller, D.M., Bose, K., Vos, T., Ferguson, J., and Mathers, C.D., 'Global Patterns of Mortality in Young People: A Systematic Analysis of Population Health Data', *The Lancet*, 2009, vol 374 (9693), pp 881-892.

[168] Asthana, Anushka, and Campbell, Denis, 'Binge Drink Scare Tactics "Do Not Work"', *The Observer*, 11 May 2008.

[169] Haggerty, 'From Risk to Precaution'.

[170] Baggott, *Alcohol, Politics and Social Policy*, pp 22-26; Burgess, Adam, 'Passive Drinking: A Good Lie Too Far?', *Health, Risk and Society*, 2009, vol 11, pp 527-540.

[171] Nick Sheron is currently secretary of the Alcohol Health Alliance and Ian Gilmore is its chair.

[172] Yeomans, *Blurred Visions*.

[173] Institute of Alcohol Studies, 'Who We Are', www.ias.org.uk/aboutus/who_we_are.html

[174] Alliance House Foundation, 'Director's Report for the Year Ended 31 March 2011', www.charitycommission.gov.uk/Accounts/Ends54/0000208554_ac_20110331_e_c.pdf

[175] Hope UK, 'Home', www.hopeuk.org/

[176] Smithers, Rebecca, 'Budget Raises Alcohol and Cigarette Prices', *The Guardian*, 22 April 2009.

[177] UK Government, *Alcohol Harm Reduction Strategy*, p 2.

[178] UK Government, *Safe. Sensible. Social.*, p 2.

[179] Ibid, p 3.

[180] Ibid, p 10.

[181] UK Government, *The Government's Alcohol Strategy*, Norwich: The Stationery Office, 2012.

[182] Hencke, David, and Sparrow, Andrew, 'Gordon Brown Rejects Call to Set Minimum Prices for Alcohol', *The Guardian*, 16 March 2009.

[183] UK Government, *The Government's Alcohol Strategy*, p 6.

[184] Cohen, Nick, 'This New Puritanism would Drive Anyone to Drink', *The Observer*, 10 January 2010; Ipsos Mori, 'No Clear Public Support for Minimum Pricing of Alcohol', www.ipsos-mori.com/researchpublications/researcharchive/2715/No-clear-public-support-for-minimum-pricing-of-alcohol.aspx; Home Office, *The Likely Impacts of Increasing Alcohol Price: A Summary Review of the Evidence Base*, London: Home Office, 2011.

[185] 'Letters to the Editor: Raising the Price of Drink Hurts the Majority While Public Disorder Goes Unpunished', *Daily Telegraph*, 15 January 2010.

[186] UK Government, *Alcohol Strategy*, p 1.

[187] Ibid.

[188] Woodhouse, John, and Ward, Philip, *A Minimum Price for Alcohol?*, London: Parliament, 2013.

[189] Von Hirsch, Andrew, 'Extending the Harm Principle: "Remote Harms" and Fair Imputation', in Simester, A.P, and Smith, A.T.H. (eds) *Harm and Culpability*, Oxford: Clarendon Press, 1996, p 259.

[190] Harcourt, 'The Collapse of the Harm Principle', p 119.

[191] There is a related academic debate here pertaining to the apparent rise of the 'precautionary principle'. Readers are directed to: Fisher, Elizabeth, 'Is the Precautionary Principle Justiciable?', *Journal of Environmental Law*, 2001, vol 13 (3), pp 315-334; Crawford, Adam, 'Regulating Civility, Governing Security and Policing (Dis)Order under the Conditions of Uncertainty', in Blad, J., Hildebrandt, M., Rozemond, K., Schuilenburg, M., and Van Caster, P. (eds) *Governing Security Under the Rule of Law*, The Hague: Eleven International, 2010, pp 9-35; Monaghan, Mark, Pawson, Ray, and Wicker, Kate, 'The Precautionary Principle and Evidence-Based Policy-Making', *Evidence & Policy*, 2012, vol 8 (2), pp 171-191.

[192] Burgess, 'Passive Drinking'; Hunt, Alan, 'Risk and Moralization in Everyday Life', in Ericson, Richard V., and Doyle, Aaron (eds) *Risk and Morality*, Toronto: University of Toronto Press, 2003, pp 165-192.

EIGHT

Conclusion: spirited measures and Victorian hangovers

Conspectus

This book began by using examples of recent regulatory changes in France and Russia to highlight the existence of significant cross-national variations in how alcohol is understood and regulated. 'Rational' explanations of these variations, which root them in levels of consumption or harm, were found to be insufficient. Chapter One further described how England and Wales have a historically demonstrable proclivity for both acute and chronic forms of public anxiety about drinking and identified that, in several scenarios at least, these anxieties were unrelated or distant from measurable levels of consumption and/or harm. Contrary to popular belief, it was emphasised that drinking is not a new, worsening or uniquely British social problem. It was insisted, therefore, that public anxieties about alcohol and related forms of governance are not the simple or exclusive products of patterns of consumption and harm, and warrant empirical attention in their own right. The book thus set out to examine the formative development of public attitudes and regulation relating to alcohol in England and Wales as well as building on the work of historians and social scientists, to consider whether the temperance movement played any role in these respective historical developments. Put simply, it is now possible to say that the problematisation of alcohol in the 19th century decisively differentiated Britain, in attitudinal and legal terms, from more permissive France and more spirits-concerned Russia. But, additionally, the book has revealed much more about how we think about and regulate alcohol in England and Wales.

Public attitudes and alcohol regulation

Chapters Two, Three and Four became occupied largely with the development and impact of the British temperance movement. Chapter Two stretched across the 18th and first half of the 19th century and argued that the temperance movement, after its teetotal turn in the 1830s, must be viewed as something historically distinct from previous expressions of anxiety about alcohol. Earlier instances of public opprobrium relating to drinking tended to be lacking in organisation, occupied with spirits or drunkenness only, and chronologically sporadic or limited in geographic spread. Hunt stresses the importance of agency, target, tactics and discourse within a moral regulation movement.[1] Using this description, it is apparent that the teetotal temperance movement that emerged in the 1830s constituted something new in regards to how drinking was understood and moralised. It was highly organised, operated through the promotion of voluntary teetotalism or prohibition and targeted all drinks and drinkers. It is this last feature, the problematisation of alcohol itself, which decisively challenged dominant discourse at the time in which beer-drinking or drinking that did not entail drunkenness were typically constructed as socially acceptable. These developments have been connected to the increasing salience of evangelical Protestantism in the first half of the 19th century. It has also been posited that, although attitudes to alcohol were already hardening and becoming more evangelical in the 1820s, the Beer Act 1830 accelerated this process as the proliferation of beerhouses prompted an enhanced recognition that beer, as well as alcoholic spirits, was a problematic substance. The advent of the teetotal temperance movement thus engendered a new and distinct project to morally regulate alcohol based around the problematisation of all forms of consumption.

Chapter Three examined how this problematisation of alcohol was effectively iterated in law between 1864 and 1872. The Licensing Act 1872 was identified as a significant piece of legislation as it normalised the idea that the law will regulate who can sell all types of alcohol and at what time it may be sold, as well as significantly advancing the criminalisation of public drunkenness, the limitation of purchase by age and police powers to enter licensed premises. In addition to these legal changes, the rhetoric of Henry Bruce, Lord Kimberley and others also made it explicit that, within these legal parameters, individuals were expected to further reform their own behaviour. The Act also, therefore, normalised the expectation that individuals will exercise self-regulation in regards to alcohol. Unlike the lax, free-trade-inspired regime of the Beer Act 1830, these legal restrictions and compulsions to self-reform applied to beer as equally as to spirits and so reflect the problematisation of alcohol advanced by the teetotal temperance movement.[2] By this point, the temperance movement had split into suasionist and prohibitionist factions. Interestingly, while prohibitionists were active in setting an agenda for licensing reforms, this governmental project of legal restriction coupled with moral compulsion towards self-reform bears much more in common with the voluntary, persuasive preferences of the moral suasionists. It is proposed that the temperance movement exercised a relatively significant amount of influence over setting the agenda for licensing reform and further contended that the character of these reforms was imbued with a fair dose of moral suasionist spirit.

This suasionist temperance spirit was found by Chapter Four to be abundantly evident within public discourse and drink regulation between 1914 and 1921. The orthodox historical view, that the issue of drink was redefined during the First World War in terms of national efficiency, was challenged through an exploration of the previously overlooked wartime pledge campaign. The pledge campaign was posited as an attempt to purify a depraved drunkard nation and thus providentially improve the nation's prospects for salvation. As well as being connected to an evangelical faith in human depravity, the pledge campaign illustrates the endurance of other Victorian temperance attitudes. Belief in the problematic nature of all drinking was reflected in the status of teetotalism specifically and self-denial generally as positive moral actions, desirable if not obligatory behaviours that had attained a heightened currency outside of the temperance movement during wartime. The extra-legal behavioural compulsion contained within the pledge campaign was accompanied by the tightening of legal restrictions on drink during the First World War. The response to war thus involved the strengthening of both aspects of the governmental model established in 1872. The Licensing Act 1921 retained some of these legal restrictions but further left behavioural space in which the exercise of self-restraint was normatively required. Chapters Three and Four showed, therefore, that the temperance movement was not an unqualified failure. Tightened legal controls reflected an acceptance of the originally teetotal idea that all types of drinking are problematic and in need of legal regulation. Broader public discourse reveals a general, hegemonic belief in the value of voluntary self-reform that relates closely to the ideas of moral suasionist temperance groups.

The next notable shift in the form of dominant modes of governing alcohol began shortly after the Licensing Act 1921. The inter-war and post-war years saw the decline of both the organised temperance movement and evangelical spirit that had done so much to sustain it. Concurrently, public alarm about drinking descended from its earlier peaks, new legal controls on drinking were barely attempted during the Second World War and, by 1961, a modest extension to the hours and premises in which alcohol sale was permissible was enacted. Nevertheless, alcohol remained the source of public concerns throughout the mid-

20th century. Significantly, this period saw the emergence of youth drinking and drink-driving as new frontiers in efforts to reform drinking habits. In some ways, this development merely revised older concerns as, for example, female drinking was reinterpreted in relation to motherhood and sexual health. But the connection of these issues, as well as male violence, to youth behaviour and alcohol consumption represents the first major historical manifestation of a specific concern for the drinking habits of young people, which is now embedded in public discourse. The subsequent direction of legal restrictions and moral compulsion at youth drinking, as well as driving, embodies the rise of more targeted forms of regulatory intervention. This was an age of partial permissiveness only, as certain forms of drinking and/ or certain groups of drinkers continued to occupy governmental attention. Alcohol remained an essentially problematic substance, even if its problematic effects were identified more within specific groups rather than all drinkers.

Chapter Six entailed a thematic look at the connection of alcohol to crime and disorder generally and a closer focus on the late 20th century onwards. After a brief survey of the association of alcohol with crime and disorder in modern history, it concentrated on how drink has been understood and regulated in the era of law and order politics from the 1980s onwards. While the trend of liberalising some aspects of licensing set by the Licensing Act 1961 has been continued by the Licensing Acts 1988, 1995 and 2003, other areas of regulation have been markedly strengthened. Chapter Five found that justifications for the regulation of youth drinking shifted from child or adolescent protection in the early decades of the 20th century to a more punitive ethos in the 1960s. Chapter Six built on this point in its analysis of targeted attempts to address drinking by young men, which were connected to football hooliganism or other forms of violent 'loutism' in the 1980s. Targeted restrictions were further implemented by the New Labour government 1997–2010 whose actions led to a proliferation of police powers and other constraints on both drinkers and drink-sellers. As well as broadening the regulation of certain types of drinking, the heightened level of contemporary public opprobrium surrounding alcohol and binge drinking in recent years has been found to equate to an intensification of the project to morally regulate alcohol. New imperatives for young people to avoid alcohol or for adults to 'drink responsibly' represent a moral regulation project in which desired codes of behaviour are promoted and behavioural alternatives are discursively devalued. Despite the relaxation of some statutory rules relating to the alcohol trade, targeted legal restrictions and moral compulsions towards 'responsibility' have been intensified. The overall picture is one of bifurcation rather than deregulation.

Encompassing issues of public health and addiction, Chapter Seven also gave a thematic overview of the whole period before concentrating more specifically on recent events. It rejects the suggestion that medical or public health models for understanding alcohol problems are morally neutral and highlights that, in public discourse, drink problems continue to be discussed in reference to individual culpability, self-control and a perceived societal moral vacuum for much of the 20th century. Recent public discourse has similarly been animated by moral regulation and this was specifically discussed in reference to the new public health position that has emerged since the 1970s. Drawing on total consumption theory and the availability theory, public health advocates have stressed that all forms of drinking entail risk and that solutions are most effective when they lower average consumption in a population instead of targeting 'problem drinkers'. The issuing of units guidance to all drinkers from the 1980s onwards and the more recent pursuit of pricing controls are evidence of the impact of this public health paradigm over some public policy. Units advice and price controls indicate an enhanced depth of government intervention in the decisions that individuals make about alcohol consumption. They also affect all drinks and all drinkers and hence show the increased breadth of governmental focus. Disillusioned with the abilities of people to effectively regulate their own drinking and convinced of the serious health risks engendered by any form of alcohol consumption, the public health model of governing drink has challenged and unsettled the dominant, targeted model.

It is thus possible to discern four main phases in the development of alcohol regulation in England and Wales within the time period studied:

1. the *pre-teetotalism phase* covering the 18th and first half of the 19th centuries. This phase was typified by a problematisation of spirits-drinking and drunkenness and, as the Beer Act 1830 demonstrated, free trade policies were feasible;
2. the *post-teetotalism phase* ushered in by legislation from 1864 to 1872, which showed an acceptance of the essentially problematic nature of all types of alcohol and the need to regulate, through legal restriction and moral compulsion, all forms of drinking;
3. the *targeted phase*, which started to emerge in the inter-war years and was consolidated in the 1960s as the regulation of drinking, through both legal restriction and moral compulsion, was relaxed for some but intensified for other social groups, notably young people;

4. the *conflict phase*, which the issuing of units guidance in the 1980s and the subsequent expanding influence of public-health-inspired, population-based ideas about alcohol and how it should be regulated have helped to create. During this phase, the governmental dominance of targeted regulation has been challenged.

This description of phased development is broad and may lack in historical nuance. But, nevertheless, the findings of this research strongly suggest that these are a fitting demarcation of the main stages in the formation of current drink regulation in England and Wales. Moreover, the importance of certain sets of attitudes, such as evangelicalism and welfarism, has been connected to these regulatory developments. But, as the next section explores further, the emergence of teetotal temperance in the 19th century heralded the most significant formative shift in how alcohol is understood and regulated.

Alcohol and moral regulation

As in the 19th century, current contention about how the law should regulate drink again pits those who see behavioural reformation as an individual, voluntary action against those who favour a societal behavioural remaking engendered by legal coercion. Whether the debates concern prohibition or price controls, the teetotal pledge or responsible self-regulation, the discursive contours are historically familiar. The way in which we think about and regulate alcohol in this conflict phase thus parallels the Victorian period. However, these are more than merely parallels at work here. The past is more than just something that precedes the present and more, in regards to the 'drink problem' at least, even than something that *has* shaped the present. Many of the arguments in this book rest on the assertion that past ideas, beliefs and values continue to construct contemporary attitudes and forms of governance. The concept of 'moral regulation' has been particularly illuminating in this regard. Broadly, it has been argued that behavioural governance and public discourse continue to be characterised by attempts to morally regulate the use of alcohol.

Chapter One defined morality as a normative judgement regarding the acceptability of certain forms of conduct and moral regulation is classified as any attempt to, in light of this normative judgement, reform a person's behaviour. The law, or at least criminal law, is therefore inextricably linked to moral regulation; it consists of regulations that problematise certain forms of conduct as well as enabling wrongdoers to be punished, their actions denounced and, perhaps, their behaviour reformed (through rehabilitative or deterrent sentences). So, as long as laws on licensing and drunkenness exist, it is perhaps not surprising to assert that *some* project to morally regulate drinking exists. However, the pertinent task then becomes looking at the specific character of moral regulation as evidenced in law at any point in time. It has been particularly argued that the provisions of the Licensing Act 1872 showed governmental acknowledgement of the problematisation of alcohol through the intensification of restrictive measures and its application to beer as equally as to spirits. Following Corrigan and Sayer's work on moral regulation,[3] it is possible to depict the teetotal temperance movement, which pioneered and promoted this problematisation of alcohol, as providing a moral ethos amenable to the expansion of the legal regulation of drink. Additionally, controversy surrounding beer-drinking and drunkenness following the Beer Act 1830 was suggested in Chapter Two to have accelerated the shift of the temperance movement towards teetotalism in the 1830s. It is worth adding, then, that certain laws may help to create a social context amenable to the emergence of new moral regulation projects.

Following Hunt and Ruonavaara, extra-legal means through which people are persuaded or encouraged to change their behavioural ways are also a central part of moral regulation.[4] Especially since the Licensing Act 1872, the law has imposed restrictions on the sale, purchase and consumption of alcohol as well as prohibiting certain types of behaviour, such as drink-driving, under-age drinking or public drunkenness. Within these legal parameters, individuals are expected to exercise self-regulation and the normative weighting of behavioural choices encourages them to do this. Politicians, journalists, doctors and others are active in the manufacture of moral imperatives and social obligations for people to avoid binge drinking or other forms of consumption viewed as unsafe and irresponsible. These irresponsible drinkers are contrasted with the 'responsible majority' of moderate, law-abiding drinkers who feature heavily in political rhetoric. The use of approved notions of respectability or responsibility to encourage certain behavioural decisions is an example of the practice of 'governing through choice' and indicative of state efforts to govern 'at a distance', as Rose and Miller would say, without necessary recourse to forms of legal coercion.[5] In the 20th century, the idea of giving individuals the information with which they can make rational informed choices about their conduct became a favourite government mantra, especially in the field of health promotion.[6] But in this analysis, choices are not free but normatively weighted as people are compelled towards socially approved outcomes.

The manner in which choices about drink are constructed further reveals affinities with the temperance movement's project to morally regulate alcohol. This is partly visible in the ongoing targeting of alcohol per se. Since government ministers echoed suasionist calls for sober self-regulation in 1872, moral compulsion has been directed by the problematisation of alcohol towards all drinkers. The rise of targeted regulation in the 20th century did indicate a governmental view that 'drink problems' were more concentrated in certain social groups or types of behaviour. But Chapters Five, Six and Seven have shown that choices about drink were not made in a context of complete permissiveness even during the mid-1900s and certainly have not been in the period since. Notably, public health campaigns, from the late 20th century onwards, have aimed at all drinkers and promoted all forms of drinking as the target of governmental action. Moreover, some of the groups involved in these health campaigns for new laws or in urging people to restrict their own consumption have organisational links to Victorian temperance. Chapter Seven recorded that Hope UK is the new moniker of the Band of Hope temperance society as well as identifying that the Institute of Alcohol Studies was formed by an offshoot of the prohibitionist UK Alliance and continues to be funded largely by a group committed to teetotalism. Some of the groups involved in attempts to regulate drinking are still connected to the Victorian temperance movement.

The active influence of Victorian temperance over contemporary public attitudes and regulation is more widely apparent within current discourse on alcohol. The construction of long-term, non-probabilistic health risks was found by Chapter Seven to equate with the slippery slope of sin, death and damnation on which temperance activists believed the drinker was positioned. Chapter Six found much of the furious reaction to the Licensing Act 2003 to be based on the 'availability theory' of alcohol consumption, in which the greater availability of alcohol necessarily entails greater consumption and greater social harm, primarily through crime and disorder. This theory was similarly found to rest on the contention that individuals cannot regulate their own drinking and their own behaviour and hence the state is required to use the law to do so instead. Increasing the availability of alcohol again places the drinker on a slippery slope, which ends in harm to themselves and others. The logic of risk and availability which structures individual choices and influences government policy displays the clear heuristic fingerprints of the Victorian temperance movement. Contemporary efforts to morally regulate alcohol are thus strongly tied to a specific historical manifestation of moral regulation.

The influence of the Victorian temperance movement over both the legal restrictions and moral compulsions that continue to regulate the use of alcohol is, therefore, significant. Importantly, the idea that all types of alcohol are essentially problematic, the conception of drinking as a slippery slope and the normative weighting of individual choices as a means to govern behaviour are no longer matters for public or personal contemplation. These historically contingent ideas, beliefs and values have become entirely orthodox, barely questioned artefacts of 'common sense' that are embedded in the national psyche. Chapter One identified a geographic and chronological association between social anxieties about alcohol, as expressed in alarmed public attitudes and strict legal regulation, and the historical occurrence of abstinence-based temperance movements. It is now possible to assert that a consistent target, enduring discursive frameworks, organisational connections and legal legacies provide the ontological substance that links the 19th-century temperance movement to the continued existence of public anxieties about alcohol in England and Wales. This might be called an attitudinal and regulatory hangover from the Victorian period but it is important to stress that these attitudes and forms of regulation are not just the backdrop to the present or a lingering relic of the past. It is argued here that the spirit of moral regulation past continues to influence measures taken, legally and extra-legally, to govern the consumption of alcohol.

Moral inheritance

To reiterate a point made in Chapter One, this book does not propose that people are subjected to some monolithic regime of pervasive governance that tightly controls how they can and cannot consume alcohol. Rose and Miller explained that 'we do not live in a governed world so much as a world traversed by the "will to govern"'.[7] Loosely, then, this book has concerned the 'will to govern' drinking. More specifically, it has traced public attitudes and the regulation of alcohol through modern British history and, in doing so, has identified persistent, ongoing attempts to morally regulate the use of alcohol. It has also emphasised the specific impact of the Victorian temperance movement in shaping these attempts to govern human behaviour. It has been apparent that how alcohol is understood and regulated has changed through time. This illustrates, to borrow from Hier, that a discursive 'volatility' within processes of moralisation is evident[8] or, to draw on Critcher, it is evidence of high and low points within existing moral currents.[9] It is also significant that, as the last section summarised, the constancy of certain discursive formations, organisational groups and the governmental model of legal restriction and moral compulsion demonstrate a discernible congruity between anxieties about alcohol past and present.

The findings of this book thus reinforce the conceptual synthesis discussed in Chapter One, in which Critcher classified moral panics as positioned within longer-term processes of moral regulation. Chapter Four explored how, when placed in historical perspective, the idea of a moral panic is slightly problematic because, in Cohen's classic formulation, episodes of panic are exceptional and temporary.[10] If this is the case, how can one outburst of public anxiety influence subsequent ideas or shape the next episode of moral panic? In this respect, moral panic theory can almost be seen as ahistorical or, to borrow Hunt's phrase, 'presentist'.[11] Within this emerging synthesis of moral panic and moral regulation theory it is important that a clear concern with the legal and discursive legacies, which certain moral panics and social movements may bequeath to their successors, is conceptually central. Elsewhere I have referred to this phenomenon as a 'moral inheritance'.[12] This moral inheritance prevents the importance of self-reform and personal agency within current drink regulation being attributed to more recent social developments. The eminence of self-regulation in alcohol governance could, for example, be subsumed within a wider political trend towards (what many people call) neoliberalism. Instead, the recognition of the moral inheritance within current efforts to regulate alcohol connects them to an older historical genealogy of governmental development. This notion of moral inheritance may, therefore, prove a useful consideration within historical social sciences and the study of social problems more generally.[13]

Of course, the conclusions here reached are contingent on the methods that have been used and the sources that have been analysed. It is possible that research using different discursive data or prioritising focus on differing time periods may produce divergent findings. Nevertheless, an extensive rebuttal of the rational model of explaining drink problems has been presented. The importance of analysing how we think about and regulate alcohol, rather than reducing these crucial phenomena to mere offshoots of patterns of consumption and harm, has been amply demonstrated. The main formative factors and moments in the development of public attitudes and regulation have also been identified. These historical forces have produced a present that is beset by public anxieties as all forms of alcohol are regarded as essentially problematic and the necessity of utilising some form of legal regulation is no longer publicly questioned. To many, these are unremarkable, common-sense positions; but 'common sense' is culturally specific rather than universally intuitive. The news stories about France and Russia cited earlier suggest that the dominant perception of beer or wine in these countries was, until recently, that they were somehow qualitatively different from alcoholic spirits and required less legal regulation. It is thus asserted that current British faith in the inherently problematic nature of alcohol and the need for its regulation (through legal restriction and moral compulsion) is the product of a historically particular configuration of factors, notably including the 19th-century, teetotal temperance movement.

It is inviting, at this stage of a historical study, to speculate on what the future might hold. The current conflict phase is characterised by tension between the dominant targeted model of regulating alcohol and the emerging public-health-inspired paradigm of governance, and so it is tempting to make some grand projection of the direction of future travel in this regard. It might be stated, for example, that the public health paradigm will either overcome the targeted governance of alcohol or fall by the governmental wayside for some reason. Perhaps the antagonism between these two opposing models of governance will cause both to be abandoned and new solutions sought. But it is equally possible that both the public health paradigm and targeted regulation will continue to co-exist indefinitely, much as they have done in recent decades, as mutually dissatisfied bedfellows. Irrespective, whatever manner in which future generations think about and regulate alcohol will have been, to a large degree, left to them by previous generations. This book has highlighted the manifold ways in which the past continues to shape the present. So, the most compelling question that remains is whether future generations are bequeathed a legacy of chronic and acute public anxiety about alcohol or whether a more reasoned, reflective approach to understanding and regulating alcohol might be forged. Using history and social science, this book is intended as a contribution to the development of just such a reasoned approach.

Notes

[1] Hunt, *Governing Morals*.

[2] It must be said that the prohibition of the under-16s from purchasing spirits for consumption on licensed premises in the Licensing Act 1872 does not support this statement. But other significant rules on licensing and drunkenness applied to all drinks during this crucial period of reform.

[3] Corrigan and Sayer, *The Great Arch*.

[4] Hunt, *Governing Morals*; Ruonavaara, 'Moral Regulation'.

5   Rose and Miller, 'Political Power Beyond the State'.

6   Davison, C., and Davey-Smith, G., 'The Baby and the Bathwater: Examining Sociocultural and Free–Market Critiques of Health Promotion', in Bunton, B., Nettleton, S., and Burrows, R. *The Sociology of Health Promotion: Critical Analyses of Consumption, Lifestyle, and Risk*, London: Routledge, 1995, pp 91-103.

7   Rose and Miller, 'Political Powers Beyond the State', pp 190-191.

8   Hier, 'Thinking Beyond Moral Panic'.

9   Critcher, 'Widening the Focus'.

10 Cohen, 'Folk Devils and Moral Panics'.

11 Hunt, *Governing Morals*, p 196.

12 Yeomans, 'Theorising Alcohol in Public Discourse'.

13 I have had helpful conversations with Dan Lett, University of Victoria (Canada), around these issues. He separates (as I understand it) moral convictions from moral rhetoric and stresses that either may change while the other remains constant.

Bibliography

Primary sources

BBC News (2003–10).
British Library's Burney Collection (1700–1800).
British Library's Catalogue of Nineteenth Century Newspapers (1800–1900).
British Library's Evanion Collection of Victorian Ephemera (1837–1901).
British Postal Museum and Archive (1851).
English Chartist Circular (1841–44).
Fortnightly Review (1893).
Hansard, House of Commons Debate, 26 November 1958, vol 596 cols 365-508.
Hunt, W., *History of Teetotalism in Devonshire*, UK: Western Temperance Advocate Office, 1841.
LexisNexis Newspaper Database (2003–10).
Orwell, George, 'As I Please', *Tribune*, 18 August 1944.
The (London) Times and *The Sunday Times* (1785–1965).
The (Manchester) Guardian and *The Observer* (1914–65).
UK Press Online (1914–65).
Wilkie, David, *The Village Holiday* (1809–11), Tate Gallery.
Windsor Magazine (1901–02).

Books and chapters in edited collections

Ayres, Ian, and Braithwaite, John, *Responsive Regulation: Transcending the Deregulation Debate*, Oxford: Oxford University Press, 1992.
Baggott, Rob, *Alcohol, Politics and Social Policy*, Aldershot: Gower, 1990.
Barr, Andrew, *Drink: A Social History*, London: Pimlico, 1998.
Bhaskar, Roy, *A Realist Theory of Science*, Hemel Hempstead: Harvester, 1978.
Bingham, Adrian, *Family Newspapers? Sex, Private Life and the British Popular Press, 1918-1978*, Oxford: Oxford University Press, 2009.
Blocker, Jack S., Fahey, David M., and Tyrell, Ian R., *Alcohol and Temperance in Modern History: An International Encyclopaedia*, Santa Barbara, CA: ABC-CLIO, 2003.
Briggs, John, Harrison, Christopher, McInnes, Angus, and Vincent, David, *Crime and Punishment in England*, London: UCL Press, 1996.

Brown, Pete, *Man Walks into Pub*, London: Pan Macmillan, 2004.

Bryman, Alan, *Social Research Methods* (2nd edition), Oxford: Oxford University Press, 2004.

Burnett, John, *Liquid Pleasures*, London: Routledge, 1999.

Cavadino, Michael, and Dignan, James, *The Penal System* (4th edition), London: Sage Publications, 2007.

Chadwick, Edwin, *Report on the Sanitary Condition of the Labouring Population of Great Britain*, Edinburgh: Edinburgh University Press, 1965.

Cohen, Stanley, *Folk Devils and Moral Panics*, London: MacGibbon and Kee, 1972.

Cook, Christopher, *Alcohol, Addiction and Christian Ethics*, Cambridge: Cambridge University Press, 2006.

Corrigan, Philip, and Sayer, Derek, *The Great Arch: English State Formation as Cultural Revolution*, London: Basil Blackwell, 1985.

Crawford, Adam, 'Regulating Civility, Governing Security and Policing (Dis)Order under the Conditions of Uncertainty', in Blad, J., Hildebrandt, M., Rozemond, K., Schuilenburg, M. and Van Caster, P (eds) *Governing Security Under the Rule of Law*, The Hague: Eleven International, 2010, pp 9-35.

Crawford, Adam, and Lister, Stuart, *The Use and Impact of Dispersal Orders*, Bristol: The Policy Press, 2007.

Critcher, Chas, 'Moral Panics: A Case Study of Binge Drinking', in Franklin, Bob (ed) *Pulling Newspapers Apart*, Abingdon: Routledge, 2008, pp 154-162.

Critcher, Chas, 'Drunken Antics: The Gin Craze, Binge Drinking and the Political Economy of Moral Regulation', in Hier, Sean (ed) *Moral Panic and the Politics of Anxiety*, Abingdon: Routledge, 2011, pp 171-189.

Davison, C., and Davey-Smith, G. 'The Baby and the Bathwater: Examining Sociocultural and Free-Market Critiques of Health Promotion', in Bunton, B., Nettleton, S., and Burrows, R. (eds) *The Sociology of Health Promotion: Critical Analyses of Consumption, Lifestyle, and Risk*, London: Routledge, 1995, pp 91-103.

Dingwall, Gavin, *Alcohol and Crime*, Cullompton: Willan, 2006.

Donajgrodzki, A.P., 'Introduction', in Donajgrodzki, A.P. (ed) *Social Control in Nineteenth Century Britain*, London: Croon Helm, 1977, pp 9-26.

Dorn, Nicholas, *Alcohol, Youth and the State*, London: Croon Helm, 1983.

Durkheim, Emile, *Suicide*, London: Routledge, 1970.

Ehrenreich, Barbara, *Dancing in the Street*, London: Granta, 2007.

Elias, Norbert, *The Civilizing Process*, Oxford: Blackwell, 1994.

Emsley, Clive, *The English Police*, London: Longman, 1991.

Emsley, Clive, *Crime and Society in England, 1750-1900*, Harlow: Longman, 1994.

Engels, Friedrich, *The Condition of the Working Class in England*, Oxford: Oxford University Press, 1993.

Ericsson, Richard V., and Doyle, Aaron, *Risk and Morality*, Toronto: University of Toronto Press, 2003.

Eriksen, Sidsel, 'Drunken Danes and Sober Swedes? Religious Revivalism and the Temperance Movements as Keys to Danish and Swedish Folk Cultures', in Strath, Bo (ed) *Language and the Construction of Class Identities*, Gothenburg: Gothenburg University Press, 1989, pp 55-94.

Foucault, Michel, *Discipline and Punish*, London: Penguin, 1991.

Foucault, Michel, *Security, Territory, Population: Lectures at the College de France 1977–78*, Basingstoke: Palgrave, 2007.

Foucault, Michel, *The Government of Self and Others*, Basingstoke: Palgrave, 2010.

Fulton Phin, Nicholas, 'The Historical Development of Public Health', in Wilson, Frances, and Mabhala, Mzwandile (eds) *Key Concepts in Public Health*, London: Sage Publications, 2008, pp 5-10.

Garland, David, *Punishment and Welfare*, Aldershot: Gower, 1985.

Glover, Brian, *Brewing for Victory: Brewers, Beers and Pubs in World War Two*, Cambridge: Lutterworth Press, 1995.

Goode, Erich, and Ben-Yehuda, Nachmann, 'Grounding and Defending the Sociology of Moral Panic', in Hier, Sean (ed) *Moral Panic and the Politics of Anxiety*, Abingdon: Routledge, 2011, pp 29-36.

Green, S.J.D., *The Passing of Protestant England*, Cambridge: Cambridge University Press, 2011.

Greenaway, John, *Drink and British Politics since 1830*, Basingstoke: Palgrave, 2003.

Gusfield, Joseph, *Contested Meanings: The Construction of Alcohol Problems*, Wisconsin, WI: University of Wisconsin Press, 1996.

Gusfield, Joseph R., 'Status Conflicts and the Changing Ideologies of the American Temperance Movement', in Pittman, David J., and Snyder, Charles R. (eds) *Society, Culture and Drinking Patterns*, New York, NY: John Wiley, 1962, pp 101-120.

Gutzke, David W., *Protecting the Pub: Brewers and Publicans against Temperance*, Woodbridge, UK: Boydell & Brewer, 1989.

Hadfield, Phil, *Bar Wars: Contesting the Night in Contemporary British Cities*, Oxford: Oxford University Press, 2006.

Haggerty, Kevin D., 'From Risk to Precaution: The Rationalities of Personal Crime Prevention', in Ericson, Richard V., and Doyle, Aaron (eds) *Risk and Morality*, Toronto: University of Toronto Press, 2003, pp 193-214.

Hall, Stuart, Critcher, Chas, Jefferson, Tony, Clarke, John, and Roberts, Brian, *Policing the Crisis: Mugging, the State and Law and Order*, Basingstoke: Macmillan, 1978.

Hames, Gina, *Alcohol in World History*, Abingdon: Routledge, 2012.

Harrison, Brian, *Drink and the Victorians*, London: Faber and Faber, 1971.

Hart, H.L.A., *Essays in Jurisprudence and Philosophy*, Oxford: Oxford University Press, 1983.

Hill, Christopher, *Puritanism and Revolution*, London: Panther, 1968.

Hilton, Boyd, *The Age of Atonement*, Oxford: Clarendon Press, 1988.

Hobhouse, Leonard, *Liberalism and Other Writings*, Cambridge: Cambridge University Press, 1994.

Hunt, Alan, *Governing Morals: A Social History of Moral Regulation*, Cambridge: Cambridge University Press, 1999.

Hunt, Alan, 'Risk and Moralization in Everyday Life', in Ericson, Richard V., and Doyle, Aaron (eds) *Risk and Morality*, Toronto: University of Toronto Press, 2003, pp 165-192.

Jennings, Paul, *The Local: A History of the English Pub*, Stroud: History Press, 2007.

Levine, Harry, 'Temperance Cultures: Concern about Alcohol in Nordic and English-speaking Countries', in Lader, Malcolm, Edwards, Griffith, and Drummon, D. Colin (eds) *The Nature of Alcohol and Drug-Related Problems*, Oxford: Oxford University Press, 1993, pp 16-36.

Lukes, Steven, *Emile Durkheim: His Life and Work*, London: Penguin, 1973.

McLaughlin, Patrick M. 'Responding to Drunkenness in Scottish Society: A Socio-Historical Study of Response to Alcohol Problems', unpublished PhD thesis, University of Stirling, 1989.

Malcolmson, Robert W., *Popular Recreations in English Society 1700–1850*, Cambridge: Cambridge University Press, 1979.

Mill, J.S., *On Liberty*, London: Penguin, 1985.

Morgan, Rod, *Summary Justice: Fast – but Fair?*, London: Centre for Crime and Justice Studies, 2008.

Muncie, John, *Youth and Crime* (3rd edition), London: Sage Publications, 2009.

Nellis, Mike, 'Humanising Justice: The English Probation Service up to 1972', in Gelsthorpe, Loraine, and Morgan, Rod (eds) *Handbook of Probation*, Cullompton: Willan, 2007, pp 25-58.

Nicholls, James, *The Politics of Alcohol*, Manchester: Manchester University Press, 2009.

Plant, Martin, and Plant, Moira, *Binge Britain*, Oxford: Oxford University Press, 2006.

Prior, Lindsay, 'Following in Foucault's Footsteps', in Silverman, David (ed) *Qualitative Research*, London, Sage Publications, 1997, pp 64-65.

Room, Robin, 'Addiction and Personal Responsibility as Solutions to the Contradictions of Neoliberal Consumerism', in Bell, Kirsten, McNaughton, Darlene, and Salmon, Amy (eds) *Alcohol, Tobacco and Obesity*, Abingdon: Routledge, 2011, pp 47-58.

Matthews, Bob, and Ross, Liz, *Research Methods*, Harlow: Pearson, 2010.

Roberts, M.J.D., *Making English Morals*, Cambridge: Cambridge University Press, 2004.

Rowbotham, Judith, and Stevenson, Kim, 'Introduction', in Rowbotham, Judith, and Stevenson, Kim (eds) *Behaving Badly*, Aldershot: Ashgate, 2003.

Rowbotham, Judith, and Stevenson, Kim, 'Causing a Sensation: Media and Legal Representations of Bad Behaviour', in Rowbotham, Judith, and Stevenson, Kim (eds) *Behaving Badly*, Aldershot: Ashgate, 2003.

Sandel, Michael J., *Justice: What's The Right Thing to Do?*, London: Penguin, 2009.

Schrad, Mark Lawrence, *The Political Power of Bad Ideas: Networks, Institutions and the Global Prohibition Wave*, Oxford: Oxford University Press, 2010.

Seddon, Toby, *A History of Drugs: Drugs and Freedom in the Liberal Age*, Abingdon: Routledge: 2010.

Sennett, Richard, *The Fall of Public Man*, Cambridge: Cambridge University Press, 1974.

Shiman, Lilian Lewis, *Crusade Against Drink in Victorian England*, Basingstoke: Macmillan, 1988.

Simmonds, N.E., *Central Issues in Jurisprudence: Justice, Law and Rights*, London: Sweet and Maxwell, 1986.

Simon, Jonathan, *Governing Through Crime: How the War on Crime Transformed American Democracy and Created a Culture of Fear*, Oxford: Oxford University Press, 2007.

Sulkunen, Pekka, *The Saturated Society: Governing Risk and Lifestyle in Consumer Culture*, London: Sage Publications, 2009.

Sumner, Maggie, and Parker, Howard, *Low in Alcohol: A Review of International Research into Alcohol's Role in Crime Causation*, London: Portman Group, 1995.

Thom, Betsy, *Dealing with Drink*, London: Free Association, 1999.

Thompson, E.P, *Whigs and Hunters*, Harmondsworth: Penguin, 1977.

Thompson, E.P., *The Making of the English Working Class*, Harmondsworth: Penguin, 1980.

Turner, Stephen, *Liberal Democracy 3.0*, London: Sage Publications, 2003.

Valverde, Mariana, *Diseases of the Will: Alcohol and the Dilemmas of Freedom*, Cambridge: Cambridge University Press, 1998.

Von Hirsch, Andrew, 'Extending the Harm Principle: "Remote Harms" and Fair Imputation', in Simester, A.P., and Smith, A.T.H. (eds) *Harm and Culpability*, Oxford: Clarendon Press, 1996, pp 259-276.

Warner, Jessica, *Craze: Gin and Debauchery in an Age of Reason*, London: Profile, 2004.

Weber, Max, *The Protestant Ethic and the Spirit of Capitalism*, London: Unwin, 1965.

Wiener, Martin, *Reconstructing the Criminal*, Cambridge: Cambridge University Press, 1990.

Wilson, George B., *Alcohol and the State*, London: Nicholson and Watson, 1940.

Winlow, Simon, and Hall, Steve, *Violent Night*, Oxford: Berg, 2006.

Yeomans, Henry, 'Blurred Visions: Experts, Evidence and the Promotion of Moderate Drinking', in Smith, Alex T., and Holmwood, John (eds) *Sociologies of Moderation: Problems of Democracy, Expertise and the Media*, Oxford: Wiley Blackwell, 2013, pp 58-78.

Yeomans, Henry, 'Theorising Alcohol in Public Discourse: Moral Panics or Moral Regulation?', in Petley, Julian, Critcher, Chas, Hughes, Jason, and Rohloff, Amanda (eds) *Moral Panics in the Contemporary World*, London: Bloomsbury, 2013, pp 101-24.

Journal articles

Anderson, Stuart, 'Discretion and the Rule of Law: The Licensing of Drink in England, c.1817-40', *Journal of Legal History*, 2002, vol 23 (1), pp 45-59.

Armstrong, David, 'The Rise of Surveillance Medicine', *Sociology of Health and Illness*, 1995, vol 17 (3), pp 393-404.

Bauman, Zygmunt, 'Social Issues of Law and Order', *British Journal of Criminology*, 2000, vol 40 (2), pp 205-221.

Ben-Yehuda, Nachman, 'Moral Panics--36 Years On', *British Journal of Criminology*, 2009, vol 49, pp 1-3.

Borsay, Peter, 'Binge Drinking and Moral Panics: Historic Parallels?', *History and Policy*, 2007, www.historyandpolicy.org/papers/policy-paper-62.html

Brown, James B., 'The Temperance Career of Joseph Chamberlain, 1870-1877: A Study in Political Frustration', *Albion*, 1972, vol 4 (1), pp 29-44.

Burgess, Adam, 'Passive Drinking: A Good Lie Too Far?', *Health, Risk & Society*, 2009, vol 11, pp 527-540.

Burroughs, A., and McNamara, D., 'Liver Disease in Europe', *Alimentary Pharmacology and Therapeutics*, 2003, vol 18 (3), pp 54-59.

Crawford, Adam, 'Governing through Anti-Social Behaviour: Regulatory Challenges to Criminal Justice', *British Journal of Criminology*, 2009, vol 49 (6), pp 810-831.

Critcher, Chas, 'Widening the Focus: Moral Panics as Moral Regulation', *British Journal of Criminology*, 2009, vol 49 (1), pp 17-34.

Dooldeniya, M.D., Khafagy, R., Mashaly, H., Browning, A.J., Sundaram, S.K., and Biyani, C.S., 'Lower Abdominal Pain in Women after Bring Drinking', *British Medical Journal*, 2007, vol 335, pp 992-993.

Fisher, Elizabeth, 'Is the Precautionary Principle Justiciable?', *Journal of Environmental Law*, 2001, vol 13 (3), p 315-334.

Greenfield, T.K., and Giesbrecht, N.A., 'Views of Alcohol Control Policies in the 2000 National Alcohol Survey: What News for Alcohol Policy Development in the US and its States?', *Journal of Substance Use*, 2007, vol 12 (6), pp 429-445.

Hadfield, Phil, and Measham, Fiona, 'After the Act: Alcohol Licensing and the Administrative Governance of Crime', *Criminology and Public Policy*, 2010, vol 9 (1), pp 69-76.

Harcourt, Bernard E., 'The Collapse of the Harm Principle', *Journal of Criminal Law and Criminology*, 1999, vol 90 (1), pp 109-194.

Hayward, Keith, and Hobbs, Dick, 'Beyond the Binge in Booze Britain: Market-led Liminalisation and the Spectacle of Binge Drinking', *The British Journal of Sociology*, 2007, vol 58 (3), pp 437-456.

Hier, Sean P., 'Thinking Beyond Moral Panic: Risk, Responsibility, and the Politics of Moralization', *Theoretical Criminology*, 2008, vol 12 (2), pp 173-190.

Hunt, Alan, 'Getting Marx and Foucault into Bed Together!', *Journal of Law and Society*, 2004, vol 31 (4), pp 596-609.

Jenkins, Philip, 'Failure to Launch: Why do some Social Issues Fail to Detonate Moral Panics?', *British Journal of Criminology*, 2009, vol 49, pp 35-47.

Jennings, Paul, 'Liquor Licensing and the Local Historian: Inns and Alehouses 1753-1828', *The Local Historian*, 2010, vol 40 (2), pp 136-150.

Jennings, Paul, 'Policing Drunkenness in England and Wales from the Late Eighteenth Century to the First World War', *The Social History of Alcohol and Drugs*, 2012, vol 26 (1), pp 69-92.

Jennings, Paul, 'Policing Public Houses in Victorian England', *Law, Crime and History*, 2013, vol 3 (1), pp 52-75.

Kneale, James, 'The Place of Drink: Temperance and the Public 1856-1914', *Social and Cultural Geography*, 2001, vol 2 (1), pp 43-49.

Lowe, Pam K., and Lee, Ellie J., 'Advocating Alcohol Abstinence to Pregnant Women: Some Observations about British Policy', *Health, Risk and Society*, 2010, vol 12 (4), pp 301-311.

Measham, Fiona, and Brain, Kevin, 'Binge Drinking, British Alcohol Policy and the New Culture of Intoxication', *Crime, Media, Culture*, 2005, vol 1 (3), pp 262-283.

Measham, Fiona, and Ostergaard, Jeanette, 'The Public Face of Binge Drinking: British and Danish Young Women: Recent Trends in Alcohol Consumption and the European Binge Drinking Debate', *Probation Journal*, 2009, vol 56, pp 415-434.

Monaghan, Mark, Pawson, Ray, and Wicker, Kate, 'The Precautionary Principle and Evidence-based Policy-making', *Evidence & Policy*, 2012, vol 8 (2), pp 171-191.

Moriarty, Kieran, and Gilmore, Ian T., 'Licensing Britain's Alcohol Epidemic', *Journal of Epidemiology and Community Health*, 2006, vol 60, p 94.

Moss, Stella, '"A Grave Question": The Children Act and Public House Regulation, c.1908–1939', *Crimes and Misdemeanours*, 2009, vol 3 (2), pp 98-117.

O'Malley, Pat, and Valverde, Mariana, 'Pleasure, Freedom and Drugs: The Uses of Pleasure in Liberal Governance of Drug and Alcohol Consumption', *Sociology*, 2004, vol 38 (1), pp 27-28.

Osterberg, Esa L., 'Alcohol Tax Changes and the Use of Alcohol in Europe', *Drugs and Alcohol Review*, vol 30 (2), pp 124-129.

Patton, G.C., Coffey, C., Sawyer, S.M., Viner, R.M., Haller, D.M., Bose, K., Vos, T., Ferguson, J., and Mathers, C.D., 'Global patterns of mortality in young people: a systematic analysis of population health data', *The Lancet*, 2009, vol 374 (9693), pp 881-892.

Reinarman, Craig, 'The Social Construction of an Alcohol Problem: The Case of Mothers Against Drink Drivers', *Theory and Society*, 1988, vol 17 (1), pp 91-120.

Rose, Nikolas, and Miller, Peter, 'Political Power Beyond the State: Problematics of Government', *British Journal of Sociology*, 1992, vol 43 (2), pp 173-205.

Rowbotham, Judith, 'Legislating For Your Own Good: Criminalising Moral Choice. The Echoes of the Victorian Vaccination Act', *Liverpool Law Review*, 2009, vol 30, pp 13-33.

Ruonavaara, Hannu, 'Moral Regulation: A Reformulation', *Sociological Theory*, 1997, vol 15 (3), pp 277-293.

Sheron, Nick, Hawkey, Chris, and Gilmore, Ian, 'Projections of Alcohol Deaths – a Wake-up Call', *The Lancet*, 2011, vol 377 (9774), pp 1297-1299.

Smith, Alexander Thomas T., 'Fear and Loathing in Kansas City', *Anthropology Today*, 2010, vol 26 (4), pp 4-7.

Sulkunen, Pekka, 'Ethics of Alcohol Policy in a Saturated Society', *Addiction*, 1997, vol 92 (9), pp 1117-1122.

Valverde, Mariana, 'Slavery from Within: The Invention of Alcoholism and the Question of Free Will', *Social History*, 1997, vol 22 (3), pp 251-268.

Warner, Jessica, 'Are you a Closet Fabian? Licensing Schemes Then and Now', *Addiction*, 2006, vol 101, pp 909-910.

Warner, Jessica, 'Temperance, Alcohol and the American Evangelical: A Reassessment', *Addiction*, 2009, vol 104 (7), pp 1075-1084.

Warner, Jessica, and Ivis, Frank, '"Damn You, You Informing Bitch": *Vox Populi* and the Unmaking of the Gin Act 1736', *Journal of Social History*, 1999, vol 33, p 4.

Warner, Jessica, Her, Minghao, Gmel, Gerhard, and Rehm, Jurgen, 'Can Legislation Prevent Debauchery? Mother Gin and Public Health in 18th Century England', *American Journal of Public Health*, 2001, vol 91 (3), pp 375-384.

Warner, Jessica, Riviere, Janine, and Carson, Jenny, 'On Wit, Irony, and Living with Imperfection', *American Journal of Public Health*, 2008, vol 98 (5), pp 814-822.

Yeomans, Henry, 'Revisiting a Moral Panic: Attitudes to Alcohol, Ascetic Protestantism and the Implementation of the Licensing Act 2003', *Sociological Research Online*, 2009, vol 14 (2), www.socresonline. org.uk/14/2/6.html

Yeomans, Henry, 'Providentalism, the Pledge and Victorian Hangovers: Investigating Moderate Alcohol Policy in Britain, 1914–1918', *Law, Crime and History*, 2011, vol 1, pp 95-108.

Yeomans, Henry, 'What did the British Temperance Movement Accomplish? Attitudes to Alcohol, the Law and Moral Regulation', *Sociology*, 2011, vol 45 (1), pp 38-53.

Young, Kevin, '"The Killing Field": Themes in the Mass Media Responses to the Heysel Stadium Riot', *International Review for the Sociology of Sport*, 1986, vol 21 (2-3), pp 253-266.

Official publications, other data sources and miscellany

Alcohol Concern, 'About Us', www.alcoholconcern.org.uk/about-us

Alcoholics Anonymous, 'The Twelve Steps of Alcoholics Anonymous', www.aa.org/en_pdfs/smf-121_en.pdf

Alliance House Foundation, 'Director's Report for the Year Ended 31 March 2011', www.charity-commission.gov.uk/Accounts/Ends54/0000208554_ac_20110331_e_c.pdf

Anderson, Peter, and Baumberg, Ben, 'Alcohol in Europe', 2006, http://ec.europa.eu/health/archive/ph_determinants/life_style/alcohol/documents/alcohol_europe_en.pdf

British Beer and Pub Association, 'Licensing Anniversary YouGov Poll – Whoops No Apocalypse', 2006, www.beerandpub.com/newsList_detail.aspx?newsId=122

'Conversation with Derek Rutherford', *Addiction*, vol 107 (5), pp 892-899.

Department for Culture, Media and Sport, 'Evaluation of the Impact of the Licensing Act 2003', 2008, www.culture.gov.uk/images/publications/Licensingevaluation.pdf

Department for Transport, 'Licensed Vehicles by Tax Class, Great Britain, Annually, 1909 to 2011', 2012, http://webarchive.nationalarchives.gov.uk/20120913084528/www.dft.gov.uk/statistics/tables/veh0103/

Donaldson, Sir Liam, *Annual Report of the Chief Medical Officer 2008: On the State of Public Health*, London: Department of Health, 2009.

Donaldson, Sir Liam, *Guidance on the Consumption of Alcohol by Children and Young People*, London: Department of Health, 2009.

Drinkaware, 'Alcohol Self-Assessment', 2013, https://www.drinkaware.co.uk/selfassessment

Drinkaware, 'Why Let the Good Times Turn Bad?', 2013, https://www.drinkaware.co.uk/good-times

Fox, Kate, 'Understanding Alcohol', 2011, *Four Thought*, BBC Radio 4, 12 October, www.bbc.co.uk/programmes/b015p86z

'Henry Bruce, 1st Baron of Aberdare', henry-bruce-1st-baron-aberdare.co.tv

Hibell, Bjorn, Guttormsson, Ulf, Ahlström, Salme, Balakireva, Olga, Bjarnason, Thoroddur, Kokkevi, Anna, and Kraus, Ludwig, *The 2007 ESPAD Report*, 2007, www.espad.org/en/Reports--Documents/ESPAD-Reports/

Hislop, Ian, *Sinful Sex and Demon Drink*, 2010, episode 3 of series The Age of the Do-Gooders, BBC2, 13 December.

Home Office, 'Alcohol – Know Your Limits', 2008, http://news.bbc.co.uk/1/hi/uk/7457746.stm

Home Office, *The Likely Impacts of Increasing Alcohol Price: A Summary Review of the Evidence Base*, London: Home Office, 2011.

Home Office, 'Tough New Powers to Tackle Alcohol Crime Announced', 2010, http://webarchive.nationalarchives.gov.uk/+/www.homeoffice.gov.uk/about-us/news/powers-tackle-alcohol-crime.html

Hope UK, 'Home', www.hopeuk.org/

Institute of Alcohol Studies, 'Who We Are', www.ias.org.uk/aboutus/who_we_are.html

Ipsos Mori, 'No Clear Public Support for Minimum Pricing of Alcohol', www.ipsos-mori.com/researchpublications/researcharchive/2715/No-clear-public-support-for-minimum-pricing-of-alcohol.aspx

National Health Service, 'Cutting Down on Alcohol', *Change4Life*, www.nhs.uk/Change4Life/Pages/cutting-down-alcohol.aspx

Office for National Statistics, 'Crime in England and Wales: Year Ending December 2012', 2013, www.ons.gov.uk/ons/dcp171778_307458.pdf

Office for National Statistics, *General Lifestyle Survey*, Newport: Office for National Statistics, 2013.

Oxford Dictionaries, 'Morality' and 'Attitude', http://oxforddictionaries.com/definition/english/morality?q=morality

Oxford Dictionary of National Biography, 'John Nicholson, *Oxford Dictionary of National Biography*, www.oxforddnb.com/view/printable/20140

Pittman, David J., 'International Overview: Social and Cultural Factors in Drinking Patterns, Pathological and Non-Pathological', 1967, www.api.or.at/akis/donauuni/pittman.pdf, p 3.

Royal College of Physicians, 'AHA Welcomes Minimum Alcohol Unit Price Consultation and Calls for 50 Pence per Unit', Press Release, 28 November 2012, www.rcplondon.ac.uk/press-releases/aha-welcomes-minimum-alcohol-unit-price-consultation-and-calls-50-pence-unit

Science and Technology Committee, *Alcohol Guidelines*, London: UK Parliament, 2011.

UK Government, *Alcohol Harm Reduction Strategy for England*, London: Strategy Unit, 2004.

UK Government, 'Licensing Act 2003 – Explanatory Notes', www.legislation.gov.uk/ukpga/2003/17/contents

UK Government, *Sensible Drinking*, Wetherby: Department of Health, 1995.

UK Government, *Safe. Sensible. Social.*, London: Department of Health, 2007.

UK Government, *The Government's Alcohol Strategy*, Norwich: The Stationery Office, 2012.

Whalley, Rachel, 'Drinking Alcohol', in Fuller, Elizabeth (ed) *Smoking, Drinking and Drug Use among Young People in England 2011*, London: NatCen Social Research, 2012, pp 121-152.

Woodhouse, John, and Ward, Philip, 'A Minimum Price for Alcohol?', *Home Affairs: House of Commons Library*, London: Parliament, 2013.

World Health Organization, *WHO Global Status Report on Alcohol*, 2004, www.who.int/substance_abuse/publications/global_status_report_2004_overview.pdf

World Health Organization, 'Levels of Consumption', *European Information Systems on Alcohol and Health*, 2012, http://apps.who.int/ghodata/?theme=GISAH&region=euro

List of statutes

Assize of Bread and Ale 1267
True Making of Malt Act 1548
Alehouses Act 1552
Act to Repress the Odious and Loathsome Sin of Drunkenness 1606
Black Act 1723
Gin Act 1729
Gin Act 1736
Gin Act 1743
Gin Act 1751
Estcourt Act 1828
Beer Act 1830
Public Health Act 1848
Licensing (Scotland) Act 1853
Vaccination Act 1853
Sale of Liquor on Sunday Act 1854
Sale of Liquor on Sunday Act 1855
Public House Closing Act 1864
Public House Closing Act 1865
Reform Act 1867
Vaccination Act 1867
Habitual Criminals Act 1869
Wine and Beerhouse Act 1869
Education Act 1870
Licensing Act 1872

Licensing Act 1874
Public Health Act 1875
Prison Act 1877
Habitual Drunkards Act 1879
Welsh Sunday Closing Act 1881
Intoxicating Liquors (Sales to Children) Act 1886
Inebriates Act 1898
Intoxicating Liquors (Sales to Children) Act 1901
Probation of Offenders Act 1907
Children Act 1908
Temperance (Scotland) Act 1913
Defence of the Realm Act 1914
Defence of the Realm (Amendment) Act 1915
Dangerous Drugs Act 1920
Licensing Act 1921
Dangerous Drugs Act 1923
Intoxicating Liquors (Sales to Persons Under Eighteen) Act 1923
Criminal Justice Act 1925
Road Traffic Act 1930
Licensing Act 1949
Licensing Act 1953
Road Traffic Act 1960
Licensing Act 1961
Road Traffic Act 1962
Licensing Act 1964
Road Safety Act 1967
Sexual Offences Act 1967
Licensing (Scotland) Act 1976
Licensed Premises (Exclusion of Certain Persons) Act 1980
Sporting Events Act 1985
Licensing Act 1988
Road Traffic Act 1988
Licensing (Sunday Hours) Act 1995
Licensing (Young Persons) Act 2000
Criminal Justice and Police Act 2001
Anti-Social Behaviour Act 2003
Licensing Act 2003
Violent Crime Reduction Act 2006
Police and Social Responsibility Act 2011

List of cases

Neale v RMJE [1984] Crim LR 485.
R v Tagg [2001] EWCA Crim 1230.
R v Bree [2007] EWCA Crim 256.
Carroll v DPP [2009] EWHC 554.

Index

Illustrations are indicated by *(figure)* following the page number. Notes are indicated by *n* following the page number and preceding the note number.

A

AA (Alcoholics Anonymous) 214–215, 216
abstinence *see also* teetotalism
  pledge campaigns 50, 108–112, 121, 245
  shift of public discourse from moderation to 43–44, 50–52, 207, 222, 224–226, 247
Act to Repress the Odious and Loathsome Sin of Drunkenness 1606: 7
advertising
  to promote alcohol 149
  to promote sensible drinking 151, 185
  pro-temperance 67, 68 *(figure)*, 85, 86 *(figure)*
  restrictions on 182, 189
affluence, impact on drinking 148–149, 175
afternoon opening hours 104, 115, 171
age legislation
  Children Act 1908: 134, 135–137
  Criminal Justice and Police Act 2001: 181–182
  Intoxicating Liquors (Sales to Children) 1886: 135
  Intoxicating Liquors (Sales to Children) 1901: 135
  Intoxicating Liquors (Sales to Persons under 18) 1903: 135–137
  Intoxicating Liquors (Sales to Persons under 18) 1923: 135–137, 161n48
  Licensing Act 1872: 74
  Licensing Act 1961: 74, 153
  Licensing Act 1964: 153, 165n164
  Licensing Act 1988: 173–174
  Licensing (Young Persons) Act 2000: 181
  Licensing Act 2003: 180, 181
  Metropolitan Police Act 1839: 92n52
  recent measures to address youth disorder 174–175, 180–182

age of drinkers, attitudes towards *see* young drinkers
agency, in moral regulation 16–17, 18
Alcohol Concern 186, 228, 239n159
Alcohol Health Alliance (AHA) 227, 228, 229, 231
alcohol industry *see* drinks industry
Alcoholics Anonymous (AA) 214–215, 216
alcoholism
  anxiety about, rise in 147, 149, 152
  classification 215
  definition 203, 212–213
  disease model 213, 216–218
  international comparisons (perceptions) 216
  legislation 99, 213
  morality, as theme in discourse about 214–215, 217–218
  treatment centres 99, 213–214, 216
ale *see* beer
Alehouse Act 1552: 7, 41, 55
Alliance House Foundation (United Kingdom Temperance Alliance) 217, 228–229
alpha alcoholism 215
Anglican Church 53, 108–109, 141
Anti-Social Behaviour Act 2003: 181
anxiety about alcohol *see* moral panics; public anxiety; public discourse
armed forces, alcohol as threat to 100–101, 105, 106–107
  see also 'treating' of military personnel
asceticism and teetotalism 52–54
Assize of Bread and Ale 1267: 6
Astor, Nancy 136
attitudes *see* public discourse
attitudes to alcohol *see* public discourse
Attlee, Clement 145
Australia 10
availability theory 172–173, 185–186, 222–223, 247
  see also 'slippery slope' of drinking

B

baby boomers 149
Baggott, Rob 8–9
Baines, Edward 76
Band of Hope (Hope UK) 62n81, 229, 250
BAPT (British Association for the Promotion of Temperance) 48, 50, 66–67
Baptist Union Assembly 142, 143
Barr, Andrew 205, 207
bars *see* pubs
Bart, Arthur 147
Batty, Robert B. 106
Bauman, Zygmunt 168
Beck, Ulrich 203–204
beer
  attitudes towards vs spirits 39, 56, 58, 104, 244
  as healthy drink 205
  patriotism and 39, 77
Beer Act 1830: 7, 35–36, 55–58, 185, 244
Beer Street (Hogarth) 37, 39
behaviour 4–6, 10–11
  see also consumption levels
Bengry-Howell, Andrew 227–228
beta alcoholism 215
'binge Britain' 186–187
binge drinking *see also* drunkenness
  anxiety about, rise in 170–171, 176, 188, 189–190, 192–194
  crime and disorder, perceived link to 168–170, 178–179
  international comparisons (perceptions) 186–187
  legislation to address 173, 174–175, 180–181, 182
  moral panic caused by Licensing Act 2003: 1–3, 167–168, 178–180, 182–185, 193, 220
  young drinkers, association with 189–190, 192
bio-politics 208–209
Black, Cyril 154–155
Black Act 1723: 14
Blair, Tony 2, 191, 229
Blair administration *see* Labour Party; Licensing Act 2003
Blunkett, David 184
Booth, Tony 179
Borsay, Peter 14, 37, 42
Brain, Kevin 171, 176
breathalysers 154
Bree, R v [2007] 183–184
Briggs, John 133, 136

British Association for the Promotion of Temperance (BAPT) 48, 50, 66–67
British Medical Association 154, 188, 210
British Teetotal Society (British Temperance League) 48
Brooke, Henry 155–156
Brown, Gordon 191
Brown, James B. 69
Brown (Gordon) administration *see* Labour Party
Bruce, Henry 80, 82, 95n128
Bunting, Jabez 53
Burgess, Adam 228
Burnett, John 205
Burns, Dawson 68–69, 71, 224

C

Calvinism 51–53
Cameron, David 222–223, 230
Cameron administration *see* Coalition Government, alcohol strategy of
Canada 10, 101
Carroll v DPP [2009] 86
Carter, Henry 142
Central Control Board (CCB) 104, 105, 112–115
  Defence of the Realm Act (DORA) 4, 123n41
'Challenge Twenty-Five' policies 182
Chalmers, Thomas 46
Chamberlain, Joseph 102
'Change4Life' campaign 224–225
children
  drinkers as threat to 99, 133–134, 142, 209
  drinking by (*see* age legislation; young drinkers)
Children Act 1908: 134, 135–137
chocolate liqueurs 154, 156
Church of England 53, 108–109, 141
Church of England Temperance Society (COETS) 49–50, 105, 107, 118–119, 168–169, 217
Churchill, Sir Winston 138
Clarke, Charles 179
Clarke, Kenneth 170
class and drinking *see* working classes
Clynes, John 119
Coaker, Vernon 191
Coalition Government, alcohol strategy of 229–230
cocoa ad (pro-temperance) 85, 86 (*figure*)
COETS (Church of England Temperance Society) 49–50, 105, 107, 118–119, 168–169, 217
Cohen, Lord Henry 209–210

Cohen, Stanley
 on 'folk devils' 13, 147
 on moral panics 14, 16, 97
Coleridge, Samuel Taylor 20
collectivism and attitudes to alcohol
 98– 99, 131–132
combustion of drinkers 48
consent and drunkenness 183–184
consequentialism 157
consumption levels (individual)
 availability theory and 172–173, 185,
 222–223
 recommended limits 219–220
consumption levels (national)
 ebb and flow of
 after Beer Act 1830: increase 185
 early 1900s: decline 5, 112, 119,
 125n82, 130, 136–137, 144
 mid to late 1900s: increase 5, 145,
 170, 178
 2000s: decline 5, 183, 227
 international comparisons 5, 130, 187
 legislation and 4–6, 41–42, 173, 185
 public anxiety levels, compared to
 correlation 130, 144, 155, 170, 178
 lack of correlation 2–3, 4–5 , 41–42,
 136–137, 183, 227
 taxation to manage 40, 99, 104, 229
 Total Consumption Theory (TCT)
 219–220, 222–223
 young drinkers 5, 136–137
Cook, Penny 220
Cookstown Temperance Society 47
Cornwall, temperance movement in
 48, 53
Corrigan, Phillip 12, 13, 20, 190, 249
court cases 86, 183–184
crime and disorder
 association between 168–170,
 178–179
 football hooliganism 172, 173, 175
 legislation 173–175, 180–182
 moral panic caused by Licensing
 Act 2003: 1–3, 167–168, 178–180,
 182–185, 193, 220
 opening hours, association with
 170–173, 177–180, 182–187
Criminal Injuries Compensation
 Authority 184
Criminal Justice Act 1925: 133
Criminal Justice and Police Act 2001:
 180–182
Critcher, Chas
 on binge drinkers 189
 on moral panics 7, 15, 42, 97–98
 on social science 16
Croydon, H.H. 100, 105, 107, 168

D

Daily Express
 on evils of alcohol 99
 on health risks 209, 210
 on magisterial powers 118
 on opening hours 116, 117
 on prohibition 102, 113
 on state ownership of drinks trade 102
 on teetotalism 108
Daily Mail, on binge drinking 184, 189
Daily Mirror
 on drink-driving laws 156
 on health risks 220
 on need for beer during wartime 139
 on VD and alcohol 210
Daily Telegraph, on binge drinking
 187–188, 189
Dalrymple, Donald 76, 82, 213
Dalrymple, Theodore 185
Darling, Alistair 229
Davis, David 185
debate about alcohol *see* public
 discourse
Defence of the Realm Act (DORA) 4,
 123n41
delta alcoholism 215, 216
deregulation, perception of recent
 legislation as 170–171, 193
Designated Public Place Orders
 (DPPOs) 181
determinism, and attitudes to alcohol
 99–100
Devlin, Lord Patrick 18, 145–146, 212
dieting 210
discourse *see* public discourse
disease model of alcoholism 213,
 216–218
diseases 209
Dispersal Orders 181
Dobson, Frank 179
Donaldson, Sir Liam 3, 220–221, 222,
 223
Dougal, Ruairi 183–184
DPP, Carroll v [2009] 86
Drink Banning Orders 181
Drinkaware (public education group)
 225
drink-driving
 anxiety about, rise in 133, 141
 legislation 75, 133, 150–151, 153–154
 premise locations and 150, 173
drinks industry *see also* off-licences; pubs
 advertising 149, 182, 189
 voluntary regulation 114, 138, 182,
 200n140
drunkenness *see also* binge drinking
 alcoholism, compared to 213

convictions, levels of 5, 130
court cases 86, 183–184
difficulty of determining 150–151
legislation 75, 174–175, 180–182
rape cases and 183–184
reported increases 145, 147, 155
Dunlop, John 47, 50
Durkheim, Emile 12, 19, 146, 212
DWI *see* drink-driving

E

economic arguments
against alcohol 52, 101, 105, 109, 119,
209
for alcohol 109–110, 170–171
Edgar, John 46–47
Edwards, Griffith 216
Edwards, Richard Passmore 53
Ehrenreich, Barbara 37
electoral reform, impact on legislation
80, 136
Elias, Norbert 17
Elliott, Matthew 189
Emsley, Clive 20, 66
Engels, Friedrich 69, 91n17
envelopes, pro-temperance 67, 68
(figure)
epsilon alcoholism 215
Estcourt Act 1828: 55, 197n62
Europe, comparisons across 1, 5, 10,
101, 186–187
evangelicalism and temperance 45–46,
53, 143, 187
evening opening hours 74, 104, 115,
137–138, 151, 152
extra-legal regulation *see* moral suasion

F

Finland 10, 101
First World War 100–112
legislation during 104–106
moral panic during 15, 97, 121–122
problematisation of alcohol during
100–101, 105–112, 121
temperance movement, role of
101–102, 111–112, 118–119
fitness, impact of alcohol 210
Flint, Caroline 229
'folk devils' 13, 41, 147, 153, 189
Foot, Isaac 140, 143
football hooliganism 172, 173, 175
Forestier-Walker, Sir Charles 117
Foucault, Michel 8, 16
France 1, 101
free trade 55, 57, 73

G

gamma alcoholism 215, 216
garages, restrictions on alcohol sales at
173
Garnier, Edward 179
Garrett, C. 70, 71
gay rights 18, 19, 145, 146
George V 108
German soldiers, portrayal of 107
Giddens, Anthony 203–204
Gilmore, Ian T. 3, 171
Gin Acts 4, 7, 40–42, 104
Gin Lane (Hogarth) 37, 67, 68 *(figure)*
gin panics 6, 7, 9, 37, 39–42
Gladstone, William 57, 73, 82, 103
Gooch, Sir T. 56
Good Templars (temperance society) 70
Gould, J.C. 117
government *see also* legislation; licensing
laws; taxation
intervention by, general increase in 66,
98–99, 100, 132, 208–209
ownership of drinks trade 10, 102,
105, 113–114, 115
Gow, Gertrude S. 108
Greenaway, John 8, 15, 97, 129
Guardian, The
coverage of alcohol 167, 194n1
on drink drivers 151
on opening hours 172
on Sunday closings 152
Gusfield, Joseph 6, 11, 13–14, 52

H

Habitual Drunkards Act 1879: 213
Haggerty, Kevin 228
Hale, Sir Matthew 44
Hall, Stuart 167–168
Harcourt, Bernard 231
Harcourt, William 67, 72, 76, 85
harm-based problematisation of alcohol
203–204, 209–210, 220–222, 247
Harris, Charles 179
Harrison, Brian, on temperance
movement
decline of 97
image of 67
legislative impact of 80
members of 48, 49, 52
overview of 9–10, 53, 54, 57
Hart, Herbert L.A. 18–19, 145–146, 230
Hayter, Diane 172–173
Hayward, K. 171
health *see also* alcoholism
historic associations with alcohol
204–209, 213–215

medicine and morality, juxtaposition of 206, 212–215 217, 218, 280
problematisation of 203–204, 209–212, 220–222, 227–229, 247
risk management approach 223–231
Heath, H. Cecil 155, 156
Heysel Stadium 173
Heyworth, Lawrence 207, 213
Hier, Sean P. 15, 98, 251
Hilton, Boyd 45, 46, 50, 52, 53, 109
Hislop, Ian 65
Hobbes, Thomas 20
Hobbs, D. 171
Hobson, Sir John 147, 148
Hogarth, William 37, 39, 67, 68 *(figure)*
homosexual rights 18, 19, 145, 146
Hope UK (Band of Hope) 62n81, 229, 250
human agency in moral regulation 16–17
Hunt, Alan
  on gin panics 6, 41
  on moral regulation 13, 54, 111, 244, 249
  on morality 19, 20
  on problematisation 14
Hunt, W. 50–51, 87, 190, 207, 213
Hurd, Douglas 174, 175

I

identification policies (of retailers) 182
Independent, The, compares international drinking 187
Inebriates Act 1898: 99, 213
inequality, and alcohol legislation 76–77, 116–118
Institute of Alcohol Studies 228–229, 250
international comparisons
  alcoholism, perceptions of 216
  consumption levels 5, 130, 187
  drinking, attitudes to 1, 10, 186–187
  legislation 5, 10, 101, 200n135
  prohibition movements 72, 101, 223
Intoxicating Liquors (Sales to Children) 1886: 135
Intoxicating Liquors (Sales to Children) 1901: 135
Intoxicating Liquors (Sales to Persons under 18) 1903: 135–137
Intoxicating Liquors (Sales to Persons under 18) 1923: 135–137, 161n48

J

Jayatilaka, Geethika 186
Jellinek, E.M. 215
Johnson, Boris 188
Johnson, William 'Pussyfoot' 113, 205

Jones, Leif 100
Jowell, Tessa 179, 185

K

Kettle, Martin 171, 177–178, 189
Kimberley, John Wodehouse, 1st Earl of 83, 85, 244
King, Ambrose 211–212
Kinnock, Neil 175
Kitchener, Horatio Herbert, 1st Earl Kitchener 108
Kneale, James 208–209, 213

L

Labour Party
  Blair/Brown era regulations 176–177, 178–183, 188
  interwar years 114
lager *see* beer
'lager louts' *see* football hooliganism; moral panics: after Licensing Act 2003
Lawson, Sir Wilfrid 53, 69, 70–71, 72, 186, 221
League of Honour (temperance society) 108
Ledermann, Sully 219
Lee, Charles A. 207
Lee, E.J. 227
legislation *see also* age legislation; licensing laws; opening hours; taxation
  alcoholics, detention of 99, 213
  availability theory and 172–173, 185
  binge drinking 173, 174–175, 180–181, 182
  consumption levels and 4–6, 41–42, 173, 185
  crime and disorder 173–175, 180–182
  drink-driving 75, 133, 150–151, 153–154
  drunkenness 75, 174–175, 180–182
  ebb and flow of
    shifts towards less restrictive 151–152, 170, 177
    shifts towards more restrictive 55, 74, 104–106, 180–183, 244–245, 247
    shifts towards targeted restrictions 144, 152–154, 158, 175–176, 246, 247
    shift back to universal restrictions 229–230, 247
  inequitable impacts of 76–77, 116–118
  international comparisons 5, 10, 101, 200n135
  licensing laws (*see* licensing laws)

moral regulation, role of in 18–20,
86–90, 121, 190–192, 248–251
as moral suasion 83–84, 86–88, 121,
190–191, 232, 245, 248–249
opening hours (*see* opening hours)
pricing 222–223, 230
public drinking 173, 180, 181–182,
188
spatial restrictions 173, 180, 181
strength of drinks 104, 115, 138
taxation (*see* taxation)
temperance movement, impact of
legislation on 35–36, 57–59
temperance movement, impact on
legislation 72–81, 86–99, 118–121,
154–157, 228–229, 250–251
'treating' of military personnel 105,
115, 123n45
Levine, Harry 10, 52
Liberal Party 72, 103
licensing laws *see also* legislation;
opening hours
Alehouse Act 1552: 7, 41, 55
Beer Act 1830: 7, 35–36, 55–58, 185,
244
Estcourt Act 1828: 55, 197n62
Gin Acts (Georgian) 4, 40–42, 104
Licensing (Scotland) Act 1853: 73
Licensing Act 1872:
moral regulation, role in 244, 249
as moral suasion 83–84, 86–88
provisions 74–75, 133
reactions to 75–79, 80–81
Licensing Act 1921: 15, 115–121
Licensing Act 1949: 145
Licensing Act 1953: 145
Licensing Act 1961: 74, 151–153, 170
Licensing Act 1964: 152, 153, 164, 165
Licensing (Scotland) Act 1976: 170
Licensing Act 1988: 31n99, 171–172,
173–174
Licensing Act (Sunday Hours) 1995:
176
Licensing (Young Persons) Act 2000:
181
Licensing Act 2003: 176–183, 198n90
moral panic caused by 1–3, 167–168,
178–179, 182–185, 193, 220
local vetoes 70–71, 72–73, 113, 132,
152, 170
Sale of Liquor on Sunday Acts (1854
and 1855) 92n48
liqueur chocolates 154, 156
liquor stores *see* off-licences
Livesey, Howard 71–72
Livesey, Joseph
'Malt Lecture' 207
on prohibition 71, 87

teetotalism and 50, 51, 52, 54, 67
Lloyd George, David 101, 103
Lloyd George, Margaret 99
local vetoes 70–71, 72–73, 113, 132,
152, 170
London
attitudes to drinking 49
ban on drinking on public transport
188
local licensing laws 74, 76, 92n52, 115,
117–118, 145, 151–152
Lowe, Pam 227
Lucas, B.G.B. 209

M

Mabane, W. 140
Mackenzie-Wintle, H. 148, 210–211
magistrates, power of 55, 117–118,
177
Mallon, J.J. 114
'Malt Lecture' (Livesey) 207
Manchester, local licensing laws 137
Manchester Guardian, The
coverage of drink-driving 133,
163n108
on drunks in air raid shelters 141
on female drinkers 142
on London licensing laws 117, 120
on state ownership 102
on Welsh licensing laws 117
on women drinkers 142
on young drinkers 134, 143
Marples, Ernest 151
Marx, Karl 49
Masham Report 172
Mass Observation 131
McKay, John 150, 153–154
Measham, Fiona 171, 176
medical issues *see* health
medicine and morality, juxtaposition of
206, 212–215 217, 218, 280
Metropolitan Police Act 1839: 92n52
military capabilities, alcohol as threat to
100–101, 105, 106–107
Mill, John Stuart 18
Miller, Peter 18, 191
Milne, F. 109
Monck, John 56
Monmouthshire 92n49, 116, 117, 152
moral panics *see also* public anxiety
definition and theory 13–16, 97–98,
121–122, 252
Georgian gin panics 6, 7, 9, 37, 39–42
during First World War 15, 97,
121–122
after Licensing Act 2003: 1–3, 167–
168, 178–179, 182–185, 193, 220

moral regulation *see also* public
  discourse
  agency in 16–17, 18
  definition 12–13, 20
  forms of 17–21, 87, 88, 190, 191, 249
  legislation, role in 18–20, 86–90, 121,
    190–192, 248–251
  moral panic theory and 13–15, 252
  as a social relation 16–17
moral suasion *see also* public discourse
  legislation as 83–84, 86–88, 121,
    190–191, 232, 245, 248–249
  prohibition vs 67–72, 81–88, 120–121,
    244–245
morality, definition 19, 248
Moriarty, Kieran 3, 171
morning opening hours 74, 112,
  198n90
Morris, Edward 54
Morrison, Herbert 137, 138
Moss, Stella 134
Myers, Edgar 216

N

National Council on Alcoholism
  (NCA) 216, 217
National Liberal Federation 72, 102
National Temperance Federation 155,
  156
National Union of Teachers 135
national/local state ownership of drinks
  trade 10, 102, 105, 113–114, 115
New British and Foreign Society for
  the Suppression of Intemperance 50
New Labour, and regulation of alcohol
  176–183, 188
New Zealand 10
newspapers *see specific newspaper*
Newton, John 99
Nicholls, James
  on Beer Act 1830 56
  on contextual factors 9
  on gin panics 37, 40–41, 59n4
  on shift from morality to science 204
  on temperance movement 9, 65
night-time economy 170–171, 176
North of England, temperance
  movement in 48, 53
Norway 10, 101
nutrition 52, 205, 207
Nutt, David 222

O

Oaten, Mark 184
Observer, The
  coverage of alcohol 160
  on legal limits 154
  on Licensing Act 1921: 119, 120

  on Licensing Act 2003: 178
  on young drinkers 134, 135, 136, 175
off-licences 152, 172
O'Malley, Pat 191
opening hours
  afternoons 104–105, 115, 171
  crime, association with 170–173,
    177–180, 182–187
  evenings 74, 104, 115, 137–138, 151,
    152
  magistrates, power of 55, 117–118,
    177
  mornings 74, 112, 198n90
  off-licences 152, 172
  private clubs 76–77, 115
  regional variations
    London 74, 76, 92n52, 115,
      117–118, 145, 151–152
    Manchester 137
    Monmouthshire 92n49, 116, 117,
      152
    Scotland 73, 113, 133, 170, 172
    Wales 73, 116, 117, 138, 152
  Sunday closings 73, 74, 92n48, 176
  theatre suppers 117
Orwell, George 143

P

Pakington, Sir John 57
Parker, Frances 105, 110
Parker, Howard 185
Parker, John 152
Parliamentary Temperance Group 155
passive drinking 220–222
patriotism
  beer and 39, 77
  temperance and 101–102, 106–107,
    110–111, 113
Pepys, Samuel 7
Perfect, P. 217
Permissive Bill (local detail) 72
persuasion *see* moral suasion
Plant, Martin 4, 185
Plant, Moira 4, 185
pledge campaigns 50, 108–112, 121, 245
Poley, David 189
police, role of in managing disorder 179,
  180–181, 198n90
Police and Social Responsibility Act
  2011: 165n164, 198n93
Pope, Samuel 68, 68–69, 221, 224
poverty 175
precautionary principle 241n191
premises *see* pubs
presentism 3–4
press, the *see specific newspaper*
pricing 222–223, 230
  see also taxation

private clubs, opening hours of 76–77, 115
Probation of Offenders Act 1907: 169
problematisation *see* public discourse
prohibition
  emergence of movement 67–72
  international comparisons 72, 101, 223
  moral suasion vs 67–72, 81–88, 120–121, 244–245
  opposition to 102, 113
prosperity, impact on drinking 148–149, 175
Protestantism
  Calvinism 51–52, 52–53
  Church of England 53, 108–109, 141
  evangelicalism 44, 45–46, 53
  puritanism 44, 46, 59n4, 152
providentialism 111
public anxiety *see also* moral panics; public discourse
  actual consumption levels, compared to
  correlation 130, 144, 155, 170, 178
  lack of correlation 2–3, 4–5, 41–42, 136–137, 183, 227
  definition 3
  historical overview 7–8
public discourse *see also* public anxiety
  ebb and flow of
    Georgian gin panics 6, 7, 9, 37, 39–42
    1820s: hardening of attitudes 42–46
    1914–1918: wartime problematisation 100–101, 105–112
    mid 20th century: limited relaxation 130, 132, 137, 139–140, 144, 158
    1960s: targeted concern 146–149
    2000s: moral panic 1–3, 167–168, 178–180, 184–185, 193, 220
  thematic shifts
    from moderation in all things to focus on drinking 38–39, 40, 45–46, 59
    from moderation to abstinence 43–44, 50–52, 207, 222, 224–226, 247
    from morality to harm produced 203–204, 209–210, 220–222, 247
    from spirits to all drink as problem 39, 40, 41, 56, 58, 247
    from universal to targeted problematisation 133–137, 144, 154, 156–158, 246, 247
    shift back to universal 219–220, 229–230, 247

public drinking 173, 180, 181–182, 188
  see also binge drinking; drunkenness
public transport, drinking ban on 188
pubs *see also* age legislation; opening hours
  improvement of 131, 134
  premise locations, drink-driving and 150, 173
puritanism 44, 46, 59n4, 152
Purnell, James 189
'Pussyfoot' Johnson 113, 205

R

R v Bree [2007] 183–184
R v Tagg [2001] 86
RAC (Royal Automobile Club) 156
Rae, John 107
Raffan, Peter Wilson 117
rape 183–184
rational model of attitudes to alcohol 3–6, 10–11, 12
regional variations
  opening hours (*see* opening hours: regional variations)
  temperance movement, strength of 48, 53
regulation *see* legislation; moral regulation
Reinarman, Craig 6, 10–11
religion and attitudes to alcohol
  alcoholism, and treatment of 214, 217
  Calvinism 51–53
  Church of England 53, 108–109, 141
  evangelism 45–46, 53, 143, 187
  puritanism 44, 46, 59n4, 152
respectability, as driver of temperance 49, 67
retailers, identification policies of 182
risk management and drinking 224–231, 233
Road Safety Act 1967: 154
Road Traffic Act 1930: 133
Road Traffic Act 1960: 150
Road Traffic Act 1962: 150
Roberts, Field Marshall Lord Frederick 106
Robinson, Victor 186
Room, Robin 213
Rose, Nikolas 18, 191
Ross, N.A. 210
Rowbotham, Judith 14–15, 21, 208
Rowse, A.L. 143
Royal College of Physicians 172, 219, 222, 225
Royal College of Psychiatrists 219, 222
Royle, Charles 153

Ruonavaara, Hannu
  on forms of moral regulation 18, 87,
    88, 190, 191, 249
  on the state and moral regulation 12,
    13
rural violence 172
Russia 1, 101
Rutherford, Derek 217, 222, 223

S

Safe, Sensible, Social 189, 190–191, 229
'Saint Monday' 3
Sale of Liquor on Sunday Acts (1854
    and 1855) 92n48
Sayer, Derek 12, 13, 20, 190, 249
Scotland, licensing laws in 73, 113, 133,
    170, 172
Scottish Prohibition Party 133
Scrymgeour, Edwin 133, 134
Seaman, Sir Owen 214
Second World War 130–131, 137–144
self-discipline *see also* availability theory;
    'slippery slope' of drinking
  British drinkers, perceptions of
    185–186
  patriotism and 102, 110–111
  temperance and 67–68, 110–111, 121,
    245
  young drinkers, perceptions of 149
Sennett, Richard 37
sessional drinking *see* binge drinking
Sheron, Nick 4, 222, 227
Shiman, Lilian Lewis
  on activities of temperance societies
    49, 67
  on decline of temperance societies 97
  on problematisation of drunkenness
    9–10
  on temperance and class 29n71, 49
Sinclair, Archibold 139
'slippery slope' of drinking 50–51, 134,
    185–186, 224–226, 250
  see also availability theory; self-
    discipline
Smith, Jacqui 185, 222
Smullen, Marion 184
Smyth, Glen 179
social class and drinking *see* working
    classes
social relations, moral regulation as 17
soft regulation *see* moral suasion
Sons of Temperance Friendly Society
    155
spatial restrictions on drinking 173, 180,
    181
spirits
  attitudes towards vs beer 39, 56, 58,
    104, 244

gin panics 6, 7, 9, 37, 39–42
Sporting Events Act 1985: 173
sports and drinking 172, 173, 175,
    196n39
Stanley, Lord Edward Henry 67, 77
state intervention, general increase in
    66, 98–99, 100, 132, 208–209
state ownership of drinks trade 10, 102,
    105, 113–114, 115
statutory limits 153–154
Stevenson, Kim 14–15, 21
Straw, Jack 190
Strength of Britain Movement (SOB)
    101–102, 113
strength of drinks 104, 115, 138
structuralism 16–17, 31n108
suasion *see* moral suasion
Sulkunen, Pekka 11, 132, 157, 200n135,
    204
Sumner, Maggie 185
Sun, The, on opening hours 184, 186
Sunday hours 73, 74, 92n48, 176
supermarkets, identification policies of
    182
Sweden 10, 101

T

Tagg, R v [2001] 86
targeted problematisation of alcohol
  shift from universal to targeted
    problematisation 133–137, 144, 154,
    156–158, 246, 247
  shift back to universal 219–220,
    229–230, 247
taxation
  as argument for alcohol 109–110
  free trade approach 55, 57, 73
  legislation 10, 40, 55, 104, 138
  to manage consumption 40, 99, 104,
    229
teenage drinking *see* age legislation;
    young drinkers
teetotalism *see also* abstinence
  asceticism and 52–54
  emergence of 50–52
  during First World War 106–112, 121
  pledge campaigns 50, 108–112, 121,
    245
  shift of moral regulation towards
    43–44, 50–52, 207, 222, 224–226,
    247
temperance *see also* temperance
    movement
  historic perceptions 38–39
  self-discipline and 67–68, 110–111,
    121, 245
Temperance (Scotland) Act 1913: 73

Temperance Council of the Christian
  Church 133, 135
temperance movement *see also*
  temperance societies
  activities of 49–50
  ebb and flow of
    emergence and growth 46–50, 244
    1900s: decline 97, 129, 132, 167, 245
    1950s-1960s: moderate revival
      154–157
    2000s: continuing involvement
      228–229
  First World War, role of during
    101–102, 111–112, 118–119
  gin panics, compared to 49–50
  legacy of 10, 86–87, 157, 187, 192,
    250–252
  legislation, impact of temperance
    movement on 72–81, 86–99, 118–
    121, 154–157, 228–229, 250–251
  legislation, impact on emergence
    of temperance movement 35–36,
    57–59
  membership, profile of 9, 48, 49,
    52–53, 54, 67
  patriotism and 101–102, 106–107,
    110–111, 113
  prohibition vs moral suasion 67–72,
    81–88, 120–121, 244–245
  religion and (*see* religion and attitudes
    to alcohol)
temperance societies *see also* temperance
  movement; UK Alliance
  Alliance House Foundation (United
    Kingdom Temperance Alliance) 217,
    228–229
  Band of Hope (Hope UK) 62n81,
    229, 250
  BAPT (British Association for the
    Promotion of Temperance) 48, 50,
    66–67
  Baptist Union Assembly 142, 143
  British Association for the Promotion
    of Temperance (BAPT) 66–67
  British Teetotal Society (British
    Temperance League) 48
  Church Of England Temperance
    Society (COETS) 49–50, 105, 107,
    118–119, 168–169, 217
  Cookstown Temperance Society 47
  Good Templars 70
  National Temperance Federation 155,
    156
  New British and Foreign Society for
    the Suppression of Intemperance 50
  Parliamentary Temperance Group 155
  Sons of Temperance Friendly Society
    155

  Strength of Britain Movement (SOB)
    101–102, 113
  Temperance Council of the Christian
    Church 133, 135
  United Kingdom Temperance Alliance
    (Alliance House Federation) 217,
    228–229
test purchasing 181–182, 198n96
Thatcher, Margaret 173, 175
Thatcher administration 171–172
theatre suppers 117
Thom, Betsy
  on actors in policy-making 8–9
  on alcoholism 9, 216
  on consumption trends 130
  on homeless drinkers 170
  on Total Consumption Theory
    219–220
Thomas, George 147
Thomas, Rhys 152
Thompson, E.P. 14, 53
Thurtle, Ernest 139, 145
Tillet, Ben 102–103
Time for Reform (White Paper) 176–177
Times, The
  coverage of alcohol 167, 194n1
  on drunkenness 43, 50, 82, 83, 114
  on early closing times 102, 116, 117,
    118
  on economic costs of drinking 209
  on football hooliganism 43, 50, 82,
    83, 114
  on health risks of alcohol 209
  on Liquor Control Board 113–114
  on prohibition 102, 103
  on restrictive legislation 56, 68, 77, 82,
    83, 84, 119, 120
  on wartime temperance 103, 105
  on young drinkers 134, 148
  'Tommy the Teetotaller' 106–107
Total Consumption Theory (TCT)
  219–220, 222–223
town centres, drinking in 178, 186, 189
'treating' of military personnel 105, 115,
  123n45
treatment centres for alcoholism 99,
  213–214, 216
True Making of Malt Act 1548: (quality
  control) 6
Turner, Charles 85, 190
'Twelve Steps' programme (AA) 214
24-hour drinking *see* licensing laws:
  Licensing Act 2003

U

UK Alliance
  aims and actions 69, 70, 71, 73, 113,
    221

on drinking and national efficiency 119, 140
Institute of Alcohol Studies 228–229, 250
legislation, reactions to 57, 81, 120
United Kingdom Temperance Alliance (Alliance House Federation) 217, 228–229
United States 10, 72, 101, 223
urbanisation, as driver of moralisation 37

V

Valverde, Mariana
    on determinism vs free will 99–100
    on government at a distance 191
    on Jellinek's classification 215
    on mixing of medicine and morality 213, 214, 215, 218
    on purification 129, 144
venereal disease 210
victims, portrayal of drinkers as 211
Violent Crime Reduction Act 2006: 181
volume of servings, legislation on 115
voluntary regulation 114, 138, 182, 200n140
Vosper, Dennis 151

W

Wales *see also* Monmouthshire
    local licensing laws 73, 116, 117, 138, 152
    local veto bills 113, 132, 152
    temperance movement in 48, 53
Warner, Jessica
    on evangelicalism and attitudes to alcohol 44
    on gin panics 7, 9, 37, 40, 41
    on prohibition movement 73
    on temperance movement 65, 70, 72
Weber, Max 51–52
weight gain, impact of alcohol 210
Welsh Sunday Closing Act 1881: 73
Wiener, Martin
    on collectivist attitudes to alcohol 98, 99
    on Henry Bruce 82
    on morality of law 20, 66
Wilkie, David: *The Village Holiday* 44, 45 *(figure)*
Williams, Garfield 140
Williams, Roger 186
wine, reduction of duties on 73
Winterton, Wilfred 216, 217
Wodehouse, John, 1st Earl of Kimberley 83, 85, 244
Wolfenden Report 145, 152

women drinkers
    child welfare, perceived link to 133–134, 142
    dieting and 210
    Georgian gin panics 37, 60n25
    historic low profile of 22
    during wartimes 108, 142
women's attitudes to alcohol
    age restrictions, support for 108, 136
    temperance and 108, 136
Woolton, Frederick Marquis, Earl of 138–139
working classes
    impact of legislation on 76–77, 116–117
    temperance movement among 49, 67
World War I *see* First World War
World War II *see* Second World War

Y

Yates, John 185
'yobbos' *see* football hooliganism; moral panics: after Licensing Act 2003
Yorkshire, temperance movement in 49, 53
young drinkers
    anxiety about
        in early 1920s 134–137
        during Second World War 141–142
        in 1960s 147–149, 153
        in 2000s 174–176, 189–190, 192
    consumption levels 5, 136–137
    crime and, perceptions of 153, 174–175
    legislation on (*see* age legislation)
    moral decline, perceptions of overall 141–142, 147–148, 155–156, 175, 211–212